1991

HEALTH SERVICES
as a
GROWTH ENTERPRISE
in the
UNITED STATES
SINCE 1875

Second Edition

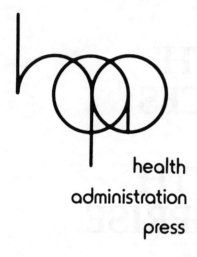

health
administration
press

HEALTH SERVICES
as a
GROWTH ENTERPRISE
in the
UNITED STATES SINCE 1875

Second Edition

Odin W. Anderson

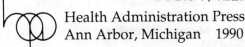
Health Administration Press
Ann Arbor, Michigan 1990

95   94   93   92   91   90   5   4   3   2   1

Library of Congress Cataloging-in-Publication Data

Anderson, Odin W. (Odin Waldemar), date.
    Health services as a growth enterprise in the United States since
1875 / Odin W. Anderson. — 2nd ed.
       p.   cm.
    Includes bibliographical references.
    Includes index.
    ISBN 0-910701-64-4 (hardbound : alk. paper)
       1. Medical care—United States—History.   2. Medical policy—United
States—History.   3. Insurance, Health—United States—History.   I. Title.
       [DNLM: 1. Health Policy—trends—United States.   2. Health Services—
trends—United States.   3. Insurance, Health—trends—United States.   W 84
AA1 A492h]
RA395.A3A   1990   362.1'0973—dc20
DNLM/DLC for Library of Congress   90-5079 CIP

Health Administration Press
A division of the Foundation of the
    American College of Healthcare Executives
1021 East Huron Street
Ann Arbor, Michigan 48104-9990
(313) 764-1380

To my father and mother, Edwin and Anna,
who died when I was too young to remember them.

Nevertheless, their relatives and friends
have made them real for me.

Contents

List of Tables

Foreword

This new edition of *Health Services in the United States: A Growth Enterprise Since 1875* is welcome and timely. Odin Anderson documents and analyzes the continued "growth" of health services over the last five or six years. He blends together a systems perspective, an intimate knowledge of the history and current operation of health services in this country, and common sense to help us understand the apparent chaos and dynamism of health care delivery and financing. While Odin Anderson's approach continues to show how basic problems of health services delivery are generic and contextual, his assessment of the most recent period suggests that it is, indeed, unusual in the rapidity of change and the magnitude of problems to be addressed.

Anderson divides the health services system's development into three periods: the emergence of the basic services of the current system (1875–1930), the era of the third party payment system (1930–1965), and the era of management and control (1965 to the present). The revised edition adds two new chapters: one describing the Reagan era and one addressing change in the structure of the system. The very terms Anderson uses for the new chapter titles—"explosions" in the Reagan era and "reshaping" the delivery system—signal the extent of change he observes.

The "explosions" emphasized in the new edition include the medical care cost escalation as well as policy dilemmas where intractable decisions must be made. Included among the latter are: the large proportion of the population without health insurance; the transplantation and supply of human organs; abortion; the multiplication of expensive medical technology; the erosion of medical care quality in the face of cost constraints and huge malpractice claims.

The last section of the book describes health services research and its role in the system. A new chapter here brings us up to date. Again the title emphasizes ferment and change as Anderson describes the "escalation" of health services research.

This book does not offer specific formulas to solve the problems of the health services system. In fact, it seems the author fears there may not be any. What the book does do is spell out the common elements of a health services system, the need to examine the larger social and political environment to understand it, and the special importance of the political process in allocating health resources since our knowledge of the contribution of those resources to the health of the population remains fragmentary. Odin Anderson's legacies for the readers of this work are a framework for understanding how the system operates; his own predictions of the system's course (which have been uncannily and disturbingly accurate in the past); and some insight into the hard choices that must be made if that course is to be altered.

RONALD ANDERSEN
Center for Health Administration Studies
University of Chicago

Chicago
September 30, 1990

Acknowledgments

Although this book is the result of quite a few years' experience and research of one person, it would not have been possible without a congenial institutional base and assistance from many individuals. The institutional base has been provided by the University of Chicago and the University of Wisconsin, Madison. More specifically, within the University of Chicago, my base has been the Center for Health Administration Studies, Graduate School of Business; within the University of Wisconsin, it has been the Department of Sociology. Since 1980, I have had academic appointments in both universities concurrently, shuttling between them. They have given me a great deal of flexibility as to time, convenience, and supporting services. I doubt that either university knew where I was most of the time, a great privilege in this bureaucratic age.

Direct financial support for research assistance and related expenditures was provided by the Blue Cross Association, then headed by Walter J. McNerney. Support for this book was an extension of an association grant for my book *Blue Cross Since 1929: Accountability and the Public Trust*, published in 1975. Indirect financial support in the form of my salary and clerical support was, of course, provided by the two universities.

I was helped considerably in library research by Larry Corder and Darwin Sawyer, graduate students in the Department of Sociology, University of Chicago. Both have since earned their Ph.D.s.

The clerical assistance needed for a book of this type, with 600 or so references, is formidable. At the Center for Health Administration Studies, University of Chicago, I gratefully acknowledge June Veenstra, Joyce Van Grondelle, Annette Twells, and Dorothy Fraser; at the Department of Sociology, University of Wisconsin, Madison, Mildred L.

Devaul, program assistant, who coordinated the typing pool, Virginia Rogers, Christy Kinney, Toni Polglase, and Christine Peters. I am very grateful to all of them.

ODIN W. ANDERSON, PH.D.
University of Chicago and
University of Wisconsin, Madison

Abbreviations

AALL	American Association for Labor Legislation
AAMC	Association of American Medical Colleges
AFDC	Aid to Families with Dependent Children
AFL	American Federation of Labor
AHA	American Hospital Association
AHSR	Association for Health Services Research
AIDS	Acquired immune deficiency syndrome
AMA	American Medical Association
APA	American Pharmaceutical Association
APHA	American Public Health Association
CAT	Computerized axial tomography
CCMC	Committee on the Cost of Medical Care
CHP	Comprehensive Health Planning
DHEW	Department of Health, Education, and Welfare
DHHS	Department of Health and Human Services
DRG	Diagnosis-related group
EMIC	Emergency Maternity and Infant Care
EPO	Exclusive provider organization
ESP	Economic Stabilization Program
ET	Expenditure target
FAH	Federation of American Hospitals
FERA	Federal Emergency Relief Administration
FSA	Farm Security Administration
GNP	Gross national product
HCFA	Health Care Financing Administration
HIP	Health Insurance Plan of Greater New York
HMO	Health maintenance organization
HSA	Health service area

IPA	Independent practice association
M.I.T.	Massachusetts Institute of Technology
NHC	National Health Council
OASDI	Old Age, Survivors, and Disability Insurance
PPO	Preferred provider organization
PPRC	Physician Payment Review Commission
PRO	Peer review organization
PSRO	Professional Standards Review Organizations
RBRVS	Resource-based relative value scale
RMP	Regional Medical Programs
RN	Registered nurse
UNAC	Universal access
USPHS	U.S. Public Health Service
VA	Veterans Administration
WPA	Works Progress Administration

PART I
The Framework

1

The Political and Economic Framework

Any attempt to trace the development of the health services enterprise in the United States from 1875 to the present time borders on the arrogant. This does not diminish the value of such an attempt, however; it is important to an understanding of both the nature of the enterprise and its implications for public policy. Because of the geometric increase in data on the health services and the interest in analyzing these data, now may be an opportune time to synthesize the political, social, and economic aspects of the health services' development. Further, I wish to evaluate the extent to which research from various disciplines has contributed to our understanding of this exceedingly complex enterprise.

THE FAMILY AND THE STATE

The care of the sick and the maintenance of healthy human beings from birth to death are the responsibility primarily of the family. In fact, it is this nurturing function that underlies many of the ambiguities we face in transforming health services from the simple palliatives provided at home to the complex and expensive technology available in hospitals.

The central dilemma is this: To what extent is the individual or family responsible for providing itself with health care (for example, by buying insurance), and to what extent is the provision of health services a public responsibility? A corollary to this is our ambivalence about profit: To what extent is it acceptable to profit from the sick?

The free market is a powerful force in Western civilization generally, and particularly in the United States, where even the nonprofit sector is suspected of profiting. Both the private nonprofit and the profit sectors of the health services have persisted to a far greater extent in the United States than in any other country. The free market concept coexists uneasily with the delivery of health services, for the profit motive tends to diminish trust in a service in which trust is essential. As recently observed by a pioneer in voluntary health insurance, C. Rufus Rorem:

> I dislike it particularly when physicians or hospital spokesmen refer to themselves as an "industry." As far as I am concerned, health care is a broad public service. It's not private property you can buy and sell over the counter—something that can be withheld from those unable to pay. It certainly isn't a private industry. More than 90 percent of the capital invested in hospitals and medical education has been provided by philanthropy and taxation.[1]

Much as I subscribe to a free market economy, I believe it is possible to exaggerate its importance in shaping social relations. As stated by Polanyi, "It means no less than the running of society as an adjunct to the market. Instead of economy being embedded in social relations, social relations are embedded in the economic system."[2]

The health services as a combination of private and public responsibility have emerged as part and parcel of the welfare state. Hence, the health services, along with other programs of social insurance, are caught up not only in simple political issues, but in moral issues as well: Who is my brother? Who is a stranger? The welfare state has institutionalized the transfer of income from those who have more to those who have less and has necessarily used coercion to do so, because most people are reluctant to help persons they do not know. As observed by theologian Reinhold Niebuhr, "All social cooperation on a larger scale than the most intimate social group requires a measure of coercion."[3] Further, since health and welfare services are inherent in the obligations of citizens to each other and hence are expressed in the political process, Niebuhr observed, "Politics will, to the end of history, be an area where conscience and power meet, where the ethical and coercive factors of human life will interpenetrate and work out their tentative and uneasy compromises."[4] Finally, I draw on the pithy (and possibly pitiless) ruminations of Thomas Chalmers, a Scottish clergyman and welfare official in the early nineteenth century: "In times like the present, the burden is not all transferred from the poor to the rich but is shared between them; it should be a compromise between the endurance of the one and the liberality of the other."[5] This grudging philosophy still finds expression in political debates on welfare issues.

Compared with other industrialized countries, the United States has shown a distinct reluctance to move into a publicly owned and financed health services enterprise. Transfer payments in the form of retirement pensions, unemployment insurance, and workers' compensation, however, are as governmentally financed and operated here as in any other industrialized country. In an emerging literature on the nature and problems of the welfare state, two theories stand out. One is the theory of financial assistance to the individual as a residual; whether it is considered a privilege or a right, the means of sustaining individuals come from social surpluses and are grafted on to the productive and distributive structure of the economic system. The individual is not financially independent (for a host of personal and impersonal reasons) and is regarded as a failure.[6] The other theory is that assistance to the individual, regardless of character or prior contribution, should promote social cohesion. Persons in need should blend inconspicuously into the social structure and therefore be free of any stigma. Both theories are oversimplifications, but they shape the policies formulated by their adherents. The tendency in parliamentary democracies is to integrate welfare recipients into the society and its economy, thus reducing stigma. Semantic examples are the replacement of the term "welfare services" by "social services" and the change from the Department of Health, Education, and Welfare (DHEW) to the Department of Health and Human Services (DHHS) after education was split off.

VALUE PERSPECTIVES AND RESEARCH

In developing the framework for this book, I wish to make clear the research perspectives I find congenial and the social and political theories I draw on in shaping my analysis and interpretation. Even though it is difficult, it is possible, I believe, for social analysts to be sufficiently value-free to perceive an independent reality. If they cannot, then social analysis becomes purely relative and subjective.

It is essential in analyzing social systems to understand the context in which problems lie.[7] The health services enterprise is an eminently social one because of the human problems it encounters. Systems analysis has a long and fruitful history in the physical and natural sciences and has had spectacular success in applied engineering, the moonshot being the favorite example. The study of social systems, however, is still in its infancy because of the complexity of human behavior. At best, then, I hope to reveal external and internal conditions shaping the development of the health services in the United States and to explore the possibilities of attaining explicit and implicit public policy objectives. As stated by Hubert M. Blalock in his presidential address to the American Sociological Association in 1979:

> Given the practical roadblocks to data collection that will continue for the foreseeable future, any piece of research will necessarily involve large amounts of missing information, thereby requiring either implicit or explicit assumptions and the neglect of numerous variables thought to be theoretically important.[8]

I also wish to show how judicious data gathering and more or less focused research have contributed to our understanding of the structure and functioning of the health services enterprise and to determine what now needs to be or can be done. In short, I am trying to continue the macrosociological approach in the tradition established by the great pioneers.[9]

Next, I wish to reveal my general ideological position. I believe that I am describing and analyzing social, economic and political reality in the United States in terms of the political philosophy we inherited from our forebears in the Enlightenment. I confess that I do not understand American society as viewed by Marxists and those who write from that point of view in the health field.[10] Our differences are based on our respective "social reconstructions of reality,"[11] which influence our analyses.

Accordingly, I accept the liberal-democratic interest-group theory of the American political system and of Western-style liberal-democratic parliamentary governments in general as a reasonable depiction of social reality in those countries. Such a framework naturally affects political values, political processes, and methods of formulating public policy.

Briefly, the Western democracies emerged in the nineteenth century in reaction to the mercantile states, which controlled virtually all important commercial transactions. A market-oriented economy and a private sector more or less independent of the state were created. The state became responsible for justice, the currency, defense, police protection, education, and minimum welfare assistance. The care of the poor was clearly a residual of the economic system; they were unable to cope within the system. The United States and the other democracies have been struggling with this concept ever since, making welfare and its beneficiaries an increasingly integral part of society.

Political values have been quite constant and similar among democracies, extending to all classes as suffrage became universal. These political values include sovereignty of the people through periodically elected representatives; one person–one vote; freedom of assembly, speech, and the press; and an independent judiciary—in other words, a government of laws not people. In general, there has been separation of powers; the judiciary, the legislature, and the executive (including the bureaucracy) have separate and relatively equal jurisdictions.

Theoretically, the citizens are supposed to work out their economic destinies in this framework with as little intervention by government as possible. The "as possible," however, has been gradually expanding as people realize that the market economy is not capable of mitigating the "slings and arrows of outrageous fortune" in the form of unemployment, disability, health services costs, premature death, and living so long that one's private resources are exhausted. Most such misfortunes are tied to the labor market in developed and industrialized countries. Lack of employment, for whatever reason, quickly results in destitution. Private resources are inadequate. Most people are either unable or unwilling to save enough for a rainy day. Increasingly, the government has become the chief agency through which to establish the welfare state. It represents the largest collective, and it is regarded as the only legitimate way to bring about a redistribution of income. The emergence of a welfare state is not peculiar to capitalist systems, however, for the same human misfortunes occur in all industrialized countries.

Almost 30 years ago Robert Dahl and Charles Lindblom set forth the twin goals of liberal-democratic political and social philosophy: (1) rational control over governments through democracy and (2) rational control over economic affairs through capitalism, or the free market.[12] A few years before that, Gerald De Gré explained the pluralistic model of checks and balances in a country with more or less equal concentrations of power, except, of course, for the residual poor. To quote from De Gré:

> ... freedom flourishes most when the relationships of groups are in a relative equilibrium determined by each other's groups having to take into account in its actions the interest, values, and powers of other groups. This is true according to the degree to which various groups are relatively equal to one another, thereby insuring the improbability of any one group's attaining a monopoly of control over the rest.[13]

This pluralist model lies between the extremes of anarchy and totalitarianism. In such a model, the individual or group is able to find a niche that is reasonable and politically tolerable in terms of efforts, abilities, and aspirations. Marxist-oriented writers, of course, would vigorously attack this description as spurious, and no amount of policies, facts, or theories can bridge the gap between the two viewpoints. The egalitarian view of society held by Marxists is, I believe, utopian.

A more realistic view of society is that there are inevitably "winners" and "losers," and, equally inevitably, the "losers" wish to minimize their losses by sharing in the resources that are produced. A pluralistic social and political system falls short of the egalitarian ideal to the extent that it allows residuals in the society—persons who are unable to function in the system because of poverty, level of education and aspiration, and discrimination. These persons are to be assisted by welfare. In a liberal-democratic society, the "losers" are generally economic losers, persons for whom economic opportunities are not available. Given some initiative, they need not be political losers, since they are enfranchised. Thus the liberal-democratic system is politically viable, but it is criticized for its lack of economic democracy, both in corporate decision making and in equalizing income and wealth. The equalization of income and wealth certainly has not been impressive in communist countries; further, political power generally rests in just one party, and incumbents in office remain there for life unless they are thrown out or liquidated first.

The purpose of these brief observations on political systems is to point out that they affect policy formulation and legislative programs. Their problem-solving and political styles range from the central decision making and five-year planning in the Soviet Union to the agitations of interest groups in the United States, where a range of interests must reach a consensus in order to assure legislation.

As described by Zbigniew Brzezinski and Samuel Huntington,* "to the Bolshevik, politics is the craft of conflict; to the American, it is the art of compromise." With respect to political issues, the Soviets ask, What is the correct line? Americans ask, What is the correct position? The authors continue:

> The difference in terminology reflects differences in political thinking. The communist "line" is the link between fundamental doctrines and stands on particular issues: it defines the meaning of the doctrines in a particular historical context and the relations between the stands on one issue and the stands on other issues. The American, however, does not have a line, there are only ad hoc positions. . . . The position which he takes on one issue may be quite discrete and unrelated to positions on other issues and to his general political beliefs. Soviet political action is justified by the line which links it to general doctrine. American political action is justified by an immediate consensus quite distinct from the consensus which may be

---

*Recent (1990) political changes in the USSR and Eastern Europe may make their observations seem obsolete to some readers, nevertheless, the polar types of political systems remain analytically appropriate. Further, the length to which the USSR will move to a Western-type liberal democracy remains to be seen.

developed on other issues and from overall agreements on the key elements of the American political beliefs.[14]

I believe it to be reasonable to use the United States and the USSR as polar extremes in styles of policy formation. There are also ranges within parliamentary democracies in degree of pluralism and access to the political process. So far, there has been more party discipline in the parliamentary democracies, enabling them to pass seemingly more comprehensive and cohesive health service legislation, than in the United States.[15]

As has been pointed out many times, the United States is a fantastically diverse social and political system. Other Western-style democracies function within a much narrower range of diversity, at least in terms of welfare and health services issues. Thus consensus is easier to reach.

PROBLEM-SOLVING STYLES

This leads us to the central characteristics of the methods of solving social problems. These have been set forth by Dahl, Lindblom, Braybrook, Grodzin and Sundquist, to name the more recent theorists who have built on the work of such men as John Stuart Mill, Hobbes, Montesquieu, and Machiavelli. Lindblom argues that, in any political system, problem solving is incremental rather than synoptic, because human beings cannot know enough about any enterprise to direct its future toward well-defined objectives. This is true even in Communist countries, where planning is a facade: sheer power is not enough to direct the affairs of human beings. In solving problems, it is necessary to learn, relearn, and shift directions as one goes along. This is particularly true of enterprises that have very few measures of input and output, such as health services, basic research, churches, universities, and all welfare state programs. All political systems must deal with the vagaries of demand, resource allocation, and price. Thus, I subscribe to the incremental concept and believe that synoptic planning is an illusion. The evidence seems to point to that conclusion, therefore we must work and live with it in formulating policy and solving social problems.

Political bargaining among interest groups is the essence of liberal-democratic governments, but it bears repeating that bargaining is much more intense in the United States because of its diverse and fluid social system. Dahl and Lindblom observe:

> In American national government, bargaining is the strategic limit on rational social action and therefore on rational political-economic action

to a degree not to be found in Great Britain, Canada, New Zealand, Scandinavia, and probably some other Western governments.[16]

The essence of social pluralism, then, is "If leaders agreed on everything, they would have no reason to bargain; if on nothing, they could not bargain."[17] In the health services in the United States, there is rhetorical agreement on equal access to health services regardless of income, race, or residence, but there is a great deal of diversity regarding method.

This chapter may be summarized as follows:

1. Organized personal health services are an extension of the nurturing function of the family.

2. Hence, in the United States, which is predominantly market oriented in its means of production and distribution, responsibility for personal health services is debated in an atmosphere of ambiguous private-public responsibility.

3. Whoever is responsible, the question is how far beyond kith and kin people will go without coercion in assuming responsibility for the care of strangers.

4. Given the relative paucity of indicators of performance, each delivery system reaches a certain equilibrium of use and expenditures, whether in market-oriented or tax-supported programs. In the market economy, price becomes the determinant of equilibrium; in public programs, taxation potential becomes the determinant of equilibrium.

5. The public policy of equal access to health care pushes the delivery system into the public sector; hence decisions about number of facilities and personnel, reimbursement, distribution, and rationing by supply rather than price are made political.

6. As more and more decisions are made in the political arena, policy formulation becomes a part of the political process and emulates that process.

7. The inability of human beings to direct long-range planning makes them rely on the incremental method of planning—limited goals over short spans of time.

8. The result is a constant tension in the body politic as to who gets what when, where, and at what cost. The players without political clout must depend on the players with clout to allocate resources according to some concept of equity.

9. Hence, the extent to which resources for personal health services are allocated equally is an expression of the depth of citi-

zens' concern for each other and of how that concern is carried out. Fundamentally, resource allocation is a moral problem.

NOTES

1. U.S. Department of Health and Human Services, Office of Health Maintenance Organizations, *Focus* 3 (October 1980):4.
2. Karl Polanyi, *The Great Transformation* (New York: Farrar and Rinehart, 1944), p. 57.
3. Reinhold Niebhur, *Moral Man and Immoral Society: A Study in Ethics and Politics* (New York: Scribners, 1953), p. 3.
4. Ibid., p. 4.
5. Quoted in Karl de Schweinitz, *England's Road to Social Security* (Philadelphia: University of Pennsylvania Press, 1943), p. 110.
6. The literature now is fairly extensive. Earlier books were Robert A. Dahl and Charles E. Lindblom, *Politics, Economics, and Welfare* (New York: Harper, 1953) and Harold L. Wilensky and Charles N. Lebeaux, *Industrial Society and Social Welfare: The Impact of Industrialization on the Supply and Organization of Social Welfare Services in the United States* (New York: Russell Sage Foundation, 1958). Others followed rapidly: Gunnar Myrdal, *Beyond the Welfare State: Economic Planning in the Welfare State and Its International Implications* (London: Methuen, University Paper Backs, 1965); Harold L. Wilensky, *Welfare State and Equality: Structural and Ideological Roots of Public Expenditures* (Berkeley: University of California Press, 1975); Arnold J. Heidenheimer, Hugh Heclo, and Carolyn T. Adams, *Comparative Public Policy: the Politics of Social Choice in Europe and America* (New York: St. Martin's Press, 1975); Gaston V. Rimlinger, *Welfare Policy and Industrialization in Europe, America, and Russia* (New York: Wiley, 1970); Morris Janowitz, *Social Control of the Welfare State* (New York: Elsevier, 1976); Richard T. Titmuss, *Social Policy, An Introduction* (London: Allen and Unwin, 1974); Robert Pinker, *Social Theory and Social Policy* (London: Heineman, 1971) and *The Idea of Welfare* (London: Heineman, 1979); Norman Furniss and Timothy Tilton, *The Case for the Welfare State: From Social Security to Social Equality* (Bloomington: Indiana University Press: 1977).
7. Kenneth E. Boulding, "Knowledge as Commodity," *Series Studies in Social and Economic Sciences, Symposia Studies Series No.11* (Washington D.C.: The National Institute of Social and Behavioral Science, 1962), p. 5.
8. Hubert M. Blalock, "Measurement and Conceptualization Problems: The Major Obstacle to Integrating Theory and Research," *American Sociological Review* 44 (December 1979): 881–82.
9. Morris Janowitz has helped me to perpetuate that tradition, which I believe continues to be sociology's major contribution to the understanding of society and its current problems. See his *Social Control of the Welfare State* (New York: Elsevier, 1976), pp. xi–xii.
10. The best known proponents of the Marxist approach to health care are Vicente Navarro, *Medicine Under Capitalism* (New York: Prodist, 1976); Bar-

bara Ehrenreich and John Ehrenreich, *The American Health Empire: Power, Profits, and Politics* (New York: Random House, 1970); and Elliot A. Krause, *Power and Illness: The Political Sociology of Health and Medical Care* (New York: Elsevier, 1977).

11. Peter L. Berger and Thomas Luckman, *Social Construction of Reality: A Treatise in the Sociology of Knowledge* (New York: Doubleday, 1966).

12. Robert A. Dahl and Charles E. Lindblom, *Politics, Economics, and Welfare* (New York: Harper, 1953). This book was reissued with a new preface by the authors: *Politics, Economics, and Welfare; Planning and Politics—Economic Systems Resolved into Basic Social Processes* (Chicago: University of Chicago Press, 1976). The authors have become considerably more sanguine since 1953 about the promise of interest groups for bringing about innovation and change "necessary for a decent, democratic society." According to their view, Americans find it difficult to correlate private and public endeavors for the common good: "In the realm of attitudes, ideas, and ideology, we Americans have an irrational commitment to private ownership and control of economic enterprises, and that prevents us from thinking clearly about economic arrangements" (p. xxvi).

13. Gerald De Gré, "Freedom and Social Structure," *American Sociological Review* 11 (October 1946): 529–36.

14. Zbgniew Brzezinski and Samuel B. Huntington, *Political Power: USA/USSR* (New York: Viking Press, Compass, 1965), p. 23.

15. See, for example, Sidney Verba and Norman H. Nie, *Participation in American Political Democracy and Social Equality* (Chicago: University of Chicago Press, 1974); James L. Sundquist, *A Comparison of Policy-Making Capacity in the United States and Five European Countries: The Case of Population Distribution*, Brookings General Series Reprint No. 345 (Washington, D.C.; Brookings Institution, 1978); Hugh Heclo, *Modern Social Politics in Britain and Sweden: From Relief to Income Maintenance* (New Haven, Conn.: Yale University Press, 1974); Gabriel A. Almond and Sidney Verba, *The Civic Culture: Political Attitudes and Democracy in Five Nations* (Princeton, N.J.: Princeton University Press, 1963).

16. Dahl and Lindblom, *Politics*, p. 344.

17. Ibid., p. 326.

2

Preview of the Development of U.S. Health Services

Personal health services have been a growth enterprise in the United States since 1875, to pick an arbitrary but accurate date. The enterprise has taken place essentially in the private sector of the economy, with a mixture of nonprofit and profit enterprises receiving increasing government support and intervention. This mixture has changed over the years, primarily in regard to sources of funding for day-to-day operations and capital funding. Americans manifest a great deal of ambivalence about who is responsible for health care, the individual or the government. Collective solutions have received mixed reactions: life insurance, fire insurance, and community fund drives for hospital construction were accepted easily a long time ago, but private health insurance foundered until people recognized that, like life and fire insurance, it was a prudent way to protect their solvency. Medical care for the poor was regarded as an expression of the noblesse oblige of the physician and the hospital, buttressed by local government and philanthropic organizations.

The personal health services system seems to fall naturally into three major stages of development: 1875 to 1930, 1930 to 1965, and 1965 to the present. I present these stages briefly, giving some attention to public health services and mental hospitals, which preceded and paralleled the growth of personal health services.

1875 TO 1930

During the latter part of the nineteenth century, physicians and pharmacists were the sole dispensers of professionally recognized health services. On the periphery were midwives, who, by the turn of the century, were beginning to be replaced by physicians. Also on the periphery were doctors of osteopathy, chiropractors, and others. Dentists developed a separate, parallel profession.

The general hospital as we know it today did not exist. Poorhouses and almshouses took care of the destitute and persons who had no family. Illnesses were treated primarily in patients' houses and physicians' offices. Physicians and pharmacists were entrepreneurs with presumably a code of ethics and professional standards. They were not motivated strictly by profit, but had an implied obligation to persons unable to pay. There were proportionately as many physicians then as there are now. They made their living treating patients for fees, and received very little income from government or philanthropic sources. In no other country have so many physicians and dentists been supported by private, fee-for-service patients. The same was true of pharmacists, who eventually established the peculiarly American corner drugstore to supplement their income from prescriptions. This income was insufficient because there were so many pharmacists and because physicians themselves dispensed drugs. Private practice and fee-for-service thus became firmly embedded in American medical care.

Surgery had become highly developed by 1875 because of operations done in the charity hospitals of the East Coast and Europe. The middle and upper classes, however, would not have been caught dead in these famous hospitals, but that changed with the advent of anesthesia and antisepsis, which made the general hospital a relatively safe and painless place for surgery. The affluent began to seek the services of surgeons, who in turn sought hospital admitting privileges. By 1900 there were 4,000 general hospitals in the United States, whereas there had been only a few score in 1875.

Hospitals were established mostly by voluntary community boards and church bodies. The church bodies, of course, had a long history of caring for the poor, and this tradition was transformed into the modern general hospital. Capital came from millionaires created by the tremendous industrial development following the Civil War. Only a small minority of general hospitals were built for the poor by municipalities. Voluntary hospitals, because of their charitable and nonprofit charters, were obliged to provide care for the poor who sought help, but by and large the poor were a minority of their patients. The burgeoning economy enabled hospitals to obtain capital funds from philanthropists and operating funds from paying patients. Physicians, particularly those who wanted to perform surgery, made deals with the hospitals to admit their private patients; these patients would pay the hospital charges and the surgeons' fees. In return, the surgeons were provided a free workshop in which to provide free care for the poor, an ideal symbiotic arrangement. American society has a long tradition of voluntary self-help on the community level, and the voluntary hospitals are prime examples of this tradition. The nurturing functions of the family found expression in the voluntary hospital when the home became unequal to the technical demands of increasingly high technology medicine.

The traditional nurturing functions of women were embodied in the trained nurse, who, in her cap and uniform, functioned as the physician's assistant. Industrial development and the growth of cities provided a respectable occupational opportunity for women from rural as well as urban areas. Florence Nightingale was an attractive model. The nursing profession became an alternative to teaching and secretarial positions for women, and it was possibly more honored because of its aura of service. Nurses' hours were long and their pay low, mostly in kind.

Dentists, like physicians, were entrepreneurs who made their way by fees from private patients. Since public concern about dental health was indifferent then, the services of dentists were not in great demand. Dentists also benefited greatly from the appearance of anesthesia and antisepsis. In fact, the first health professional to use ether was a dentist, thus ushering in the use of anesthesia.

During the nineteenth century, most physicians were trained through apprenticeships with practicing physicians. There were also so-called diploma mills, which were established by physicians to train several students at a time in rather primitive arrangements. Later, private and public universities established medical schools. Dentists also had first proprietary schools and eventually schools in universities. Nurses were trained by hospitals, which benefited from the inexpensive labor. Student nurses were under virtually total supervision, reflecting the view of young women's roles at that time. As medical science advanced, a variety of other types of personnel began to appear.

All this took money, but money became available with the growth of the economy. The surplus was increasingly poured into personal health services, which, until the 1930s, Americans bought without the help of government or private insurance. Thus the infrastructure of the personal health services as we know them today—the voluntary hospital and the privately practicing physicians, dentists, and pharmacists—was in place by the 1930s.

Public health services and mental hospitals were not wanted services in the same sense as personal health services. Before 1875, cities and counties had begun to establish health departments because effluents were contaminating the water and causing epidemics of cholera. Later, when communicable diseases in children could be controlled by immunization and pasteurization, the health department expanded its function based on bacteriology and epidemology. The public health nurse for mothers and infants was created by adding public health training to the registered nurse's curriculum. Public health separated itself early from the private practice of medicine. Public health officers were not allowed to practice medicine.

The building of mental hospitals (usually out in the country) preceded the development of personal health services. Mental hospitals were—and continue to be—more or less separate from personal health services. Mental hospitals were and are largely publicly owned and operated. Like public health departments, they are not a wanted service, judging from the public funding they receive relative to the magnitude of the problem they deal with. Personal health services, through sheer demand and popularity, have cornered the available funding.

This was the situation in 1930, and it is the situation today. The system was shaped by hospital owners, physicians, and philanthropists. Government, except by issuing licenses and setting standards, did nothing to influence the system. The public presumably approved of the structure because they used and paid for it in increasing numbers. The government helped the system indirectly by permitting hospitals to be tax-exempt enterprises. In addition, capital gifts to hospitals were tax-exempt and interest-free. In other words, the private sector subsidized the construction of hospitals, an interesting mixture of nonprofit and profit enterprise that was accepted by the body politic as natural. The personal health services, which are oriented toward acute care, were stimulated enormously by the dynamics of medical science, technology, and money. In the 1930s, this system was poised for even more dynamic expansion than it had experienced since 1875. Relative to the personal health services, public health departments and mental hospitals have barely held their own.

1930 TO 1965

While the period from 1875 to 1930 witnessed the development of the health services infrastructure, the period from 1930 to 1965 is characterized mainly by the emergence of a third party to pay the day-to-day expenses.

The rise of the third party payer was undoubtedly stimulated by the Depression of the 1930s, when both hospital and personal income fell, but it is likely that the third party would have emerged eventually anyway. Hospitals could operate better with a steady income, and families could more readily meet the increasing costs resulting from improved medical technology. Hospitals began to sponsor prepayment plans, which eventually became known as Blue Cross plans. In fact, after 1933, the health services resumed their growth, as reflected in the proportion of the gross national product (GNP) directed to them. Hospital stays were relatively costly and lent themselves well to insurance, since a predictable number of individuals in the population would incur hospital expenses in a year.

At the same time, prepayment for physicians' services in the hospital, mainly surgery, began to appear in the late thirties. Sponsored by state medical societies, these became known as Blue Shield plans. Surgery was also a relatively costly procedure and lent itself to the principle of insurance. State governments continued to sponsor health services for the poor, and eventually a shared program between the federal government and the states emerged. The Emergency Maternal and Infant Care Program for the wives and dependents of servicemen during World War II represented the first national health services program for a conspicuous segment of the population. Congress felt it could do nothing less for our soldiers.

During the forties and into World War II, private insurance companies discovered from the experience of the Blue Cross and Blue Shield plans that hospital care and surgery were insurable. Congress gave the voluntary plans a financial boost by decreeing that health insurance (and pensions) were fringe benefits and thus exempt from the wartime freeze on wages. This is another example of government encouragement of the private sector, since the portion of health insurance paid by the employer is a tax-exempt business expense. Further, signing up for fringe benefits became a condition of employment; this form of compulsion was acceptable, whereas any compulsory government program would have been taboo. After the passage in 1935 of the Social Security Act, which mandated mainly pensions and unemployment insurance, legislation proposing compulsory health insurance was put on the back burner of the congressional stove until 1952, the last year of Truman's presidency.

The Blue Cross and Blue Shield plans and the private insurance companies were spectacularly successful. They went far beyond their own expectations in enrolling employee groups in the major industries, and by 1952 over one-half of the population was covered by some form of health insurance, mainly hospital care and physician services in the hospital. With the election of Dwight Eisenhower in 1952, the venomous controversy over voluntary versus compulsory, government-sponsored health insurance subsided. Eisenhower would not support government health insurance.

A salient aspect of the rise of third party payers is that the organizational structure of health services that had emerged since 1875 was taken as a given; the insurance agencies and the government were concerned with paying its charges. In the case of hospitals, the concept was charges or costs, whichever was lower, since hospital accounting systems were underdeveloped and not uniform. Physicians were paid by voluntary health insurance according to generous fee schedules negotiated by Blue Shield plans. There were no direct negotiations at all with private insurance companies because there were no contracts with them. These reimbursement methods seem irresponsible in retrospect, but then money flowed freely in a rapidly expanding economy. The public was exhorted by public health departments to "See your doctor early," and maternal and child health programs were promoted. Encouragement was scarcely needed for either major or minor surgery. Admissions to hospitals and visits to physicians increased dramatically between the late thirties and the sixties: hospital admissions increased from 90 per 1,000 persons in the population per year to 145; the percentage of the population who saw a physician in a year increased from 39 to 65. The supply of hospital beds and physicians increased, but not in relation to demand. Physicians became very busy and prosperous. Hospital occupancy rates went up, and hospitals also became more prosperous, their chronic deficits notwithstanding.

To add to the stock of hospitals and beds, particularly in rural areas, Congress in 1946 passed the Hospital Survey and Construction (Hill-Burton) Act. This act was supported by such diverse interests as the American Hospital Association (AHA), the American Medical Association (AMA), and labor organizations, which ordinarily worked at cross-purposes in efforts to enact government health insurance. The act was designed as a one-shot grant to hospitals, both public and voluntary, for start-up costs, with grant funds to be matched by the hospitals. Each state for the first time took an inventory of its hospital beds, and grants were made to hospitals within the framework of a loose plan. The act supplied around 25 percent of the expenditures for hospitals, which in turn generated a considerable amount of money from private and public sources, mainly private. The main object of the act, which was very successful, was to buttress the voluntary hospital. The old sources of capital, philanthropy and community fund-raising drives, were diminishing, and public hospitals were regarded as outside the mainstream of the hospital system. This is another instance of government supporting the private, nonprofit sector. The voluntary hospital is an integral part of community life and interweaves the private and public sectors so closely as to make it difficult to differentiate between the two.

By the early 1950s, an engine of finance had been established from private sources for the day-to-day operation of the hospital and physician services and from public and private sources for the supply of hospital beds, physicians, and other personnel. The general economy and the health services economy were booming. The existing health services infrastructure continued to be accepted as a given.

Within the relatively private, nonprofit health services economy, however, there rose a development that was concerned directly with restructuring the delivery of physicians' services and indirectly with hospital care. This was the group practice prepayment plan, which attempted to compete with solo-practice fee-for-service medical delivery, engage a range of specialists on a salary, provide a full range of physician services, from curative to preventive, and serve a known population. The Kaiser-Permanente plans were established in the West, and the Health Insurance Plan of Greater New York (HIP) was established in the East. In cities like Washington, D.C., Seattle, St. Louis, Minneapolis–St. Paul, similar plans were established on a more or less cooperative, consumer-owned basis. Initially, opposition on the part of medical societies to these new arrangements was fierce. Gradually, however, they began to take their place in the spectrum of types of health services delivery and in some areas came to be regarded as options in labor-management negotiations for fringe benefits. Their influence appeared to be out of all proportion to their pace of growth (involving around 4 percent of the population), since they became reference points for quality health services at a "reasonable" price. It seems that only in the United States was this diversity of delivery types possible. American physicians have an entrepreneurial propensity, and an ability to raise capital, unlike physicians in any other country. The concept of private group practices, in which physicians live on fees, undoubtedly inspired the concept of group practice prepayment, in which physicians live on premiums divided among the physicians on salaries.

The private engine of finance was probably aided by the public engine with the passage of the Medicare Act for the aged and the Medicaid Act for the poor in 1965. Medicare is a federal program and Medicaid is a shared federal-state program. Medicare takes the cost of care of the aged off the backs of families and the private sector, and Medicaid, along with assuaging the national conscience, takes the cost of care of the poor off the shaky revenue structure of the states and tries to equalize care for the poor across states. By 1965, private and nonprofit insurance agencies were supplying 40 percent of the cost of day-to-day operations of hospitals and 30 percent of physicians' services. Government, mainly the federal government, was paying for 50 percent of the hospital costs and 20 percent of the physicians' services. The stage was set for a spectacular increase in price and use. There were no serious built-in controls on costs. The health services enterprise had become accustomed to being paid what it asked, and the funding sources did not demur because employees, employers, and Congress did not demur either. From 1950 to 1965, expenditures as a percent of GNP rose from 4.6 to 5.9. Expenditures per capita for all services rose from $78 to $198, not accounting for inflation, which was moderate during that period. The private insurance agencies and the government teamed up, as it were, to assure a health service where cost would be of no consequence.

Concomitantly, the proportion of people age 65 and older was increasing, particularly those 75 to 80 and older. Ineluctably associated with aging are chronic illness and disability and the increasing financial helplessness that overtakes families with aged members. By the fifties, expenditures on nursing homes became a visible portion of the national medical dollar, but only a small portion of this cost could be expected from direct-pay patients. Public medical assistance for the indigent in nursing homes became a prime source of funding for day-to-day operations, and it was buttressed greatly after 1965 by Medicaid. True to the American tradition, the market for nursing homes was met largely by the private sector, both profit and nonprofit, and standards were set by the states together with Medicaid and Medicare. Government was unable or unwilling to supply enough nursing home beds to meet the demand and need. As usual, government bought services from the private sector and paid pretty much what the nursing homes were charging.

1965 TO THE PRESENT

It was not until the latter sixties that there began to be general concern by the big buyers of services—government, employers and labor unions, and insurance and prepayment agencies—over rising expenditures for personal health services. It was the pace of the increase that was alarming, with costs rising faster than the general economy as reflected in the consumer price index and the GNP. The public was mainly interested in reducing out-of-pocket expenditures, and the buyers of services were interested in keeping insurance premiums and reimbursements to providers low. Hospital expenditures were rising at the dizzying pace of 15 percent annually. Expenditures for physicians' services were close behind. Providers said the increase in expenditures was justified in large part because of improved services and increased use, as well as rising labor costs in this labor-intensive enterprise. No one knew what constituted an appropriate level of expenditures, but there seemed to be general agreement that the current level was too high. Theories of costs and expenditures were equally primitive.

This period, then, is characterized by an intense concern with how to manage the health services enterprise so that buyers know what they are buying and providers know what they are offering. The practice of simply paying what the providers asked was being seriously questioned. Further, the payment mechanism was to be used to manage the system. Three methods of doing so emerged, largely in this order: (1) monitoring physician decision making in hospitals, (2) control of hospital beds, and (3) control of hospital reimbursement rates.

Attempts at rationalization of the personal health services, to use an economic term, were expressed mainly in group practice prepayment plans. These were set up not simply to save money, but to provide high quality and comprehensive services efficiently and conveniently. It seemed that saving money was a secondary although acknowledged consideration. Likewise, the scores of hospital planning councils that were established in major cities, sponsored by local hospitals and funded in large part by DHEW, were aimed less at saving money than at systematizing hospital relationships and cooperation on the local level. The councils were intended to serve as information clearing-houses on hospital beds and equipment in local areas, the presumption being that the hospitals would recognize their own interests. These councils may have had other effects, but the evidence shows that reducing duplication of services or stabilizing the bed supply was not among them.

The seeming lack of success of the hospital council concept led to the federal program called Comprehensive Health Planning (CHP). This program was to be concerned with facilities planning through the states and incorporated many of the hospital planning councils as agents of the state. Another federal endeavor through the states at this time, the Regional Medical Programs (RMP), was aimed at the delivery of services for heart disease, cancer, and stroke (and related diseases). It attempted to connect practicing physicians to medical schools and major medical centers so physicians could benefit from the latest knowledge concerning these diseases and refer their patients more rapidly. Saving money was not the primary concern, integrating physicians' services was. Both CHP and RMP failed in terms of the nonexistent performance standards implicit, but certainly not explicit, in the legislation. In the meantime, expenditures increased apace; the internal and external dynamics of this tremendous growth enterprise were indeed awesome. Two prestigious government commissions were formed, one on so-called hospital effectiveness (1968) and one on Medicaid and medical care for the poor

(1970), the latter actually expanding its vague charge to consider the entire delivery structure and planning. The tone in both reports was confusion and frustration, as well it might be: the commissions were ambiguous about planning, although advocating it, and distressed by the prospect of further government intervention, although helpless to suggest anything else. The Medicaid report began to refer to competition among delivery systems as a means of containing rising expenditures.

More specific attempts at containing expenditures, however, were made in the Medicare Act; these also applied to Medicaid. The Medicare Act mandated reviews of physicians' decisions regarding length of stay in hospitals—that is, direct monitoring of professional decision making. From the profession's viewpoint this was a radical step.

On the state level, legislatures began to pass laws calling for certificates of need for hospital beds. The building of new hospitals and the expansion or renovation of old hospitals had to be approved by a state planning agency, a control on supply. State legislatures also began to regulate hospital rate setting, a control on price.

As a result of its 1965 mandate, Congress passed a law in 1972 requiring utilization review of hospital care (that is, physician decision making) on an areawide basis by committees of physicians. These groups were called Professional Standards Review Organizations (PSROs). To cap all these developments, Congress passed the Health Planning Act, which mandated the creation of over 200 health planning areas; these were administered by health services agencies, whose boards of governors were made up primarily of consumers. Consumers were to be appointed on the basis of race, ethnic background, income, and geographic area. The health services agencies were to determine the appropriateness of hospital construction, distribution, and renovation and the acquisition policies of hospitals regarding expensive equipment such as CAT scanners. Further, the health services agencies were to work up masterplans of the health needs in their areas according to federal guidelines. Plans were then passed on to the appropriate state and federal agencies for review and consideration. Congress intended to place determination of needs and control over the construction of facilities on the local level. Local needs, as determined by health services agencies, would be communicated to upper levels of government, particularly the federal government, which could then negotiate on a long-term basis. Congress and perhaps even the bureaucracy are exceedingly chary of imposing a blueprint on the states and local areas, preferring instead to set up fairly loose guidelines for discussion in order to reach consensus. It was apparently Congress' intent to put a planning apparatus in place before the enactment of some form of national health insurance in order to have a handle on costs and to direct the development of personal health services. Certificates of need and rate control, although functions of the states, became part of the health services agencies' decisions and therefore a concern of the federal government, which can withhold payment from hospitals that do not comply. Even so, the current planning apparatus does not seem to have a firm place in national political policy and continues to exist on sufferance.

Americans look suspiciously at structures, boundaries, and budget caps. It is hoped that the monitoring of physician decision making will lead to a rational, justifiable volume and quality of services at reasonable costs within the planning framework briefly described here.

The latest concept being tried to contain escalating costs is the Health Maintenance Organization (HMO). Old as a concept but relatively new in terms of government support, HMOs embody several types of prepayment plans that attempt to monitor physician decision making, set a fixed premium for comprehensive services, and serve a known population. These plans have shown that they use hospital services less than the fee-for-service system and hence tend to cost less. Competition is thus being carried over to health services delivery, encouraging a choice of plans among employed groups in hopes of tempering the rise in health services costs.

In the meantime, the personal health services economy is growing, expenditures continue to rise, and attempts to manage the system do not seem to have much effect as yet. Between 1965 and 1980, the percent of the GNP spent for all health services increased from 5.9 to 9.0, and per capita expenditures increased from $198 to $865. By 1990, the estimated percent of GNP spent for health stood at 12 and per capita expenditures at $2,511. The ultimate weapon, of course, is in the hands of the big buyers of services, who can refuse to provide more money. The pluralistic nature of funding, however, makes such a course difficult, even though the federal government is now the source of 40 percent of all expenditures for personal health services.

Some years ago I wrote a book on the private and public financing of personal health services, called *The Uneasy Equilibrium*. The uneasy equilibrium between private and public control and financing continues, but in a much more intense form. The government still does not own, nor does it want to own, the hospitals. It does not want to make physicians into salaried employees, nor would Congress enact such a plan in the foreseeable future. Thus the private sector, if it is politically astute, is playing on Congress' reluctance to set up a highly structured system. The private sector may well continue to be an effective balance to government intervention—a term implying that government is intervening in a normal situation—because the American people want choices, easy access, and the latest technology rather than low cost. To the public, the relationship of health services expenditures to the GNP is an abstraction that has no bearing on their daily lives.

3

Systems Elements of a Health Service

The health services enterprise lends itself to systematization because its various parts are interrelated. Even though our understanding of the degree and nature of those relationships is fragmentary so far, it is reasonable to assume that they are in fact interrelated. The continuing problem is to uncover patterns in the system. There are entry and exit points for patients, there is a hierarchy of personnel and facilities, and there are various sources and destinations of funding. It is a highly valued enterprise, as evidenced by its persistence, growth, and apparent durability into the future. Two major characteristics peculiar to this enterprise are (1) that the people who use it are by and large sick and (2) that the sick person seeks the help of a trained professional, the physician. The self-definition of illness, which leads patients to seek assistance, is exceedingly varied in time and place. The judgment of the physician regarding what the ill person needs once help is sought is also exceedingly varied in time and place. The result is an enterprise with few systematic indicators of performance. The economist's desire to get the most output for the least input founders because there are no measures of efficiency. The best that has been done so far, a compromise between economics and the behavioral sciences, is to relate input and output to Herbert Simon's concept of "satisficing"—that is, maximizing and balancing the expectations of patients, the professional judgments of physicians, and the resources available in some kind of tolerable and temporary equilibrium.

In the middle of the nineteenth century, the health services enterprise was very simple, but volatile. It had the same elements of a sick person and a designated professional (a physician) but no complicated facility like the modern hospital with its resource-devouring capacity.

Physicians charged fees for each service, and legend had it that services were frequently free to low-income people, since physicians charged on a sliding scale. Society expected but did not formally enforce this practice. The house and office were the primary treatment sites. Normally, physicians did not have even receptionists to act as facilitators or barriers between themselves and their patients. In home care, physicians delegated nursing duties to an appropriate adult. Relationships were informal, although the authority of the physician was undoubtedly recognized and accepted.

With antisepsis and anesthesia came a hospital setting, requiring nurse attendants, kitchen help, janitorial service, an administrator, and, in the case of voluntary hospitals, boards of trustees. The community became informed about the hospital through the boards of trustees. Relationships were established with philanthropic sources of capital. The physician-surgeon needed an efficient, nurturing figure who could sustain sick people under the physicians' guidance. The nurse became the bridge between the administrator and the physician. Physicians spontaneously and effortlessly became the power center of the hospital because of their monopoly on medical knowledge. The community provided the resources and the patients, the physicians provided the skills, and a tripartite division of power and responsibility emerged among the board, the administrator, and the physician. The administrator might be a senior nurse, a minister (in the case of church-sponsored hospitals), or a bookkeeper. The hospital took on a hierarchical structure quite naturally because of the life-and-death decisions that were always latent. Its several layers of personnel could not be entered from the bottom up, only laterally. Hospitals immediately had as wide a range of unskilled to skilled to professional personnel under one roof as existed anywhere then or now, with the nonprofessional staff considerably outnumbering the professional staff. The professionals wore white coats or other types of uniforms, nonprofessionals did not. The administrator, if a man, wore a white shirt, tie, and business suit; if a woman, usually a nurse's uniform. The board and the administrator controlled the resources, but, as public demand rose in the increasingly affluent society, physicians seemed generally to get what they said they needed for high quality care.

Resources were increasingly poured into the specialties, which required high technology and surgical equipment, resulting in further differentiation among technical personnel. Physicians themselves established a hierarchy, usually with the surgeon at the top and general practitioners on the bottom. Each laboratory skill and each medical specialization formed its own association. These structures became more and more impermeable, and the board and the administrator found themselves dealing with more and more entities. Physicians established informal referral patterns with each other, which are obscure to this day, but these patterns are at the core of physician behavior.

The hospital's financial management was exceedingly simple—in effect, one drawer in the administrator's desk for income and another for outgo. Cost accounting was not considered, because the hospital was a nonprofit, charitable institution whose surpluses were an embarrassment and whose deficits, within reason, were considered normal. The care of sick people was beyond price, and there were no indicators of performance anyway. The hospital was an extension of the home, where cost accounting is not generally practiced. Thus, it is not surprising that there are little data on the structure and operation of the health services enterprise between 1875 and 1930. The structure was known only as a conglomeration of hospitals, beds, expenditures and capital funding, number of physicians by specialty and their incomes, nurses and their incomes, and so on. It is remarkable that this tremendous health services infrastructure was able to develop with so little operational information to guide it.

Other types of practitioners, who were outside the mainstream of medical practice—for example, naturopaths, chiropractors, faith healers, and osteopaths—grew up during this period. The osteopaths' one-cause, one-therapy philosophy eventually acquired the major characteristics of mainstream medicine. The extent to which these alternative practitioners were sought out by the general public is not known, but it is reasonable to assume that it was considerable, since they depended on fees from private patients. It may also be reasonable to assume that the emerging mainstream, scientific medicine, began to absorb the major share of health care practice by the early twentieth century. The dental services emerged as a separate system and did not need hospital facilities until much later.

A considerable and unmeasured contribution to the medical establishment was care provided by the members of patients' families and patients' self-care. Even today little is known about the substratum of care given by nonprofessionals, that gray area between the official medical establishment and the community and family support structure. It is on the periphery of the system.

In order to bring out the systems nature of the health services, it is necessary to develop statistical indicators of the structure and process of the enterprise. National data on physicians and dentists were published routinely by 1850, and data on nurses by 1900. These listed gross number of personnel, number of training institutions, and number of graduates. Systematic data on hospitals and beds did not become available until around 1909. Not until 1946 were aggregate data on expenditures for health services published annually or even sporadically. The system was in full swing before there was any knowledge of how much it was costing, who was getting services, what kind of services, or for how much. By this time, however, data on vital statistics and population had been well-developed by the U.S. Census Bureau and state health departments, the latter mainly for reportable diseases. The Census Bureau was the source for data on mortality. Only fragmentary data on morbidity in the general population had been collected. The prevailing and plausible assumption was that there must be a relationship between mortality, morbidity, and the presence or absence of health services. The general mortality rate was, of course, going down, as were many of the reportable diseases, and the leading causes of death were being turned upside down. Tuberculosis, pneumonia, and gastroenteritis were being replaced by heart disease, cancer, and stroke.

From 1928 to 1933, however, the most massive national study of the extent of morbidity and the use of and expenditure for personal health services by families ever attempted by any country was conducted. This was primarily a private endeavor and was funded by six foundations. Twenty-six studies were published on many phases of personal health services, from morbidity to delivery systems. The most important one from the standpoint of the general public's relationship to personal health service was the household survey. For the first time, a contour map of the public's problems was juxtaposed with national data on facilities, personnel, and expenditures. It now became possible to base public policy on facts.

Quantifying the elements of the health services enterprise precisely is a never-ending task. Because of the difficulties of defining and measuring need, demand, and professional judgment, discussion and debate on a "good" or "efficient" health services enterprise become largely matters of informed opinion and experience on the part of decision makers. This situation results in administrative and political platitudes implying a precision and certainty that cannot exist. Happily, however, reliable indicators of performance are beginning to appear.

As a beginning, it is necessary to set forth the usual indicators of general tendencies and ranges so that a single system can be compared with itself and with other systems over time. The comparative approach, both in time and across space, is about the only one available, because the performance indicators appear to have no internal reference points such as the chemical composition of water or the body temperature of a normal human being. Our daily lives are suffused with "indicators" we take for granted—temperature and humidity, driving speeds, baseball batting averages, prices, air pollution indexes, and so on. Indicators are also being used more and more often in the health field, for example hospital admission rates, number of visits to physicians' offices, and the proportion of the GNP being allocated to the health services.

The following indicators are not exhaustive, but they are probably detailed enough for a global approach to the personal health services system. Analysis of the functioning of a department in a hospital or of a particular specialty practice will need much more detailed, specific indicators.

OUTLINE OF ELEMENTS OF A HEALTH SERVICES SYSTEM

Types of Facilities

General Hospitals. The general hospital is mainly a facility for patients with acute conditions. This seeming precision of definition, however, is illusory. Convention has it that patients remaining in a general hospital fewer than 20 to 30 days are short-term patients. Any patient remaining longer is long-term and constitutes a significant and worrisome minority to payment agencies. Thus, the definition of acute is fuzzy. Length of stay is also a function of the relationship of the hospital to the home and long-term facilities, not to mention physicians' practice habits.

Treatment units are usually organized according to type of care—medical-surgical, obstetric, pediatric, psychiatric, and emergency. This mix has changed considerably over time and will continue to do so in the face of new technology and specialties. The rising costs of hospital care may drive patients with "minor" conditions into physicians' offices. The care of the elderly is becoming a large gray area straddling acute and long-term care, the latter being given in various sites.

Treatment sites are also determined by type of accommodation, private, semiprivate, or ward. Private always means one patient in a room, semiprivate can mean from two to four patients in a room, and ward can mean many more patients in a room. These kinds of accommodations were originally a product of the patient's class, with little regard for medical condition. Popular cant was that the quality, that is, the technical quality, of care did not vary among patients in the different types of accommodations. Amenities improved, however, with privacy. With increasing egalitarianism, particularly in countries with universal health insurance, patients came to be placed in accommodations on the basis of the severity of their conditions: the more severe the condition, the greater the amount of privacy.

The European pattern of accommodation has been largely open wards (with a very small component of private rooms for the upper classes), but in this country there has always been a relatively large number of private and semiprivate rooms. Since World War II, the proportion of private and semiprivate beds has exceeded that of ward beds, a function of rising standards of living and increasing desire for privacy. Privacy is expensive and becomes more desirable with rising affluence.

Finally, administrative units are determined by the type of technical equipment and facilities required—operating room, delivery room, pharmacy, laboratory, and x-ray department. In a very large hospital there are others. These are the so-called ancillary services, that is, ancillary to bed, board, and general nursing services. Ancillary services have become an increasingly larger component of the charges, reflecting the growing technology of medical care. Many hospitals have outpatient departments for out-of-hospital consultation and emergency departments for trauma. These are regarded for administrative purposes as separate components.

Mental Hospitals. These institutions have generally been separate from general hospitals. The unusual and unpredictable behavior of their patients set mental patients apart, and they were usually established before general hospitals. The philosophy of therapy is also vastly different in mental hospitals and involves less complicated technology. Mental hospitals are often located out in the country in order to isolate patients. It is not as easy to classify mental patients by administrative type, whether in relation to the degree of freedom given them within the hospital building and on the grounds or by diagnosis (schizophrenic, manic-depressive, alcoholic, and so on). Since World War II, there has been an attempt to establish psychiatric units in general hospitals for initial observation and therapy, to build community mental health clinics, and to deemphasize institutional care. The trend is toward bridging the traditional gap between psychiatric patients and the mainstream of medicine. Naturally, this creates further difficulties in classifying patients across institutions and tends to blur the purity of institutional types for measuring purposes. The population of mental hospitals has been decreasing over the years.

Tuberculosis Hospitals. These hospitals represent one of the very few instances of serving a special and relatively well identified disease entity. Demand for beds has been decreasing for many years, largely because chemotherapy and earlier case finding have resulted in shorter stays.

Long-Term Care Facilities. Long-term hospitals, nursing homes, and rehabilitation centers provide care after discharge from general hospitals for patients with chronic illnesses that do not require the high technology usually available in general hospitals. Nursing homes have been the fastest growing component of long-term care for the last 20 years. They fall somewhere between the general hospital and the home. The nursing home is adding to administrative complexity in regard to standards, costs, and services. For example, nursing homes are supposed to classify patients by the intensity of care given in order to determine costs.

Other Facilities There are many other facilities serving people with health-related problems, but they have a large "social" component. These facilities may employ social workers or simply housekeepers in addition to professional health personnel. Homes for the aged who need primarily custodial care are examples, as are residential schools for the blind and deaf. A relatively new type of institution has emerged in the past few years in response to the increasing number of terminally ill people who need support and relief from pain—the hospice. The relationship of the hospice to the mainstream of the health services enterprise is not yet clear. Health professionals in hospices are skilled in relieving pain and giving psychological support; clergy are also present.

Uses of Facilities

This group of conventional indicators refers to events that measure access to facilities, length of stay and eventual discharge, and expenditure.

Admissions. For general hospitals, the rate of admissions is measured as the number of people per 1,000 persons in the population admitted during a year. A further refinement is the proportion of the population with one admission, two admissions, and so on in a year.

The conventional measurement for mental and tuberculosis hospitals is number of admissions per 100,000 population in a year. As with general hospitals, a refinement is the number of first admissions, second admissions, and so on. Readmissions are particularly important indicators of patient problems, in these hospitals.

For nursing homes and other long-term care facilities, there seems to be no standard measure of admission rates. Rather, the usual measure is the number of patients in these facilities at a given time. The assumption is that patients stay a very long time, most of them until they die. If admission rates were used at all, it is likely that they would be expressed per 100,000 persons.

Expenditures. Care must be taken to differentiate between expenditures and costs. Expenditures simply reveal what the system is charging. Costs are supposed to reveal how much it actually costs to produce a given service. There is a great deal of ambiguity and controversy surrounding costs as facilities are increasingly being reimbursed by third-party payers. The usual gross measurement is of total expenditures per fiscal year, refined by per diem, per case, or per bed measures, or combinations of these. Within the facility, expenditures can be divided by room into bed, board, general nursing, and the combination of ancillary services mentioned earlier. They can also be broken down by type of labor and goods; this breakdown reveals the exceedingly labor-intensive nature of the health services.

Age, Sex, and Diagnosis. All of the foregoing indicators need to be related to age, sex, and diagnosis of the patient. Case mix is an important factor in comparing costs across hospitals, because patients with some diseases are much more expensive to treat than others. Individual hospital costs are being codified so that they can be compared for accounting and reimbursement purposes by a method known as diagnosis-related groupings (DRGs) of disease. In order to understand the relationship between a facility and the community, we must also measure the educational and income levels, places of residence, and ethnic characteristics of patients—that is, their place in the social structure.

Types and Uses of Personnel

Physicians. The physician is a distinct occupational type. He or she almost always has an M.D. degree, but a visible minority of osteopathic physicians (D.O.s) also belong in this category. Beyond the basic criterion of a medical degree there are great variations. There are roughly 35 specialties in addition to general, or family, practice, which is also regarded as a specialty. There is great variety among practice organizations, from so-called solo practitioners to large group practices. Sometimes these group practices are single-specialty groups, at other times multi-specialty groups. Methods of payment also vary, the predominant one being fee-for-service; some physicians are on salary, and many have a combination of income sources and methods of payment. They are, in effect, entrepreneurs.

The usual measures of physicians' services are units per person per year, which in this country appears to range between four and five. The other is the proportion of the population that sees a physician in a year. The current proportion is between 70 and 75 percent, a considerable increase since 1940. These indicators can be related to home, office, and hospital calls and to time of day. A more detailed measure of utilization is type of procedure performed, diagnostic or therapeutic. Therapeutic procedures can be divided into medical and surgical treatment and all their variants, with a rough measure of surgical treatment being number of operations performed per 1,000 persons per year. These hardly exhaust the possible measures, and more and more information is being gathered on types of operations, the range and proportion of illnesses, and conditions for which people seek care. Finally, the number of physicians per 100,000 population or the number of people per physician roughly indicates supply and potential utilization. The supply of physicians should be divided into specialties available in a given area. Physicians are mainly men, although the proportion of women is increasing.

Nurses. The usual classification of nurses is headed by registered nurses (RNs) and their various specialties (public health, surgical, and clinical). There is a lower-level category called licensed practical nurses and a large group of nurses' aides. In recent years another RN specialty has emerged—the nurse practitioner, who takes over many of the physician's patient assessment and therapeutic procedures under the physician's supervision. Nurses are overwhelmingly female, but some male nurses are beginning to appear. Another type of practitioner that has emerged, although more as an extension of the physician's role than of the nurse's role, is the physician assistant. These nurses are usually male. Naturally, these new types add to the complexity of role relationships among the health services personnel.

Dentists. Dentists are a distinct occupational type and are concerned with dental and mouth diseases and dental surgery. They have a D.D.S. degree. They have differentiated themselves from physicians ever since dentistry developed as a health service in the middle of the nineteenth century. Dentists are also specialists to some degree. The site of service is usually the private office, although a relatively small amount of hospital work is done for multiple extractions of teeth and oral surgery. The overwhelming majority of dentists are general practitioners, but a few specialize, usually in orthodontics or oral surgery. Types of procedures performed can be divided roughly into preventive (checkups, tooth scaling) and treatment (fillings, extractions and replacements). Dentists are usually paid on a fee-for-service basis, although a few may be salaried. The utilization of dentists' services is measured in number of visits per 1,000 persons per year. As usual, age, sex, and procedure performed are necessary variables in assessing the use of dental services.

Pharmacists. The pharmacist is also a distinct professional type and has a Registered Pharmacist degree, R.Ph. The usual site of service is the retail pharmacy, but hospitals and clinics are becoming common sites. The usual method of payment in a retail pharmacy (unless the pharmacist is the owner) is by salary. Pharmacists may also be paid per prescription filled.

Support Personnel. The wide range of technical support personnel includes laboratory and x-ray technologists, physical and occupational therapists, and social workers. New types seem to be constantly emerging, for example, inhalation therapists.

Levels of Health

If human beings were not prey to disease, disability, and premature death, there would obviously be no health services enterprise as we know it today. Hence, health services are charged with managing, curing, preventing, rehabilitating, or at least palliating disease. There is a common-sense assumption that somehow health services affect public health. This is by no means clear. What is clear is that professionals and the public believe there is. In only a relatively small proportion of instances is it possible to establish a direct relationship, for example in the control of diabetes or the prevention of smallpox. What is quite clear is that at any time and in any place there is a disease and mortality pattern and this pattern is related to the social and economic environment, including health services. The ecology of disease is exceedingly complex: there are multiple reasons for a disease and mortality pattern at any given time.

Mortality. The conventional measurements of mortality are as follows:

— Crude mortality rate—the number of deaths per 1,000 persons per year
— Age-specific mortality—the number of deaths in a given age group per 1,000 persons in that group per year
— Cause-specific mortality—number of deaths due to a given diagnosis per 1,000 persons per year
— Age specific cause-specific mortality—deaths related to age at death and diagnosis simultaneously
— Survival curve at given ages out of each 100,000 persons born alive

- Curve of expectation of life—years of life remaining at given ages
- Average life expectancy (other variables such as sex or race can and should be introduced, depending on the problem to be examined)
- Infant mortality—the number of deaths of infants under the age of one year per 1,000 live births. Refinements are perinatal mortality (number of deaths within one week after birth per 1,000 live births) and neonatal mortality (number of deaths within four weeks). Definitions vary, but the primary criterion is the viability of the fetus before and a few days after birth.

The foregoing variables can be differentiated by sex, cause, number of previous births to the mother (parity), birth order, and age of the mother. Neonatal mortality is largely biological in origin, whereas post-neonatal mortality has a large environmental component. Biological causes of mortality are much less amenable to control than are environmental ones. This is why the greatest reductions in infant mortality have occurred among infants between the ages of one and twelve months.

Morbidity. Morbidity rates are regarded as much more refined measures of health status than mortality rates alone. Only a small proportion of illnesses results in death, thus a measure of the illness in a population can be regarded as a measure of its health status. Other measures of health status that involve illness are number of days in bed per year and absence from work or school. Statistics on mortality and its causes are usually routinely recorded by public agencies. Morbidity is much more difficult to measure than mortality because it is open to a variety of definitions whereas mortality is a discrete event. Thus appropriate need-demand relationships to use of services are difficult to specify.

During the past 20 years, great efforts have been made to measure morbidity; the main ones are:

- Household surveys asking about symptoms and conditions
- Physical examinations of a sample of the population by a medical team
- Existing records on reportable diseases, physicians' records, hospital records, insurance companies' experience, and others.

The kinds of morbidity rates in general use are similar to the mortality rates, that is, morbidity by age, sex, and cause. It is difficult to differentiate between acute and chronic morbidity, leading to arbitrary definitions of duration. The statistical convention is that a condition lasting less than three months is acute, one lasting more than three months is chronic.

Indicators of mortality and morbidity relate primarily to the biological characteristics of the individual, for whom it is hoped that health services will pay off in terms of longer life and decreased morbidity. As the survival rate from acute disease increases, there will be more chronic illness. Thus other indexes of payoff need to be used to evaluate the effectiveness of a health service. These indexes must involve relief of pain and anxiety, measures of satisfaction, and accommodation to the disabilities inevitably accompanying aging. These are measures of quality rather than quantity of life and will require far greater conceptual and methodological sophistication than we now have. The biological indicators are no longer adequate—if they ever were—for affluent, industrialized countries.

Expenditures

Not surprisingly, the most common and popular indicators are the expenditures on the entire health services enterprise, the costs of its components, and sources of payment. It is difficult to learn much about resource allocation and results from these indicators, but money does give some idea of society's priorities. Expenditures also give some indication of the limits of political and private market tolerance. In an overall approach, it is customary to break down the major components of the personal health services into the so-called medical dollar, as follows:

— Hospital care, both short-term and long-term
— Physician care
— Dental care
— Drugs
— Appliances
— Nursing home care
— Other

Since these components are more or less freestanding, one can determine the differential expenditures on them and the interplay among them. For example, there has been intense concern about expenditures for general hospital care, which absorbs more of the medical dollar than any other single component. Physicians, it is estimated, are responsible for about 80 percent of the medical dollars spent, since, in addition to their own fees, they control hospital use and prescribed drugs and they influence the purchase of many nonprescription drugs as well as appliances and nursing home care.

Other conventional measures of expenditures are percent of GNP a country allocates to health services and percent of family income spent on health services. Finally, sources of funds for health services, such as government, private insurer, employer, employee, or direct payment, indicate potential sources of control over the operation of the health services enterprise.

BOUNDARIES

I have dealt so far chiefly with the components of the health services enterprise that are professional and official. They constitute the boundaries of a relatively easily defined system with entry and exit points, hierarchies of personnel types, and patients, all of which are necessary to a systems approach.

The system's indicators are so closely related that a change in one produces unpredictable results in the others. In probably no other human enterprise do so many unintended consequences result from attempts at change. Politicians and policy makers are driven wild because they can find no convenient or effective handles. The unexpected and unintended consequences flow from the facts that (1) the "customers" are sick and therefore relatively irrational and (2) those from whom they seek help, the physicians, require a great deal of discretion and authority, given the nature of medical practice. The enterprise is thus inherently volatile and must be managed, if it can be managed at all, with a great deal of looseness. All the indicators in this chapter help us to understand the workings of the enterprise, and so far these are all we have.

PART II

The Health Services, 1875–1930

4

Public Health and Personal Health

Any history of the development of American health services must draw on a great many secondary sources, for no one author can research the entire field. I hope, however, to place these secondary sources in my own framework. In addition, I can bring my own primary research to bear on various aspects of the development of the health services. Such a synthesis has not been attempted before. In the process, I will reveal the evolution of scholarship in this field.

Although there has been endless talk of integrating public health and personal health services, they started out separately and they remain separate, coming together operationally, if at all, in primary and family care practices. There are structural reasons for this separation: public health deals with problems that individuals are unable to cope with—pure water, pure milk, communicable diseases, occupational diseases, and air pollution—and personal health services deal with the illnesses and disabilities of individuals. Public health deals with masses, whereas personal health services are essentially a one-on-one relationship between a patient and a physician or other personnel. Public health evolved largely from engineering and chemistry and later from bacteriology and the study of communicable diseases. Clinicians have always had a trained incapacity to think in community or group terms; they are understandably and necessarily oriented toward the pathologies of the individual. Clinicians should not confuse the individual and the mass, and the obverse is true: public health personnel should not confuse the mass with the individual. The clinician sees individuals; the public health officer sees statistics. Nevertheless, both types of practitioners must work within the resources that public policy determines.

Aside from the early infirmaries for the indigent sick, public funding in the field of health started with public health problems. The public treasury is the sole source of funds for public health activities; separate funding for public health programs and the emerging personal health services took place later. Sources of funding for personal health services became largely private, a fact that has greatly influenced the relative affluence of the two sectors. Public health was grudgingly funded.

Until the middle of the nineteenth century, responsibility for the health of the public rested with local government, which dealt with epidemics or foul-smelling effluents. The state became involved later, primarily in response to near-crises. Local slaughterhouses were smelly, but the states did not act until the smell became statewide. As Harry S. Mustard says, "The state as a whole did not smell the odor of a local slaughterhouse."[1] State legislatures were preoccupied with the maintenance of order and the encouragement of commerce. They had no interest in formulating broad-gauged well-defined social and health programs. The foul smells had not yet been connected with the emerging theory, backed by scientific evidence, that bacteria cause many of the scourges of mankind. That came later in the nineteenth century.[2] Not surprisingly, therefore, there was a three-generation gap between the establishment of local boards of health and state boards of health. The first state to establish a board of health was Massachusetts, in 1869.

THE FEDERAL ACTIONS

There was no national responsibility for public health, because the states had not ceded it to the federal government in the Constitution. Further, the states had not ceded their traditional responsibility for the destitute, which went back to the Poor Laws of 1601. During the nineteenth century, as cities grew, there were periodic and deadly epidemics of cholera and typhoid fever. These disrupted interstate commerce and threatened the stability of the entire economy. During such epidemics, the federal government, despite the opposition of the states, sent teams of sanitary investigators to port cities and up the Mississippi River, which was teeming with commerce and consequently with people and their effluents. The federal government exercised its constitutional power to maintain commerce, both domestically and internationally, by quarantining ships and ports in order to control the spread of epidemics.[3] Health problems as such were more or less incidental.

Federal-state relations continued to be sticky, but Congress enacted laws in 1878, 1879, and 1893 giving the federal government more power to control epidemics directly. The Marine Hospital Service was given the responsibility for enforcement in 1878. It was the logical agency because it was concerned with waterborne commercial traffic and ports, the apparent loci of epidemics.[4]

In 1879, another group was making itself felt. A nucleus of physicians in the American Public Health Association (APHA), which had been organized in 1872, advocated a national department of health. This idea was also supported by a nucleus of physicians in the AMA. It can be said that medical interest was piqued when the bacteriological causes of many scourges were discovered. They joined forces with the early sanitarians and sanitary engineers. In 1879, the National Board of Health was created, and the power to enforce interstate quarantine laws was taken away from the Marine Hospital Service and given to it. This board, however, was given a legal life of only four years, apparently because it was opposed both by the Marine Hospital Service and by many of the health officers in the South, who had strong, traditional convictions about states' rights. Quarantine duties were returned to the Marine Hospital Service, and in 1890 Congress passed a law that gave the Service authority to propose and enforce regulations for the interstate control of cholera, yellow fever, smallpox, and plague.

Apparently, specific diseases were designated in order to limit federal action as much as possible. This may be inferred from an act passed in 1893 granting the Service additional power in interstate quarantine: to the clause that conferred authority to prevent the "introduction of infectious or contagious diseases into the United States from foreign countries" was added "or from one state or territory . . . into another state or territory." Further, instead of listing specific diseases in the act, the expression "cholera, yellow fever, or other contagious diseases" was used. It was thus possible to be flexible through regulations stemming from a basic law without specific authority from Congress. In 1912, however, the Marine Hospital Service became the U.S. Public Health Service (USPHS) by an Act of Congress.

A brief history of the Marine Hospital Service from its establishment in 1878 to its demise in 1912 is pertinent here because of federal actions in health services. Following precedents set by Great Britain in providing care for seamen, Congress in 1798 passed legislation authorizing the establishment of the Marine Hospital Service. The United States was also concerned with the welfare of its merchant seamen, because it was preparing to engage in world commerce and might face naval clashes in the intense competition for territory and commerce. Sailors came into port with no one directly responsible for those among them who were sick or destitute. Several of the coastal states had so-called hospitals for seamen, but in the Act of 1878 Congress attempted to make the care of seamen a federal responsibility. As an example of congressional parsimony, the original act deducted 20 cents a month from the payroll of all seamen, with no supplements from the national treasury. In 1799, the benefits of the act were extended to naval personnel, and 20 cents a month was likewise deducted from their pay.

The creation of the Marine Hospital Service marked the first time that federal, state, or local governments dealt with special groups and problems rather than general health programs. From the perspective of today, it may be easy to exaggerate the extent to which the Marine Hospital Service was a health service rather than a home away from home; the state of the art in health care was fairly primitive at that time. The Service seems to have set no precedents for federal action in the health field. For example, it would seem to have had no effect on the agitation for compulsory health insurance in 16 states between 1916 and 1918 or on similar agitation for compulsory national health insurance since 1939.[5] As observed by Mustard:

> As a fact accomplished, the Act of 1798 was in the nature of insurance, and it was compulsory. But in the light of the problems, thoughts, and attitudes then current, it would appear questionable to attribute to the Fifth Congress, in admiration or in condemnation, an intent to institute a medical insurance scheme as such schemes are today regarded.[6]

The Act of 1884, however, seems to be more germane to current public policy. That Act eliminated the seamen's required financial contributions to the Marine Hospital Service. Funding came from a special tonnage tax and general revenues. The tonnage tax was eliminated in 1905, and thereafter the Marine Hospital Service was supported entirely from general revenues. This may have set a precedent for financing the medical care of veterans after World War I, since their care is paid for completely from general revenues.

STATE AND LOCAL ACTIONS

Cities grew in size and number in the early nineteenth century. Public health activities were simple in organization and limited in scope; between 1800 and 1830, only five major cities established boards of health.[7] By 1900, however, every state had established a board of health. The establishment of the U.S. Public Health Service represented a solidification of official public health development and suggested that a national concern was emerging. Growth was from the grassroots up, in characteristic American style. Congress' intent was apparently to have a federal agency oversee national and interstate public health affairs. Much later, grants-in-aid were given to states for specific diseases and populations.

Also established in 1912 was the Children's Bureau in the Department of Commerce and Labor (later the Department of Labor). This bureau was the result of increasing concern about child labor laws and the general welfare of children. Before long, the Bureau became engaged in health-related activities such as maternal and child welfare, and particularly infant mortality, in seeming competition with the USPHS. The Bureau was mainly a fact-gathering agency and a clearinghouse for all matters relating to child welfare. Beginning in 1906, it had the support of a variety of influential interest groups promoting reform in child welfare. This reform was sparked by a cadre of women working in settlement houses in the city slums, notably Lillian D. Wald, who founded the Henry Street Settlement in New York City. She made the first appeal for an agency for children to President Theodore Roosevelt in 1906.[8]

During the early nineteenth century, the majority of physicians took little interest in sanitary reform. The conventional explanation for this lack of interest is that the problem of sanitary reform did not call on any special medical knowledge or unit directed toward any particular disease. The data needed were social and statistical, and engineers and statisticians, who think in terms of systems and large numbers, played a larger role than did persons with medical-clinical training. For example, Shryock observes, "The whole spirit in public health work, indeed, was the antithesis of the prevailing emphasis in medical science in the study of specific diseases."[9]

As commonly happens, early sanitary reformers subscribed to the wrong theory, but they applied the right methods to make the cities safer and more pleasant places in which to live. At that time, it seemed reasonable that the garbage, manure piles and open sewers gave off vapors which poisoned the air. These vapors were exceedingly smelly, and their removal very likely received community support for that reason alone, since the poisonous effects were difficult to measure. Consequently, early public health measures, before the advent of bacteriology, were concerned mainly with cleaning up the streets, alleys, and backyards.

Three deservedly famous reports were published in the middle of the nineteenth century: those by J. C. Griscom[10] and Elisha Harris[11] working in New York City, and the one by Lemuel Shattuck[12] in Massachusetts. These reports promoted a new concept—that many deaths are preventable by better sanitation. Griscom's report embodies the principles and objectives of American sanitary reform for decades to come. He pointed out that (1) there was a relationship between illness, premature death, and poverty; (2) they were to a large extent unneccessary and avoidable; and (3) they produced great moral evils which, from an economic point of view, warranted correction on the assumption that the result would be a more productive work force. The latter was important in a country and period that gave economic development a high priority. Even so, the concept of spending public funds for long-term sanitary benefits was unpopular. Logical and dazzling as these early reports appear in hindsight, the difficulty of implementing them has been documented in several histories of public health departments. Barbara Gutman Rosenkrantz, for example, in a sweeping view of public health in Massachusetts, observes that the early pioneers were motivated by religious and moral principles which equated health with a "perfect balance of physical functions achieved by adherence to old-time virtues of cleanliness and morality."[13] Even so, as she remarks, the religious and moral implications of the Shattuck report did not impress the Massachusetts politicians, who were naturally more concerned with the voting behavior of the immigrant poor than with their hygienic habits. Studies of other state and city health departments reveal parallel stages of development, from sanitary control to communicable disease control and the inevitable embroilment of public health in local politics.[14]

Shortly after the APHA was organized, in 1872, the AMA established its Section on State Medicine and Hygiene. The first session of the Section was held during the 1874 annual meeting of the AMA. According to Wilson Smillie, there was misunderstanding and much discussion about the meaning of the term "state medicine."[15] The term is not precise today either, but one may easily infer that physicians were fearful of government intervention in medical practice early on.

Accordingly, the official public health agencies evolved outside the mainstream of personal health services. Until about 1890, public health departments were established as a direct result of the sanitary reform and quarantine movement. Within about ten years, however, as specific causes of epidemic diseases became known, these shotgun efforts became more targeted. The new methods, of course, were a direct result of the burgeoning research in bacteriology. The public health laboratory became the vehicle for government responsibility for the people's health insofar as such responsibility dealt with communicable diseases. In fact, and as Rosenkrantz pointed out, by the beginning of the twentieth century, sources of infection "were shown to be more often people than things, and it became difficult to determine at what points public health encroached upon the duties of physicians or the rights of patients."[16] Further, one might ask, to what extent was public health encroaching on the private practice of medicine through maternal and child health programs?

In 1911, one of the great pioneers in public health, Herman Biggs, then Commissioner of Health of New York City, formulated the motto: "Public health is purchasable. Within natural limits, a community can determine its own death rate."[17] This optimistic motto seemed reasonable because communicable diseases, rampant at the time, and infant mortality were seemingly controllable and direct intervention might well have some effect. Subsequent trends have borne out this optimism, but there is now debate as to what other factors may have had a bearing on the decline of communicable diseases, for example, nutrition, housing, and better living conditions generally.

By 1915, all states had health departments, as did many of the large cities. In addition, many states and cities had established public health laboratories, a sure sign of enlightenment among state legislatures. Health departments were undoubtedly expensive, and they had to start from nothing. Their growth paralleled that of the personal health services, particularly the growth of hospitals. Public health departments seem to have evolved from the top down, for it was not until after 1915 that the recruitment of full-time county health officers was underway. In view of the fact that there were around 3,000 counties, although not all of them with a population large enough to warrant a full-time department, there was great potential in public health work for both physicians and nurses.

Before 1915, public health personnel were recruited mainly from schools of engineering, medicine, and nursing. The first university degree in public health was established at the University of Michigan in 1910. Training in public health was at first a spinoff of engineering because of its early involvement with sanitary issues. As an example, in 1912 a program in sanitation was organized at the Massachusetts Institute of Technology (M.I.T.). A few years later, when it became clear that the environmental aspects of public health were only one of many, the M.I.T.-Harvard School of Public Health was formed. Later, Harvard separated from M.I.T. and established its own school of public health. Other private and state universities followed suit over the years, thus establishing the basic framework for the field of public health.

FEDERAL AND STATE COLLABORATION

The Children's Bureau, on the basis of its extensive research on infant mortality, prompted the formulation and passage of the Sheppard-Towner Act in 1921. This Act, which was outside the mainstream of official public health, set up grants-in-aid to the states for maternal and child health programs aimed at reducing maternal and infant mortality. I elaborate on maternal and child health activities because, of all the traditional public health activities, these have the greatest potential effect on the private practice of medicine and curative medicine. The Public Health Service objected to the Children's Bureau's being entrusted with the implementation of a program that logically belonged to public health, even though the PHS apparently had little to do with the formulation or passage of the act. In this regard, it is the opinion of V.O. Key, a student of the grant-in-aid concept, that the Bureau had gained control over the program "by right of discovery and occupation and that the Public Health Service had been derelict in not promoting this type of work with sufficient vigor to maintain its belated claim to jurisdiction."[18] A further reason for the Bureau's retention of this program was expressed by Robert D. Leigh, an authority on federal health activities before the Social Security Act:

> The Children's Bureau is based not only on the administrative theory of the special population group, but also upon the political conviction held by large groups of women and social workers that child and maternal welfare problems were, before its creation, suffering from comparative neglect, and since its creation have obtained at the hands of its essentially feminine personnel a sympathetic and progressive development.[19]

As the Bureau evolved, the health aspects of its program became the most important and politically visible, hence the inevitable clash with the PHS. The federal government granted $1.24 million a year to the Children's Bureau for grants-in-aid to states and $50,000 a year for administration. The states could accept or reject aid as they saw fit, but the opportunity for money was so tempting, as the act intended, that 45 of the 48 states submitted programs for approval. The Sheppard-Towner Act was in effect for seven years and was not renewed. Reasons for this are not clear, but federal intrusion in state activities appeared to be the main one. A sympathetic observer of the program wrote that "no Federal law has been so consistently misrepresented nor so frequently accused of making possible Federal domination."[20]

Evaluation of the impact of the Sheppard-Towner Act is not easy, as is true of any service program, but it seems clear that the act laid the groundwork for a national maternal and child health program administered by the states. This program was eventually given permanent life in Title V of the Social Security Act, which was passed in 1935. Although the Sheppard-Towner Act represented the first long-range grant-in-aid program for maternal and child health, the grant-in-aid concept itself had precedents in federal grants for the improvement of agricultural practices. The shift of federal interest from farm animals and crops to people came rather late, because the Constitution limited jurisdiction of health and welfare to the states.

NOTES

1. Harry S. Mustard, *Government in Public Health* (New York: Commonwealth Fund, 1945), p. 91.
2. See George Rosen, *A History of Public Health* (New York: MD Publications, 1958).
3. Mustard, *Government*, p. 57.
4. The Merchant Marine Hospital Service is described by Robert Straus, *Medical Care for Seamen: The Origin of Public Medical Service in the United States* (New Haven, Conn.: Yale University Press, 1950) and Ralph C. Williams, *The United States Public Health Service, 1798–1950* (Bethesda, Md.: U.S. Public Health Service, Commissioned Officers Association, 1951), pp. 31–32.
5. Milton Terris, "An Early System of Compulsory Health Insurance in the United States, 1798–1884," *Bulletin of the History of Medicine* 15 (May 1944): 433–44.
6. Mustard, *Government*, p. 27.
7. Rosen, *History*, p. 234.
8. See the story in Nathan Sinai and Odin W. Anderson, *EMIC (Emergency Maternity and Infant Care): A Study of Administrative Experience* (Ann Arbor: School of Public Health, University of Michigan, 1948), pp. 7–17.
9. Richard H. Shryock, *Medicine and Society in America, 1660–1860* (New York: New York University Press, 1960), pp. 164–65.
10. John H. Griscom, *The Sanitary Condition of the Laboring Population of New York, with Suggestions for Improvement* (New York: Harper, 1845).
11. Elisha Harris, *Report of the Council of Hygiene and Public Health of the Citizens Association of New York on the Sanitary Conditions of the City, 1865,* reported in Rosen, *History*, p. 245.
12. Lemuel Shattuck, *Report of a General Plan for the Promotion of Public and Personal Health . . . Relating to a Sanitary Survey of the State, 1850* (Cambridge, Mass.: Harvard University Press, 1948).
13. Barbara Gutman Rosenkrantz, *Public Health and the State, Changing Views in Massachusetts, 1842–1936* (Cambridge, Mass.: Harvard University Press, 1972), p. 35.
14. See John Duffy, *A History of Public Health in New York City, 1866–1966.* (New York: Russell Sage Foundation, 1974) and Judith Walzer Leavitt, *The Healthiest City: Milwaukee and the Politics of Health Reform* (Princeton, N.J.: Princeton University Press, 1981).
15. Wilson G. Smillie, *Public Health, Its Promise for the Future: A Chronicle of the Development of Public Health in the United States, 1707–1914* (New York: Macmillan, 1955), p. 307.
16. Rosenkrantz, *Public Health*, p. 129.
17. Quoted in C. E. A. Winslow, *The Life of Herman Briggs* (Philadelphia: Lea and Febiger, 1929), p. 230.
18. Valdimer O. Key, *The Administration of Federal Grants to States* (Chicago: Public Administration Service, 1937), p. 208.

19. Robert D. Leigh, *Federal Health Administration in the United States* (New York: Harper, 1927), p. 528.
20. Austin F. Macdonald, *Federal Aid* (New York: Crowell, 1928), p. 223.

5

Hospitals and Physicians

The growth of mental hospitals preceded by quite a few years that of other hospitals. In addition, mental hospitals and psychiatric care in general evolved independently of curative personal health services because of inherent differences between mental and somatic illness. Although Sigmund Freud himself was originally a neurologist, even he was unable to bridge that gap.

Mental hospitals were the responsibility of the states. They were usually founded in association with county poor farms (now called health centers*). The main surge in the building of mental hospitals took place after 1840 and before the great wave of construction of general hospitals. The treatment of mental disease and the construction of large mental hospitals resulted mainly from the humanitarian movement, which discarded the devil theory of human behavior and mental illness, rather than from specific developments in the medical sciences.[1] Most mental hospitals were built in rural areas, where wide expanses of countryside presumably provided a quiet, salubrious environment for patients. Dorothea Dix is regarded as the originator of this movement. Undoubtedly the increasing difficulty of harboring unpleasant and unpredictable people in large cities contributed greatly to the rise of mental hospitals.

The superintendents of institutions for the mentally ill, although usually physicians, were generally custodians rather than clinicians. This continues to be true. Since they were supported by general revenues, the mental health services were not lavishly funded. It seems that,

---

*This is an example of the post–World War II tendency to improve the image of an activity by changing its name rather than its substance.

although mental disease eventually came to be regarded as such, the intractable problems it presented were behavioral; hence patients were removed from society so as not to jeopardize its functioning. Public policy regarding mental hospitals remained static for a hundred years. During that time there was one snake-pit revelation after another, a situation inherent in mental hospitals and prisons. Fundamental reforms are difficult because the mentally ill require a great deal of community forbearance and tolerance.

The real action during those years took place in the acute and curative sector of somatic disease, represented by the general hospital and surgery; interest in mental disease remained quiescent until the 1950s. The seemingly sudden emergence of the general hospital and surgery was based on a long history of scientific and medical discoveries. The mass practice of surgery was not possible until research had isolated bacteria as specific causes of many infectious and communicable diseases and had developed anesthetics to control pain. The bacteriological discoveries made surgery, which had become highly refined in the world's famous charity hospitals, less risky. Postoperative infection was dramatically reduced, and the previously high death rate declined. Concurrently, the hospital became a far safer place for treating the sick because it reduced the danger of cross-infection as well.

Medicine in the latter nineteenth century was primarily a search for specific causes of disease. It took this form because of work in normal anatomy done by Italian physicians during the Renaissance and because of later work in morbid anatomy. The concern with morbid anatomy led to the medical specialty of pathology, the identification of diseases and their causes. Medical historians point out that this required 300 years of basic research. Many leaders in public health medicine, such as Herman M. Biggs, William H. Welch, and William Osler, were originally pathologists. They reached professional maturity as German pathologists, and particularly Virchow began to disseminate their findings.

Following the clear description of disease came bacteriology, which traced the causes of humankind's worst scourges—typhoid, tuberculosis, syphilis, diphtheria—to specific bacteria. When individual physicians combined their knowledge of pathology with bacteriology, the effect on the future of medical practice and the structure of health services was profound and unpredictable. This occurred at a time when there were about as many physicians per capita as there are now. Many medical schools existed, but the few general hospitals were dangerous and primitive. The application of bacteriological discoveries and anesthesia changed all this.[2]

Although the practice of medicine in the United States was generally in a sorry state before 1875, the basis of future medical service was there—the privately practicing physician, whose skills ranged from downright dangerous to state of the art. Since medical practice was exclusively private and solo, the method of payment was fee-for-service. Although care of the poor was implicit in public policy, emergency care for the indigent was usually provided through contracts with individual physicians in a county or township.

For the general public (the poor in America being in the minority, unlike the poor in Europe), physicians' services were bought and paid for as private transactions, with no government payments or private health insurance. As Mark S. Blumberg observes, there was a great deal of competition between physicians:

> ... the productive potential of physicians in most areas of this country was greater than the effective demand for their services. Hence, the doctors' primary problem in such areas was to obtain an adequate number of patients, to keep them, and to get the patients to pay.[3]

Blumberg continues: "Understandably, physicians had a great fear of price-cutters, and this led to formal fee schedules."[4] The fees adopted by medical societies from the early nineteenth century on were minimums set to avoid cut-rate competition. Blumberg found that, as medical societies were founded, their first order of business was the adoption of a fee schedule.[5] This practice may be viewed cynically, but the physicians had to make a living. The public bought their services, and the number of private practitioners increased steadily. There were, of course, scarcely any hospital visits at that time, chiefly office visits and house calls. Although we may wonder what physicians had to offer before surgery in the hospital, a review of the many procedures listed and the fees reveals a great variety of palliatives, bone setting and wound treatment. A very dismal picture of nineteenth century medicine, however, is painted by John Duffy, a medical historian and physician: "Until the twentieth century, medicine consisted largely of bleeding, blistering, purging, vomiting, and sweating."[6] There are no data on the number of visits to physicians, but there must have been enough to sustain them on at least a modest and genteel level.

The economics of medical practice is not much better understood now than in the nineteenth century, but income reporting is better. Physicians are undoubtedly earning much more money today than they did in the nineteenth and early twentieth centuries, even discounting payment in kind.

Eventually, private practitioners, particularly those developing surgical skills, arranged admitting privileges with the hospitals. It seems reasonable to assume that by 1915 it was necessary for a physician to have some sort of hospital appointment in order to conduct a successful practice. The hospitals were chartered as nonprofit institutions and were obliged to provide care to charity patients. Physicians agreed to provide a modicum of free care in return for admitting privileges, which enabled them to charge their private patients fees.

Consequently, the essentially private practice of medicine and the voluntary general hospital became the vehicle for the application of scientific medical knowledge. As Shryock observed:

> The encouraging results attained in medical practice, especially after 1900, were bound to affect the whole spirit of the medical profession. The revolution in surgery, the services of endocrinology and dietetics, the value of serum and chemotherapy, the accomplishments of hygienic procedures—these in themselves were sufficient to banish the nihilism of 1850. The negative enthusiasm of that day, which found its chief service in disclosing the uselessness of traditional remedies, was now replaced by positive amelioration and care.[7]

Even by the turn of the century, many advanced procedures in medicine were performed in offices that had only a table that could be used as a laboratory and a medicine cabinet, sofa, or examining table.[8]

The hospital naturally became the place where the expensive new equipment associated with surgery and radiology was introduced. Hospitals were a center for fund raising, and they engendered community pride akin to schools, churches, and baseball teams. Technical innovations were increasing rapidly, and medical staffs were clamoring for them. Even as early as 1903, John Fehrenbatch, in his presidential address to the Conference of Association of Hospital Superintendents of the Central States and Canada (later the American Hospital Association), encouraged hospitals to acquire as quickly as possible all "mechanical devices that help in healing."[9] He recognized the problems that practitioners in their private offices might have in gaining access to capital funds by remarking:

> But as the introduction of machinery and mechanical devices into private practice involves considerable enlargements of office quarters and a considerable outlay of money, it is incumbent upon the American Hospital to take the lead. The hospital has the room and the facilities for the successful operation of all kinds of mechanical devices and machinery for the treatment of disease and surgery.

In these early days, physicians were suspected, as they still are, of asking for too much technical equipment. Fehrenbatch felt moved to counter this feeling in the same address:

It is sometimes said that many things done in the hospital are for the benefit of doctors. In reply to this I can only say that if the doctors are not benefited, the money spent in the hospital in taking advanced steps in the treatment of the sick and injured is not only spent in vain, but is simply wasted.

It is obvious that no alarm was raised during this period by the gradual shift of medical practice to the hospital. The cost of health services was being increased thereby, but it was apparently absorbed by the great industrial and economic expansion of that period. Between 1873 and 1909, the number of hospitals in the United States increased from 178 to almost 4,400, and the number of beds from about 50,000 or 60,000 to 421,000, a 1,000 percent increase.[10] In 1870 the population of the United States was estimated at 40 million and in 1910 at 92 million, an increase of a little more than 100 percent. In 1873, then, there were only about 0.14 beds per 1,000 persons, but by 1909 there were 4.0 beds per 1,000. (The bed complement currently is over 6 per 1,000.) I estimate that there were fewer than 4 admissions per 1,000 population in 1873. (The current rate is 150 to 160 per 1,000.)

There is no way of determining precisely what proportion of hospitals built between 1873 and 1909 was financed by taxation and what by private capital. They were predominately general hospitals, however, and it is reasonable to assume that they were financed largely through private philanthropy and community fund drives. E. H. L. Corwin observed that a primary social policy during this important developmental period was that the voluntary hospital was to be funded by private subscription rather than by general revenues.[11] Wealth must have been accumulated rapidly in those days. Many newly made multimillionaires such as John D. Rockefeller, Johns Hopkins, Stephen Harkness, and Cornelius Vanderbilt gave generously to the major hospitals and medical centers. With the westward growth of the country, many lesser millionaires were created. Their gifts, along with community fund drives for the voluntary hospitals, made the general hospital the backbone of the hospital system in the United States; this is true of no other country. These early multimillionaires were Calvinists in their outlooks and gave to the community ventures in health and education in order to create opportunities for self-improvement for everybody rather than acting as lady bountiful to individual poor families.

There was a great increase in wealth during the last half of the nineteenth century, and it spilled over into health and educational endeavors. Lee Soltow estimates, for example, that there were 41 millionaires in 1860 and 545 in 1870.[12] An analysis of trends in the American economy in the nineteenth century by Robert Gallman reveals that, as measured by commodity output per capita, the output in 1839 was $64, rising steadily to $154 in 1899. The decennial rate of change in percent per capita was 11 in 1849 and between 1879 and 1880; it leaped to 35 in 1884, fell to 30 in 1889, and dropped to 13 in 1899. These are impressive gains, but perhaps they can be made more understandable by quoting Gallman: "Over the last six decades of the nineteenth century, American commodity output increased eleven fold, or at an average decade rate of 50 percent."[13]

A social surplus was created, and it spilled over into health, education, and welfare services. Personal discretionary income also expanded. Merle Curti *et al.* estimate that philanthropic contributions in Western Europe for all purposes—education, social work, religion, scientific research, and art—amounted to less than 0.5 percent of the annual national income, whereas in the United States they amounted to 2 percent of national income.[14] In all likelihood, the American percentage was computed from a larger per capita national income than obtained in Western Europe at that time.

The rapidly expanding economy transformed the traditional concept of hospitals as purely charitable institutions; patients began to have to pay, and they were undoubtedly increasingly able to do so. This change in custom had several important effects on the characteristics of hospitals in this country. To paraphrase Corwin:

1. It contributed to the rapid expansion of general hospitals by disassociating them from charity and low- or no-income patients. Paying patients were encouraged to utilize the emerging voluntary hospital through referrals from their own private practitioners.

2. It discouraged the growth of hospitals as a private business for profit. Patients who could afford to pay did not go to private nursing homes or special private beds in the famous charity hospitals, as they did in England; they went to hospitals that provided free care to those who could not pay and who were thus a minority and not "permeating the entire institution."

3. It assured a quality of care commensurate with the expectations of the middle class, making hospitals a matter of general community concern and not just of well-intentioned people interested primarily in the welfare of the indigent.[15]

It is reasonable to assume that hospitals built in the heady developmental environment of the West and Midwest in the 1890s could more easily adopt the concept of serving paying patients than could the old, established hospitals of the East.

An important example of the philosophy of catering to paying patients was the construction in the 1890s of St. Mary's Hospital in Rochester, Minnesota, in connection with the Mayo Clinic. The nuns who were to build St. Mary's Hospital naturally thought in terms of the conventional charity hospital, even providing a door for dispensing alms to beggars. The Mayo brothers, being both brilliant surgeons and business entrepreneurs, quickly disabused the worthy Sisters of this concept and persuaded them to build a hospital that would attract primarily paying patients. Caring for charity patients would be a subsidiary, not a dominant function. The Mayo brothers wanted to appeal to the large middle class, which had enough discretionary income to buy their own care and sustain the emerging private practices of medicine and nonprofit hospitals. The Sisters complied.

After the hospital was in operation, one of the first uses to which extra money was put was to make the rooms "homelike," resembling bedrooms in small-town and urban middle-class homes. Appropriate beds and bedding were purchased, followed by rocking chairs, dressers, pictures, and mirrors. Dainty china and silverware were used to make the serving trays attractive. The importance of these amenities is reflected in the hospital records. For example, on September 21, 1891, the first half-dozen silver knives and forks were bought; they were carefully wrapped up and stored between meals.[16] Though the hospital and health services continued their vigorous growth, undoubtedly exceeding the GNP of the time, nobody paid any attention. By 1918 there were over 5,000 hospitals and 612,000 beds in the United States; by 1923 there were almost 7,000 hospitals and 802,000 beds.[17]

There appear to be no systematic data on the operating income of hospitals before 1923 (in fact, not until a 1946 study that was retrospective to 1929), but a Bureau of the Census report revealed that two-thirds of the operating income for hospitals in 1992 was derived from paying patients. The average per diem rate was $4.15.[18] From the same report it could be estimated that the national admissions rate to hospitals per 1,000 population was 38, the average length of stay was 12.5 days, and the number of patient days per 1,000 population was 500. (The estimates for 1980 are, respectively, 150, 8, and 1,200.)

When medicine began drawing on the basic sciences, the character of medical education and medical schools changed, but the full effect was not felt until long after 1900. During the last quarter of the nineteenth century, some university-affiliated medical schools in the United States began to emulate British and European schools. Many medical students studied in Europe and returned to infuse the latest scientific discoveries into American medical education. Between 1880 and 1900, the number of medical schools increased from 100 to 160, and the number of students increased from 11,800 to 25,000. Graduates increased from over 3,000 to over 7,000.[19] Clearly, the number of schools and students was increasing appreciably faster than the population. The proprietary medical schools, operated by physicians who took students for a fee, continued to compete. They offered lower standards and shorter training periods than were required by the university-affiliated schools.

Attempts to improve the quality of medical education resulted in a net decrease in the number of schools. These attempts started as early as 1876, when 22 schools joined the newly formed Association of American Medical Colleges (AAMC). For a while it did not appear to have any effect, but in 1891 it set minimum requirements for admission to membership. By 1896, 55 of the existing 155 medical schools had been admitted.[20]

Many states had no licensing laws, thus only a minimum of training was needed before physicians could set up their own offices. Physicians with M.D.'s began to support licensing laws in order to protect themselves from the stiff competition offered by quacks and charlatans, as well as, it is hoped, to protect the public. By the end of the nineteenth century, healing groups outside the mainstream of allopathic medicine had evolved; these make for interesting reading, particularly as fissures developed among them. One of these groups was osteopathic medicine, which managed to gain both patients and relative respectability.[21]

By 1896, 26 states had enacted medical licensure laws. The remaining states did so within a few years as a result of the efforts of the AAMC. The AAMC issued an ultimatum in 1904 requiring its 60 member schools (160 schools were then in existence) to withdraw from the Association if they did not require a minimum standard of high school graduation as a prerequisite for admission. Also in 1904, the AMA established its Council on Medical Education, which coordinated the efforts of all state and county medical societies to support higher standards for medical education. Surveys of the medical schools were undertaken by the AMA Council. The first one, conducted in 1906, resulted in the classification of schools into A, B, and C grades. The *Journal of the American Medical Association* reported the findings, which caused a furor, presumably among the Bs and Cs.[22]

Hard on the heels of this exposé, the Council on Medical Education invited the Carnegie Foundation for the Advancement of Teaching to evaluate medical education in the United States and Canada. It was felt that a survey conducted by an agency independent of medicine would have more credibility than one carried out by the Council. In addition, the surveyor was not a physician, but an educator, which presumably assured some objectivity. Apparently it seemed possible in those days for an educated layman to evaluate the general characteristics, curriculums, and equipment of medical schools. The result was the Flexner report, which has become enshrined in the history of medical education.[23] Abraham Flexner delegated nothing and visited personally all the existing medical schools. He made an inventory of each of the vital elements such as faculty, enrollment, standards, and equipment and facilities. In terms of today's sophisticated survey techniques, his survey was crude. It did not have reference points for standards or any evaluative statistics whatsoever. For his purposes, however, a more refined survey was not necessary. Apparently Flexner found consensus among highly regarded medical educators about what range of specialization should be represented in a medical faculty, what kind of laboratory equipment and classroom space were desirable, how long the training period should be, what level of education an applicant to medical school should have, and whether or not patients were available for teaching purposes.

Flexner evaluated the general status of the 135 schools then in existence. About 30 schools had closed since 1900, indicating that pressures to upgrade schools were already in operation. His report was credited with being directly responsible for the closing of 29 schools between 1910 and 1914. More were closed when state licensing boards accepted the final list of 66 schools approved by the Council on Medical Education.[24]

The Flexner report was given credit for dealing the final blow to medical schools that did not meet the standards of the AAMC and for promoting generally higher standards for medical schools in the United States. Ultimately, of course, it affected the standards of medical practice in general, since graduates of approved schools accounted for increasing proportions of practicing physicians. According to John Dietrick and Robert Berson, the decades of 1910–1929 marked the establishment of medical education as a university-sponsored endeavor with university standards of training.[25] It was undoubtedly the fusion of medical education onto the broad scientific base that was emerging by this time that led Lawrence Henderson, M.D., to remark, "I think it was about the year 1910 or 1912 when it became possible to say of the United States that a random patient with a random disease consulting a doctor chosen at random stood better than a fifty-fifty chance of benefiting from the encounter."[26]

Raising the standards of medical care naturally increased the costs of both medical practice and medical education; however, it is almost impossible to document these increases. The medical schools that adopted the higher standards required more capital, higher student fees, and greater investments of time in training before graduates could earn a living. Undoubtedly, the large endowments that were accumulated between 1875 and 1915 helped considerably in establishing outstanding, modern medical schools.

Previously, medical schools had in large part been adjuncts to private practice. It seems that legislators were inclined to grant charters for medical schools to any physicians who desired them. As Shryock observes about the economic and political milieu of the country at the time: "Wasn't the United States by this time a free society in which competition was the life of trade and also of professions, which—if not actually trades—were something close to them?"[27] Business shaped the ethics of the profession, short of making them tradesmen.

In pre-Flexner days, professors of medicine earned the bulk of their incomes from private practice. Thus, many schools needed little financial support from taxes and required few facilities. "Everyone," says Shryock, "was happy about such arrangements except those who worried about standards."[28] It is little wonder, considering the added cost of maintaining medical schools, that the number of schools decreased so rapidly after 1910. Upgrading all the medical schools then in existence was simply out of the question—the standards mandated were too expensive. Economists have raised the question of hidden agenda in the drive for improved standards.[29] Mainstream physicians obtained a clear monopoly on the practice of medicine, both through licensure and the upgrading of medical school standards. The supply of physicians shrank from 146 per 100,000 population in 1910 to 125 per 100,000 in 1930.[30] Undoubtedly, the overall quality of physicians improved during that period.

As the number of medical schools and medical students grew, there was an increased demand for patients, who were known as "clinical material," a term being used less and less. Low-income and destitute persons, particularly immigrants living in cities, used outpatient services, which were usually free, and dispensaries for particular diseases and age groups. Michael M. Davis and Andrew W. Warner defined a dispensary as "an institution which organizes the professional equipment and special skill of physicians for the diagnosis, treatment, and prevention of diseases among ambulatory patients."[31] There were only 100 dispensaries in 1900. By 1914, however, an estimated 750 to 800 dispensaries had been established in the United States, 400 of them general dispensaries, 300 for the care of tuberculosis, and 60 for specialty services such as eye, ear, nose, and throat. New types of dispensaries emerged with new programs established by public health departments. Over 425 venereal disease dispensaries were reported, and 500 were designated for infant and child hygiene. Industries alone reported having 450 dispensaries.[32]

The dispensary movement is significant because dispensaries served the poor in large cities, filling a gap between hospitals and private medical practitioners. It was estimated in 1914 that 75 percent of dispensaries were set up in cities with populations of 100,000 and over.[33]

It is conceivable, and the medical profession has claimed, that before 1900 and the development of expensive medical equipment, the poor received free care in physicians' offices and hospitals. As medical practice required greater capital investment and a higher overhead, more dispensaries were established for the poor, either as outpatient units of general hospitals or as independent facilities. Many physicians provided free care, and public and private contributions built and maintained the facilities. People who might need a physician at the hospital could be referred to the outpatient department or dispensary. Hospitals provided diagnostic and laboratory services.

To some, the dispensary promised to be the nucleus of a new system of organizing physicians' services. When the dispensary movement was in full swing, Davis and Warner, enthusiastic proponents, were moved to observe that:

> . . . in medicine, as in industry, specialization requires organization to develop maximum efficiency. With the advance of medical science, and the use of specialties, there has begun to develop medical organizations. We see this most concretely incorporated in the hospitals, dispensaries, and public health departments.[34]

The industrial model—specialization, salary, central budgeting and bookkeeping, fixed hours, technical and clerical support personnel, access limited to one primary physician—has intrigued many people interested in health services delivery. Indeed, it began to emerge as private group practice clinics. Some of them, such as Health Insurance Plan of Greater New York and Kaiser-Permanente in California, combined group practice and prepayment. In the early days, however, the medical profession was never enthusiastic:

> The general public and a number of physicians do not as yet understand the nature and advantage of this new type of medical work. They still think of the hospitals as a medical hotel, and look down upon the dispensary as the medical soup kitchen.[35]

Logical and compelling as the dispensary seemed to nonphysicians, it did not really find a niche in the mainstream of medical care. It acted as a buffer to protect the mainstream from those who could not afford to pay for private physicians' services. By 1922, dispensaries were handling a volume of service approaching 30 million units a year.[36] The population of the United States was then 106 million. Assuming two visits to physicians per person per year (less than one-half today's average), dispensaries provided 14 percent of the total care, a not insignificant proportion.

In 1914, the Committee on outpatient work of the AHA expressed a great deal of dissatisfaction with the character of dispensaries:

> With all the problems that had been made in dispensary service, the outstanding problems today are in general much the same as those of five, ten, or fifteen years ago. The hospital world needs today, just as those needed in the past, to give more serious attention to outpatient work. The dark horse, the Cinderella, the step-child, the poor relation, are terms which have been and in many instances can still be truthfully applied to this important member of the hospital household . . . far too many outpatient departments today are poorly housed, poorly equipped, inadequately staffed, poorly organized and abominably supported. Hospital trustees have not demanded of their outpatient departments the same degree of medical efficiency, or administrative efficiency, as they have from the so-called hospital proper.[37]

As has been alluded to previously, the health services delivery system that came to fruition in the 1920s was based on the assumption that it was a pay-as-you-go system, at least for day-to-day care. Free services for the poor—a residual—were grafted onto the main system by private donation, taxation, and care provided without charge by practitioners who depended for their livelihood mainly on fees from private patients.

NOTES

1. See, for example, Richard H. Shryock, *Medicine and Society in America, 1660–1860* (New York: New York University Press, 1960). pp. 290–91.
2. Ibid., p. 147.
3. Mark S. Blumberg, "Physicians' Fees As Incentives," in *Proceedings of the Twenty-First Annual Symposium on Hospital Affairs*, June 1979 (Chicago: Graduate Program in Hospital Administration and Center for Health Administration Studies, Graduate School of Business, University of Chicago, 1980), pp. 20–26.
4. Ibid., p. 21.
5. It appears that only two descriptions of fee schedules in the nineteenth century have been published: Mary Louise Hall, "Some Nineteenth Century

Fee Bills," *Bulletin of the History of Medicine* 6(1938):62–80 and George Rosen, "Fees and Fee Bills: Some Economic Aspects of Medical Practice in Nineteenth Century America," *Bulletin of the History of Medicine Supplement No. 6,* 1946.

6. John Duffy, *The Healers: The Rise of the Medical Establishment* (New York: McGraw-Hill, 1976), p. 98.
7. Richard H. Shryock, *The Development of Modern Medicine: An Interpretation of the Social and Economic and Scientific Factors Involved* (London: Gollancz, 1948), pp. 256–57.
8. Bernard J. Stern, *American Medical Practices in the Perspective of a Century* (New York: Commonwealth Fund, 1945), p. 20.
9. *The National Health Hospital Record* 7 (December 1903):9.
10. The first national survey of hospitals in the United States was conducted by the U.S. Bureau of Education in 1872–3 and was reported in *Transactions of the American Medical Association* 25(1873):314–33. The next national survey was coordinated by the American Medical Association in 1909.
11. Edward H. L. Corwin, *The American Hospital* (New York: Commonwealth Fund, 1946), p. 2. See also Charles E. Rosenberg, *The Care of Strangers: The Rise of America's Hospital System* (New York: Basic Books, 1987), particularly Chapter 4, "Expanding A Traditional Institution: Social Sources of Hospital Growth 1850–1875," pp. 97–121, about the time before the post-1875 take-off in growth.
12. Lee Soltow, *Men and Wealth in the United States, 1850–1870* (New Haven, Conn.: Yale University Press, 1975), p. 112.
13. Robert E. Gallman, "Commodity output," in *Conference on Research in Income and Wealth. Trends in the American Economy, Studies in Income and Wealth,* vol. 24 (Washington, D.C.: National Bureau of Economic Research, 1960) p. 19.
14. Merle Curti, Judith Green, and Roderick Nash, "Anatomy of Giving: Millionaires in the Late 19th Century," *Political Review Quarterly* 75 (March 1960):87, see also *American Quarterly* 15 (Fall 1963):415–35.
15. Corwin, *American Hospital,* pp. 62–63.
16. Helen Clapesattle, *The Doctors Mayo* (Minneapolis: University of Minnesota Press, 1941), pp. 261–62.
17. *Historical Statistics of the United States, Colonial Times to 1970,* Bicentennial Edition, part I (Washington, D.C.: U.S. Bureau of the Census, 1975), p. 79.
18. *Hospitals and Dispensaries,1923* (Washington, D.C.: U.S. Bureau of the Census, 1925), p. 4. It should be noted that in 1891 St. Mary's Hospital in Rochester, Minnesota, reported a per diem rate (calculated as a weekly rate) of approximately $1.50. In 20 years that rate had tripled.
19. *Historical Statistics,* pp. 75–76.
20. John E. Dietrik and Robert C. Berson, *Medical Education in the United States at Mid-Century* (New York: McGraw-Hill, 1953), p. 12.
21. The definitive work on osteopathic medicine is Norman Gevitz's *Osteopathic Medicine in America* (Baltimore: Johns Hopkins University Press, 1982).
22. American Medical Association, *The Story of America's Medical Schools* (Chicago, 1960), pp. 8–10.

23. Abraham Flexner, *Medical Education in the United States and Canada: A Report to the Carnegie Foundation for Advancement of Teaching* (New York: Carnegie Foundation, 1910).
24. American Medical Association, *Story*, p. 8–10.
25. Dietrik and Berson, *Medical Education*, p. 13.
26. Credited by Alan Gregg in his *Challenge to Contemporary Medicine* (New York: Columbia University Press, 1956), p. 13.
27. Shryock, *Medicine*, p. 141.
28. Ibid., p. 141.
29. See, for example, Reuben A. Kessel, "The AMA and the Supply of Physicians," *Law and Contemporary Problems* 35 (Spring 1970):267–83.
30. U.S. Department of Health, Education, and Welfare. *Health U.S. 1978*. Series B275–290, pp. 75–76, Table 120, p. 337.
31. Michael M. Davis and Andrew W. Warner, *Dispensaries: Their Management and Development* (New York: Macmillan, 1918), p. 27.
32. George Rosen, "The First Neighborhood Health Center Movement—Its Rise and Fall," *American Journal of Public Health* 61 (August 1971), 1620–37.
33. American Hospital Association, Report of the Committee on Outpatient Work, *Transactions of the American Hospital Association* 16 (1914):74, 312–28.
34. Davis and Warner, *Dispensaries*, p. 350.
35. Ibid., p. 353. It should be noted that what might be called "super private practice" had already been established at the Mayo Clinic in Rochester, the Ochsner Clinic in New Orleans, the Lahey Clinic in Boston, and the Crile Clinic in Cleveland.
36. American Hospital Association, Report of the Committee on the Outpatient Work, *Transactions of the American Hospital Association* 24 (1922):100.
37. Ibid., pp. 102–3.

6

The Cost of Personal
Health Services as a Risk

Not long after the turn of the century, costliness of illness began to find expression in concern for the middle-class patient. Frederick Brush, medical superintendent of New York Post Graduate Medical School and Hospital, observed at the eleventh annual meeting of the AHA in 1909:

> The hospitals were for the poor. They are now largely for the rich. In time, they may be for all. An old question presents, "Has the middle class patient who can for a term pay the family physician, a right to expect hospital treatment in time of stress?" In the years of disrupting controversy over hospital abuse, it has often been nearly decided that he has not! . . . Consciously or not, all concerned in hospital management are daily working out the beginning of this great extension—hospital provision for the Third Estate.[1]

The third estate—that is, the middle class—became the seedbed for some form of hospital insurance, whether sown by the government or private agencies. Traditionally, no general social reform succeeds in the United States unless the middle class is activated. Precursors of national health insurance were the worker compensation laws enacted in many states between 1910 and 1916.

WORKER COMPENSATION

Although worker compensation was originally concerned with cash payments to workers for time lost from work due to injuries and disease associated with their occupations, it became relevant to personal health services when the costs of medical treatment and rehabilitation became fringe benefits.[2] This led naturally to direct government involvement with the providers of health services. At issue were scope of services, reimbursement methods and amounts, choice of physician and hospital, and standards of quality. Reimbursement methods and amounts became the most important issues, and disagreements about them were exacerbated by lack of precedents for government as a source of payment. Thus, worker compensation may be regarded as the first general government-sponsored program to involve hospitals and physicians; it went beyond government's traditional concern for the indigent, the mentally ill, and groups under its auspices, such as seamen and servicemen.

Before the relationship of employee to employer became complex, an employee, according to common law, assumed the risks associated with the job. The prevailing theory was that, since the employee was presumably aware of the conditions of his chosen work, personal liability was also assumed. The employer assumed no liability whatsoever for accidents or illnesses associated with the occupation. Eventually, the employer became liable for all job-related injuries and illness, regardless of cause. Social policy had it that industrial accidents and illnesses were a legitimate part of the cost of production. That cost, in turn, was assumed by society at large, through higher prices. Increased productivity made it possible to shift the cost from the employee to the employer and the larger society. Early laws establishing the employer's complete liability were enacted in Germany in 1871, Great Britain in 1889, Alabama in 1885, and Massachusetts in 1887.

In time, however, even the concept of employer liability proved inadequate: it resulted in long-drawn-out expensive litigation, since employers were inclined to contest the claims in court. The concept of worker compensation took the place of employer liability. Definitions of benefits, injuries, and occupational illnesses were systematized and standardized, funds were pooled by employers, and legal issues were simplified. Litigation was forsworn by both parties, although not avoided altogether because of the due process tradition of our legal system. Worker compensation clearly established a no-fault basis for occupational injuries and illnesses.

By 1910, most industrial workers in Europe were covered by worker compensation. In the United States, the period from 1900 to 1916 was one of study and investigation, the familiar preliminaries to action. Thirty-one states and the federal government appointed commissions to investigate and report. At the same time, many states enacted worker compensation laws: by 1915, 30 states had such laws; by 1920, 42 did.

Worker compensation was and is essentially a means of ameliorating and correcting the conditions arising from an industrial society. As described, it was the master-servant relationship redefined under modern industrial conditions. It recognized the fact that, if there were a break in family income, the family would become destitute. Since occupational injuries and illnesses were regarded as inherent in the production system and beyond the control of the worker, worker compensation represented the first clear break with public assistance laws and the assumption that anyone unable to make a living was somehow personally at fault.

Like employer liability, worker compensation shifted the blame for and the economic burden of unemployment from the worker to the employer and society. It was believed that employers would be induced to improve working conditions, thereby minimizing accidents and illness, in order to keep their compensation costs as low as possible. "Safety first" became a selling slogan.

In sum, then, worker compensation was essentially a reform movement within the free-market economy to cushion the harmful side effects of a production system in which workers had little control over their work environment. Instead of threatening and changing the going economic and production system, it really served to support it.

HEALTH INSURANCE

The rapid enactment of worker compensation laws stimulated agitation for government health insurance in 16 states between 1915 and 1920. Because of the federal-state division of labor regarding health and welfare, federal action was inconceivable at this time. Further, because health insurance did not have a broad base of support among the middle class, it was unable to withstand the attacks of its well-organized opponents.

The American Association for Labor Legislation (AALL) which had led the successful drive for worker compensation spearheaded the drive for health insurance for the general population. Organized in 1906, the AALL grew out of the International Association of Labor Legislation meeting in Paris in 1900. Steps were taken to organize an American association at the annual meeting of the American Economic Association held in Baltimore in 1905. A leading economist and social reformer, Richard T. Ely, professor of economics at the University of Wisconsin, became the first president. The first secretary, also an economist at the University of Wisconsin, was John R. Commons, a social reformer and early student of labor economics.

The AALL grew steadily from 165 members in 1906 to a peak of over 3,300 in 1913. Its members were economists, social workers, sociologists, and political scientists with a common interest in social reform. Although regarded as radicals by the business community, the members of AALL supported the basic framework of representative and constitutional government. Government was a regulatory power for the public good. Members believed in improving the existing form of government, not in overthrowing it and starting anew. They believed in individual initiative and freedom and that people maintain self-respect by earning their own way. They also recognized, however, that the system was faulty, for example in creating unemployment because of problems inherent in the labor market. This was a radical concept at that time. It was nonetheless a concept that could be adopted without changing the fundamental characteristics of the economic system. In 1913, about the time that the states were beginning to debate compulsory health insurance, the officers and members of the administrative council of the AALL were familiar names in American politics.*

The first annual meeting of the AALL was held in Madison, Wisconsin, on December 30–31, 1907. The association formulated plans for the investigation of industrial accidents, diseases, and poisons, stressing both present and future social and economic losses caused by illness and premature death. As reflected in the states' legislation by 1915, AALL was overwhelmingly successful. It established branches in Illinois, Minnesota, New York, Pennsylvania, Ohio, Michigan, and Missouri. In 1909, permanent headquarters were established in Madison, Wisconsin (and later moved to New York City), and members, numbered 903. The AALL was supported entirely by membership fees and voluntary subscriptions. Considering that peak membership was 3,300, AALL members must have represented the elite among social scientists of the period.

Health insurance was considered the logical next step after worker compensation. Compensation protected workers from loss of wages due to illness and accidents related to employment; health insurance would protect workers against the cost of illness and accidents outside employment. This goal seemed fairly easily attainable after the unexpectedly easy victory in worker compensation. It seems, however, that compulsory health insurance was a reform whose time had not yet come.

The public was becoming aware of conditions in the emerging industrial complex that resulted in accident, disability, and premature death. The reformers were caught up in the Progressive movement

---

*Jane Adams, Louis D. Brandeis, Richard T. Ely, Samuel Gompers, John B. Andrews, Woodrow Wilson, Sophonisba B. Breckenridge, Edward A. Filene, Lee K. Frankel, Andrew Furuseth, Florence Kelley, Roscoe Pound, I. M. Rubinow, F. W. Taussig, C. E. A. Winslow, Paul U. Kellogg, and Carol E. Perry.

headed by Theodore Roosevelt in his bid for the presidency through a third party in 1912. His platform expressed the mood of the Progressives:[3]

> The supreme duty of the nation is the conservation of human resources through an enlightened measure of social and industrial justice. We pledge ourselves to work increasingly in state and nation for: Effective legislation looking to the prevention of industrial accidents, occupational disease, overwork, involuntary unemployment, and other injurious effects evident in modern industry. . . .

The Progressive party platform alluded to health insurance in rather general terms: "The protection of home life against the hazards of sickness, irregular employment, and old age through the adoption of a system of social insurance adapted to American use. . . ." This was apparently an oblique endorsement of health insurance, but it was presented in the framework of occupational hazards in industry. The Republican and Democratic platforms of 1912 made no mention of social insurance.

The social reformers of this period were not good political strategists or tacticians. They assumed that facts and logic would prevail, as they had seemed to in the case of worker compensation. Health insurance, however, involved a proud profession, not simply the writing of a check for disability pensions. (Health services for recipients of worker compensation came later and exhibited similar administrative problems.) Further, the forces that would arise to oppose government health insurance were not visible in 1909. This created the feeling among reformers that the concept would simply succeed on its own merits. It did not take long for them to be disabused of this notion.

In 1912, the AALL established the Committee on Health Insurance, the first of its kind in the United States. Three members also served on the Social Insurance Committee established by the AMA in 1915 apparently as a spinoff of the AALL committee. They were Alexander Lambert, I. M. Rubinow, and S. S. Goldwater, all physicians and the latter a well-known administrator.

The AALL organized the first American Conference on Social Insurance, held in Chicago in June 1913. At that conference, Rubinow delivered what was probably the first paper to be presented on health insurance in this country. Drawing on his experience, he predicted developments as follows:

> A new movement for a social policy must meet its strongest opponent in the fetishism of self-help. Even after the advantages of [compulsory] insurance over individual provision became apparent, voluntary health insurance remains the creed for some time. Thus the earliest efforts of or-

ganized society in Germany were for regulation of voluntary benefit societies, so as to make them safe and efficient.

The next step is to subsidize these voluntary insurance institutions,
and thus to stimulate their growth. The fetishism of free self-help is still
strong, and the subsidy is granted not without misgivings.

But all these systems of "assisted liberty" are only the first steps
toward a well-planned social policy.[4]

Rubinow was advocating skipping the voluntary stage and going immediately to a government system of health insurance. He might well have
believed this to be feasible because the United States had no voluntary
health insurance to speak of. But Rubinow underestimated the "fetishism" of self-help.

At the seventh annual meeting of the AALL, held in Washington,
D.C., in December 1913, Joseph P. Chamberlain delivered a paper laying the groundwork for consideration of health insurance, should the
states take action. He recommended a government-sponsored health
insurance system. At the same time, Lee K. Frankel, of the Metropolitan
Life Insurance Company, suggested that standard reporting forms be
distributed to fraternal orders, trade unions, and insurance companies
so that statistics on illness in the United States might be obtained. There
were no data, either on morbidity or on use of health services, on which
to base use and cost estimates. At about the same time, the AALL sent
Olga S. Halsey to Great Britain to study its health insurance system,
which was enacted in 1911. Outside a few fraternal and benefit associations, there was no administrative experience with health insurance in
the United States on which to base a health insurance scheme. Halsey
might better have gone to Germany, which had experienced government health insurance since 1883.

In seemingly short order, the Committee on Social Insurance of
the AALL adopted preliminary standards for drawing up a health insurance proposal.[5] This proposal set a pattern for implementing the concept of health insurance. It stated that:

1. The system should be compulsory, with contributions from employer, employee, and the public. (Compulsory contribution
   was a radical idea for its day, but the tripartite source of contributions was conservative: it was not thought advisable to rely
   completely on general tax funds, although some persons believed that taxes would provide the most equitable means of
   distributing the burden.)

2. Persons who are not in groups that are covered should be able
   to join the system voluntarily. (Although it was recognized that
   payroll deductions would make it difficult and sometimes im

possible to enroll persons who were self-employed, it was still thought desirable not to rely solely on general taxation, in which all groups would be automatically covered.)

3. There should be a supplementary disability insurance so that both the cost of health services and the loss of income due to illness would be covered.

4. The system should be administered by employers and employees under public supervision. Private insurance carriers, properly supervised, might be utilized. (Even proponents of compulsory health insurance did not feel that public administration was necessary.)

5. Wherever possible, prevention of illness should be emphasized. (This principle reflects the growing public health philosophy of immunization, early diagnosis, and routine physical examinations.)

Curiously, the scope of services to be covered was not spelled out. Presumably hospital services and all physician services, regardless of site, were to be covered, since they were implicit in the cost problems facing families. There was also confusion, which continues to this day, about whether health insurance was to be a means of promoting the general health of the public or a means of paying for expensive medical contingencies. Mitigation of economic hardship seems to have been given the most emphasis, but some people felt that the primary purpose of health insurance was to reduce illness and premature death. The contingency concept was easy enough to prove (it was known anecdotally at the time and proven statistically later), but the public health concept underlying the control of communicable diseases was not. There was also controversy over the use of terms, such as sickness insurance or health insurance. Purists uninterested in public relations insisted that so-called health insurance was insurance against the costs of sickness and had nothing at all to do with health. Pragmatists trying to sell the concept said that sickness insurance sounded morbid, whereas health insurance had a positive note. (The same controversy occurred over insurance against untimely death: death insurance became life insurance.)

A subcommittee of the AALL Committee on Social Insurance was appointed in 1913 to study health insurance and to draft a bill in preparation for an active campaign in the states. Over a year later, the Executive Committee of the AALL voted unanimously that the Committee on Social Insurance should be encouraged to prepare a model health insurance bill to be introduced in several state legislatures in January

1916. This was done, and copies of the bill were exhausted within a month. A second edition of 5,000 copies was printed in the middle of December. At the same time, it was reported that the AMA had appointed a committee to cooperate with the AALL Committee on Social Insurance "in putting the finishing touches in the medical sections of the bill. . . ."[6]

Several other leading organizations had appointed committees early in 1916 to study the AALL proposal. With seemingly firm support from the top echelons of relevant interest groups, the secretary of the AALL optimistically wrote in the annual report: "The opportunity now appears good for a big educational campaign for the conservation of health, with fair prospects for legislative commissions to investigate in 1916 and for compulsory health insurance legislation in this country in 1917."[7]

The opposition to the AALL's model bill was not yet apparent, particularly since the proposal seemed to have the approval of the AMA committee. It should be noted, however, that action for approval or disapproval had not yet been taken by the AMA House of Delegates, the final policy making body, or the board of trustees. The AMA as a body had not really been faced with this kind of profound policy issue before—a policy that would shift the primary source of physicians' income from individual patients to the government and that would introduce into the patient-physician relationship a fiduciary third party.

The AALL went gaily on its way with no particular political strategy for creating coalitions in the state legislatures. A popular slogan, "health first," was coined because proponents assumed that an emphasis on illness prevention would reduce the cost of health insurance.

In the general enthusiasm, extravagant claims were made for the indirect social benefits of health insurance. For example, Irving Fisher of Yale, in his presidential address at the tenth annual meeting of AALL in December 1916, said that the United States had the "unenviable distinction" of being the only great industrial nation without compulsory health insurance. He attributed Germany's comparative freedom from poverty, reduction in death rates, and physically fit soldiers (judged by their performance in World War I) in great part to health insurance.[8]

This 1916 meeting of AALL saw a crescendo of discussion on the subject. Joint sessions were held with the American Economic Association, the American Sociological Society (now Association), the American Statistical Association, and the American Political Science Association. Rubinow summed up the status of the drive for health insurance at the 1916 meeting. Drawing on European stages of development, he said:

Essentially the health insurance movement spreads along the same lines of development as did the [worker] compensation movement seven or eight years ago. But the states of agitation, private committees, government commissions, and preparation of bills follow one another in such rapid succession that they appear to go on at the same time.[9]

At this early stage in the debate on health insurance, public administration was not a given, although government would be prepared to underwrite the program and negotiate with private carriers to administer it. There were precedents in worker compensation. Thus contractual relationships with the private and public sectors have an early, pragmatic connection with health services.

As long as compulsory health insurance was only under study and discussion, potential opponents paid no heed to it. However, when state commissions were established to study the subject and make recommendations, and particularly once bills resulting from such reports were introduced, opponents expressed vehement disapproval. Proponents were surprised, bewildered, and defenseless in the face of the opposition's gathering strength. The AALL had no political strategy worthy of the name, no money for lobbying, and no bell ringers to arouse the citizenry. Controversy surfaced within the Committee on Social Insurance itself, the citadel of support for compulsory health insurance legislation. One committee member, Frederick L. Hoffman, a statistician and high-level staff member of the Prudential Insurance Company of America, resigned when the committee went on record in 1916 in support of a form of government-sponsored health insurance. His company and other insurance companies would lose income from disability insurance, some insurance against medical services, and burial costs.

Hoffman took to the road as an articulate and vigorous opponent of government-sponsored health insurance. He and Rubinow, his counterpart among the proponents, became symbols of the debate. They were articulate, and they traveled and lectured extensively.

By the end of 1918, the movement reached its peak. Some support had developed: many organizations had formed special committees to consider health insurance,* ten states had established commissions to

---

*The AHA, AMA, Actuarial Society of America, American Association of Industrial Physicians and Surgeons, American Association of Mechanical Engineers, American Institute of Homeopathy, American Association of Public Health Nursing, American Pharmaceutical Association, American Nurses' Association, National Association of Casualty and Society Underwriters, National Association of Manufacturers, National Conference of Charities and Corrections, and the National Convention of Insurance Commissioners.

study the subject,* and 16 states had introduced health insurance bills.†
During this time, the United States had also entered World War I, although there appeared to be no slackening of the momentum for reform.

There was also some activity on the federal level. Early in 1916, a
resolution was introduced in the House of Representatives (H.R. 159)
"for the appointment of a commission to prepare and recommend a plan
for the establishment of a national insurance fund for the mitigation of
the evil of unemployment." The resolution also included sickness and
disability. Hearings before the House Committee on Labor were held
in April of that year.[10]

Only one witness, Samuel Gompers, president of the American
Federation of Labor (AFL), appeared to oppose the resolution. The
treasurer and vice-president of the same organization, John B. Lennon
and James O'Connell, respectively, favored government-sponsored
health insurance. Another labor supporter was the president of the
Order of Railway Conductors, Austin G. Garretson. Gompers was
afraid that the commission would be prejudiced in its findings and
recommend compulsory health insurance. Being an old-line trade un-
ionist, he was suspicious of government involvement in health and
welfare for workers; he urged a study of voluntary methods.

After the hearings in April, H.R. 159 was reintroduced as H.R.
250. On July 1, 1916, the Committee on Labor recommended to Congress that the resolution be passed.[11] The commission to be appointed
by the president was to make a study of the causes of unemployment
and to investigate methods of insurance against the hazards of unemployment, sickness, invalidity, and old age. It was further recommended that the commission report on the advisability of establishing
a comprehensive federal insurance system; if one were considered prac-
ticable, the commission should prepare rules and regulations for its
administration. Although committee members recognized that a number of states had already appointed commissions to study the subject,
they believed that Congress should encourage study from the national
standpoint. The vote on the resolution, with only 40 minutes of discussion on the day of adjournment, fell considerably short of the two-thirds
majority necessary for passage.

Late in 1917, another resolution to establish a federal commission

---

*California in 1915; Connecticut, Illinois, Massachusetts, New Hampshire, New Jersey,
Ohio, Pennsylvania, and Wisconsin in 1917; and Indiana in 1919.

†New York, Massachusetts, and New Jersey in 1916; and California, Colorado, Connecticut, Illinois, Maine, Michigan, Minnesota, New Hampshire, Ohio, Oregon, Pennsylvania, Washington, and Wisconsin in 1917.

to study social insurance was introduced in the House by the same member who was responsible for the previous resolution.[12] This resolution (H.R. 189) was also reported favorably by the Committee on Labor and was considered by the House on January 16, 1918. It encountered serious opposition and did not pass, presaging the end of activity to promote compulsory health insurance on either the federal or state level during this early period. Scarcely anyone at this time would have guessed that Congress would do a complete turnabout 20 years later and pass the Social Security Act.

THE MEDICAL PROFESSION

At the 66th annual session of the AMA in June 1915, the Judicial Council published a lengthy report describing worker compensation in the United States and abroad as well as government health insurance abroad. It also explored the possibility of establishing some form of government health insurance in the United States. Sympathetic study was advised, and the report was referred to the Reference Committee on Reports of Officers.[13] This committee, in turn, recommended acceptance of the report and urged that state medical associations bring the question of health insurance before their constituent county societies. The chairman of the council was Alexander Lambert, also an influential member of the Committee on Social Insurance of the AALL.

That same year, the *Journal of the American Medical Association* announced the publication of the model health insurance bill drafted by the Committee on Social Insurance of the AALL. In regard to it, a prophetic editorial read:

> It is hoped that physicians will take advantage of this opportunity and that it will be possible to avoid that lack of cooperation between physicians and legislators which, for a time, marred some of the foreign legislation. If physicians will study this important and rapidly developing problem and help to work out an equitable method of furnishing medical care and relief for working men, much dissatisfaction later can be avoided.[14]

At the request of the AALL, the Council on Health and Public Instruction of the AMA immediately appointed a committee to assist in drafting a health insurance bill to be introduced in the state legislatures in 1916. This was an important policy matter and one that had not been cleared with the board of trustees of the House of Delegates of the AMA. The members of the AMA committee were prestigious physicians: Alexander Lambert, from New York City; Henry B. Favill, from Chicago; and Frederick J. Cotton, from Boston. The consensus was that "cooperation is desirable and opportune."[15]

This body became the Committee on Social Insurance. It was appointed under the power vested in the Council on Health and Public Instruction, whose chairman was Henry B. Favill, in cooperation with the Judicial Council. On February 9, 1916, the board of trustees confirmed the appointment of the committee, indicating an open mind on the question of compulsory health insurance:

> ... the purpose and duty of the Committee be understood to be the careful compilation of information regarding social or health insurance and the relation of physicians thereto; and to do everything in their power to secure such construction of the proposed laws as will work the most harmonious adjustment of the new sociologic relations between physicians and laymen which will reasonably result therefrom, and that this Committee be authorized to carry on its work wherever seems more desirable.[16]

I. M. Rubinow became executive secretary. According to him, the committee intended to (1) educate physicians in the essential part they had to play in any successful adaptation of health insurance legislation to American conditions, (2) make statistical studies for policy formulation, and (3) appear before legislative bodies to bring about a friendly understanding among all parties concerned and to protect the legitimate economic interest of the profession. It was further hoped that the considerable bitterness that existed between physicians and politicians in England might be avoided by appropriate and timely action.[17]

Two months after Rubinow's report, there was an editorial in the *Journal of the American Medical Association* about the committee:

> ... it will probably require two or three years' work to collect the necessary data and arrive at definite conclusions as to what is to be the position of the medical profession of this country in the ultimate solution of the problem. In the meantime, it is urged that individual physicians and medical organizations refrain from isolated active efforts, either for or against social insurance bills in state legislatures, in order that the attitude of the profession in this subject may be harmonious and that its influence may be exerted unitedly and effectively.[18]

The editorial counseled reasonableness, assuming that high stakes could be discussed or debated rationally. In the meantime, Lambert, the chairman of the Committee on Social Insurance, submitted a long report to the House of Delegates at the 1916 annual session of the AMA. The report was referred to the Reference Committee on Legislation and Political Action, which approved it and urged the House to endorse both the report and the committee. It also recommended that each state association be requested to establish a committee on social insurance to work with the parent committee. The House of Delegates did so. Thus studying the question of compulsory health insurance and counseling state legislatures became official policy of the AMA.

The issue was beginning to surface for the rank and file of physicians in the United States, at least for those who read the *Journal of the American Medical Association*. For example, Lambert published an article in the journal on health insurance and invited reactions.[19]

At the 1917 annual session of the AMA, the committee offered to the House of Delegates a resolution that recommended, among other matters:

> That the House of Delegates instruct its Council on Health and Public Instruction to insist that such legislation shall provide freedom of choice of physician by the insured; payment of the physician in proportion to the amount of work done; the separation of the functions of medical official supervision from the function of the daily care of the sick; and adequate representation of the medical profession on the appropriate administrative bodies.[20]

The house took no action on this resolution, and it is difficult to figure out why. In any case, physicians were beginning to enunciate the classic demands of the profession everywhere in response to third party payers: (1) free choice of physician, (2) fee-for-service payment, and (3) significant, if not majority, representation on administrative bodies. Physicians at that time were in full charge of their own practices and had a major influence on hospital policy. The hospital was known as the "doctor's workshop." Naturally, changing the source of payment and possibly the method of payment from the individual patient to a potentially powerful and monopolistic third party was viewed with concern.

World War I began in April 1917, and the Committee on Social Insurance was discontinued for the duration of the war. Nonetheless, there was a great deal of activity on the state level, as revealed in journals of the state medical societies. This is understandable, in that the state legislatures were considering the question of compulsory health insurance, but their seriousness was not easy to determine. The fact that legislation based largely on the model bill of the AALL was being promoted at all was impressionistic evidence that something was going on.

The reactions of state medical associations seemed mixed. The AALL model bill was endorsed by the Wisconsin and Pennsylvania medical societies, and there were indications of support from the medical societies of California and Illinois. The bill failed, however, to win endorsement from the Massachusetts Medical Society.

As observed by Donald L. Numbers:

... judged by most criteria AALL's state-by-state campaign was a success. No state had passed the model bill, but several had set up commissions to study needs for it. No state medical society had taken a stand against insurance, while two had officially endorsed it and at least six more had established health insurance committees.[21]

The ultimate criterion, however—enactment of any legislation—was not achieved. Numbers believes that the great mass of the profession remained apathetic. If so, it was not for long, as can be seen when the state medical society delegates gathered at the annual meeting of the AMA in 1919 and 1920.

The two leaders of the national organization, Alexander Lambert and Frank Billings, the latter chairing the Council on Health and Public Instruction, joined the armed forces. When Lambert returned from Europe in early 1919, the work of the Committee on Social Insurance was resumed. The committee was reorganized, and new members were added: M. L. Harris, one-time member and secretary of the AMA board of trustees and chairman of the Judicial Council, Chicago; S. S. Goldwater, a prominent hospital administrator, New York; and Frederick Van Sickle, Olyphant, Pennsylvania. Lambert continued as chairman and was also president-elect of the AMA. Thus support for a judicious examination of health insurance was indeed present in the inner circles of the AMA. Further, the interest was sympathetic, or at least neutral.

At the annual meeting of the AMA in June 1919, Lambert presented to the House of Delegates a report that avoided making any definite recommendations on health insurance. The house accepted the report and simultaneously referred to the Reference Committee on Legislation and Political Action a resolution against government-sponsored health insurance.[22] The Reference Committee tabled the resolution because " ... the evidence for and against is far from complete,"[23] a rational enough conclusion under the circumstances. New York State was in the middle of a legislative fight, and delegates from that state were reflecting it. Further, grassroots physicians, through their state associations, were beginning to react negatively to the sympathetic reports of the Committee on Social Insurance. The heat generated by the committee was great enough to move Victor G. Vaughan, chairman of the Council on Health and Public Instruction and Dean of the School of Medicine, University of Michigan, to admonish the delegates in his report to the house:

> The attitude of the majority of physicians to date has been one of an unqualified and often unreasoning opposition, without any effort to study the question or to consider the argument I put forward in favor of the proposed plan. Unreasoning opposition or sweeping and often erroneous

general arguments against the measure will not prevent its adoption nor will it enhance the influence of the physicians. It is of the utmost importance to the medical profession at present that we give this question the most careful, painstaking, patient and disinterested study, that we qualify ourselves as authorities instead of allowing this function to be exercised by the active proponents of social insurance.[24]

This came from an academic dean who, with other essentially nonpracticing physicians, was trying to infuse some rationality into a situation in which it seemed unreasonable to expect practitioners to be reasonable: their style of practice and their livelihood, which they viewed as professional freedom, would be changed by a monopolistic, third party payer.

By the time of the annual session in April 1920, almost a year later, the reaction of the state associations to academic physicians and top officials of the AMA was gaining momentum. Vaughan's pleas for an objective appraisal were not heeded, nor have they been heeded by the medical profession since. A small but passionate group of delegates was going to the New Orleans session "to get Lambert," as they put it. Most opposition came from delegates from New York, Michigan, Illinois, and California, the states where legislative activity was most intense. Vaughan reported again to the House of Delegates:

The House of Delegates has not yet seen fit to commit the Association to any position on this question, evidently feeling that the time has not yet come for the Association going on record either for or against social insurance.[25]

Vaughan went on to explain that, although many of the AMA members through their state journals wanted the Council on Health and Public Instruction to go on record against health insurance, it was not the council's function to enunciate policy.

The council was quickly relieved of any necessity for taking a stand on policy, because at the same meeting the House of Delegates formulated an unequivocal official policy that stood like Gibraltar until 1965, when the AMA equivocated on Medicare. Such consistency can be admired or condemned, depending on one's viewpoint, but opponents of the AMA position always knew clearly where the organization stood (although at times they found it hard to believe the AMA really meant what it said). This classic policy states:

Resolved, that the American Medical Association declares its opposition to the institution of any plan embodying the system of compulsory contribution insurance against illness, or any other plan of compulsory insurance which provided for medical services to be rendered contributors or their dependents, provided, controlled, or regulated by any state or the Federal Government.[26]

Thus ended this early period of health insurance as far as the AMA was concerned. The grass-roots battles, however, continued to be fought in several states, particularly in New York and California, where the state medical associations were extremely active in opposition. Furthermore, in California the health insurance proposition lost resoundingly in a state referendum.[27]

The United States' entry into World War I added another seemingly rational reason to oppose health insurance: it was made in Germany under Bismarck in 1883. An example of the intensity of the opposition as expressed by a physician from New York, follows:

> Conceived in iniquity, nurtured in hypocrisy, struggling for deliverance at the frantic behest of socialist doctrines, compulsory health insurance should die a-borning. Nowhere has the fiendish greed of the debasing propaganda of state socialism been more brazenly exposed than in this merciless attempt to steal the livelihood of the most unselfish profession in the world.[28]

Equally purple in his prose and his opposition was Samuel Gompers, whose AFL was a federal of skilled trade unions and the elite of the labor movement. He testified in 1916 before the House Committee on Labor in reference to H.R. 159, the resolution to establish a federal commission to study social insurance:

> I am apprehensive that the attempts of government under the guise of compulsory social insurance for the workers in cases of unemployment, sickness, and disability will result in every Government agent going into the houses and lives of the workers as a spy. We have enough already of spies and detectives coming into the lives and workshops of the toilers. After centuries of struggles, during the past twenty years we concentrated our efforts in an agitation that has gone through the whole country to secure from the hands of Congress a larger liberty of action than has ever been accorded to the working people of any other country on the face of the globe in the entire history of the world. As long as there is one spark of life in me, my mentality, whatever that may be, of my spirit, I will help in crystallizing the spirit and sentiment of our workers against this attempt to enslave them by the well-meaning siren songs of philosophers, statisticians, and politicians.[29]

It is apparent that, with the help of the House of Delegates of the AMA, Gompers' wish was fulfilled. In 1916 his memory of government's antilabor actions in the form of lockouts and injunctions against strikes was still fresh. The prevailing trade union philosophy was to strike for higher wages and better working conditions so that workers could solve their own problems as private collectives.

In retrospect ten years later, a California physician wrote that the health insurance bill proposed in California:

> ... was a good one, as such laws go, and yet its approach was exceedingly tactlessly handled. It was born in propaganda, bred and spread by a man of Russian name [concurrent with the Russian Revolution in 1917]. It developed without any organized effort to win over the leaders in the medical profession.[30]

It seems doubtful that more tact would have made any difference. The profession was not ready for legislation of this kind, and it never has been anywhere. Membership in the AMA was increasing, strengthening the influence of the private and predominantly solo type of practice and fee-for-service method of payment. A solid front was established, as expressed by the House of Delegates at the annual meeting in 1920.[31]

There has been some speculation as to why the AMA leadership did not continue to push for health insurance after the adamant resolution of the House of Delegates in 1920. One might ask, Who would dare? John Gordon Freymann believes that the increase in full-time clinical positions freed many academics from the struggle for economic survival and that the growth of specialization had caused medical scientists to turn from state and local medical associations to specialty societies.[32] Numbers' statistical analysis of the composition of the House of Delegates in 1917 and 1920 appears to show otherwise. The new delegates were neither less academic nor less scientific than their predecessors. In fact, between 1917 and 1920, the percentage of academics among state delegates increased from 15.4 to 18.3, while general and small-town physicians lost representation.[33] Also, throughout the early 1920s the presidency of the AMA was filled by an academic-scientific elite.

Numbers seems to be arguing that the medical profession in general is profoundly guarded regarding its rights, privileges, and prerogatives, and this characteristic became increasingly salient as more of the rank-and-file physicians were exposed to the implications health insurance had for them. Certainly, the predominant physician type was the general and solo practitioner, to whom the leadership paid heed in characteristic American fashion. Despite the apparent perpetuation of an academic and speciality leadership, the grass roots of medicine on the state and local levels effectively pulled the AMA leadership away from the issue of health insurance, even away from studying how to accommodate it in the profession's interest.

The intellectual and political spearhead of health insurance, AALL, was attacked from many quarters, a new experience for that organization. The members were called uplifters or do-gooders. In the wartime hysteria of 1918, it was claimed that AALL was not really an American organization because it was affiliated with a number of similar organizations in foreign countries and many of its members had been born in central Europe. Although President Woodrow Wilson was a member, it was remarked that even he could make mistakes.[34]

NOTES

1. Frederick R. Brush, quoted in *Transactions of the American Hospital Association* 11 (1909):182.
2. Most of the material on workmen's compensation insurance was obtained from Clarence W. Hobbs, *Workmen's Compensation Insurance, Including Employers' Liability Insurance*, 2nd ed. (New York: McGraw-Hill, 1939) and Herman M. Somers and Anne R. Somers, *Workmen's Compensation: Prevention, Insurance, and Rehabilitation of Occupational Disability* (New York: Wiley, 1954).
3. Progressive National Committee, *A Contract with the People*, platform of the progressive party adopted at its first national convention, Chicago, August 7, 1912, p. 5.
4. I. M. Rubinow, "Sickness Insurance," *American Labor Legislation Review* 3 (June 1913):162–71.
5. *American Labor Legislation Review* 4 (December 1914):595–96.
6. *American Labor Legislation Review* 6 (March 1916):104–5.
7. *American Labor Legislation Review* 6 (June 1916):155.
8. Irving Fisher, "The Need for Health Insurance," *American Labor Legislation Review* 7 (March 1917):9.
9. I. M. Rubinow, "Health Insurance Through Local Funds," *American Labor Legislation Review* 7 (March 1917):69.
10. U.S., Congress, House, Committee on Labor, *Hearings on J. Res. 159*, 64th Cong., 1st sess., 6 and 11 April 1916.
11. U.S., Congress, House, *Social Insurance and Unemployment: Report No. 914 to Accompany J. Res. 250*, 64th Cong., 1st sess., 1 July 1916.
12. U.S., Congress, House, *Report No. 218 on J. Res. 189*, 64th Cong., 2d sess., 15 December 1917.
13. Proceedings of the 66th Annual Session of the American Medical Association, June 21–24, 1915, San Francisco, in *Journal of the American Medical Association* 65 (3 July 1915):74–92.
14. Editorial, *Journal of the American Medical Association* 65 (20 November 1915):1824.
15. *Journal of the American Medical Association* 65 (25 December 1915):2247.
16. I. M. Rubinow, "Social Insurance," *American Medical Association Bulletin* 11 (15 March 1916):250.

17. Ibid., p. 251.
18. Editorial, *Journal of the American Medical Association* 66 (6 May 1916): 1469–70.
19. Alexander Lambert, "Health Insurance and the Medical Profession," *Journal of the American Medical Association* 68 (27 January 1917):257–62.
20. *Journal of the American Medical Association* 68 (9 June 1917):1755.
21. Donald L. Numbers, *Almost Persuaded: American Physicians and Compulsory Health Insurance, 1912–1920* (Baltimore: Johns Hopkins University Press, 1978), pp. 46–48. This book gives a well-documented account of this period. I am not persuaded, however, that American physicians were "almost persuaded": only a few of them were.
22. *Journal of the American Medical Association* 72 (14 June 1919):1832, 1936.
23. Ibid., p. 1836.
24. Ibid., p. 1750.
25. *Journal of the American Medical Association* 74 (1 May 1920):1241–42.
26. Ibid., p. 1319.
27. See Numbers, *Almost*, pp. 75–84. See also Arthur J. Viseltear, "Compulsory Health Insurance in California, 1915–1918," *Journal of the History of Medicine* 24 (April 1969):151–82.
28. W. P. Cunningham, "Health Insurance," *New York Medical Journal* 106 (13 October 1917):683.
29. U.S., Congress, House, Committee on Labor, *Hearings*, p. 185.
30. Philip K. Brown, "Organized Medicine's Interest in a Health Insurance Plan for Small Wage Earners," *New England Journal of Medicine* 205 (1931):1287.
31. See James Burrow, *A.M.A.: The Voice of American Medicine* (Baltimore: Johns Hopkins University Press, 1963) pp. 27–53.
32. John Gordon Freymann, "Leadership in American Medicine: A Matter of Personal Responsibility," *New England Journal of Medicine* 270 (1964):710–15.
33. Numbers, *Almost*, pp. 110–11.
34. *Journal of the Maine Medical Association* 9 (September 1918):16.

7

Lack of Political Consensus in the Third Estate

Although the leadership of the AMA and the AALL seemed to be assuming that somehow their support of compulsory health insurance would succeed on its merits, they undoubtedly found it hard to predict how the political protagonists would line up. They found out soon enough. Besides the AMA and the AFL, other interest groups opposing compulsory health insurance were the insurance and pharmaceutical companies, business and industry, the AHA, the nursing profession, and the U.S. Public Health Service.

ORGANIZED LABOR

Without the united support of organized labor from 1915 to 1920, the political chances of compulsory health insurance were nil. Its supporters had no single, strong interest group leadership. Indeed, the outright hostility of Samuel Gompers came as a surprise to them. Some individual labor leaders looked on compulsory health insurance favorably, but Gompers' adamant opposition blunted labor support. Twenty-one state federations of labor supported health insurance, the most important being the New York federation. In addition, 29 national trade unions expressed support.[1]

The reluctance of the AFL to take any action whatever is revealed in the tone of its deliberations at annual conventions between 1918 and 1921. Health insurance did not reach the level of the executive council of the AFL until its convention in June 1918, when it authorized a committee to study health insurance and recommend a course of action. The executive council's tone, although favorable to the study, was suspicious:

> Whereas during the past few years great efforts have been made to obtain approval and support of organized labor to a scheme of Social Health Insurance, *promoted by persons and organizations who have no affiliation with the Labor movement;* and whereas, owing to the intensive and costly campaign which the promoters of this scheme have carried on during the last two years, at one time seeking to have this legislation adopted in twenty-eight states, suspicion has been aroused that this scheme is supported by those who, for years, have sought to disrupt and retard the cause of the workers [emphasis added].[2]

During this period, social reformers, economists, sociologists, public health experts, and other intellectuals represented in the AALL were unable to gain the confidence of either medicine or labor: they were outsiders to both groups, and their assistance was not sought until 15 to 20 years later. Ideological positions were taken quickly and intuitively by everyone, including the intellectuals. It was not until the 1930s that ideological positions and definitions were further clarified and a factual foundation laid on the basis of massive studies.

In 1919, the executive council of the AFL decided to continue the study of health insurance before declaring the federation's position.[3] Interest must have been desultory, because at the 1921 convention there was no report. At the 1922 convention, health insurance was not mentioned at all: it had become a dead issue. The AMA had established a policy, but the AFL had not. It was another 20 years before the issue was joined, when the two "natural" organizations for taking polar positions did so, and health insurance as a political issue reemerged. The AFL's position seems curious today, but at that time health insurance was not a bargaining issue between labor and management. One wonders how even relatively well paid skilled workers paid their medical bills. Perhaps the incidence of high-cost illness was not yet great enough for a groundswell to develop among them.

INSURANCE COMPANIES

Private insurance companies were first among the interest groups opposing government-sponsored health insurance to attack the AALL model bill in 1916. They were alert to its implications for themselves, and they reacted so swiftly that they thought at first they were alone. In retrospect, it seems curious that they did not anticipate the opposition of organized medicine. The insurance companies assumed that organized medicine would see an increased income in health insurance. William G. Curtis, president of the National Casualty Company, stated in September 1916: "The Medical Fraternity wants it [health insurance] because it will mean at least two or three times as much for medical treatment of wage earners."[4] Curtis was also president of the Insurance Economics Society, which was organized by insurance companies in 1916 to combat compulsory health insurance. From 1916 to 1919, 13 expository reports were written, most of them by Curtis. One was written at the request of Royal Meeker, Commissioner of Labor Statistics; it was to be read before the Conference on Social Insurance in Washington, D.C., on December 7, 1916. When Meeker saw it, he said it would neither advance the purpose of the conference nor help foil the plans for social insurance. One of its sentences confirmed his impression: "When compulsory Health Insurance enters the United States, Socialism will have its fist upon the throat of the nation."[5]

After Frederick L. Hoffman resigned from the Committee on Social Insurance of the AALL in 1916, he wrote and lectured extensively against government-sponsored health insurance. As chief statistician for the Prudential Insurance Company, he presumably had its sanction to lecture to numerous professional and scientific associations, medical societies, and business and citizen's groups. The extent to which irrationality can displace considered judgment in a time of extreme partisan stress is revealed in his statement that health insurance had not benefited Germany, because suicide rates in Berlin rose from 2.3 per 10,000 population in 1900 to 3.8 in 1913, while in the Bronx and Manhattan rates decreased from 2.4 to 1.8 per 10,000 population during the same period.[6] Irving Fisher of Yale believed the opposite—that compulsory health insurance was responsible for Germany's military preeminence. Disagreements among experts can result in bizarre conclusions having no relevance to the issues.

Hoffman's counter proposal to government-sponsored health insurance embodied the viewpoint of all opponents then and since: provision of health services for the poor; increased facilities and access for all; measures to combat and care for persons with occupational disease; and better sanitation, nutrition, and other extra-health service factors. He also felt that the standard of living of the average worker was sufficiently high that costly illnesses occurred relatively infrequently. Attacking the members of the AALL, his former colleagues, Hoffman said that industrial insurance companies might with greater justification than the AALL claim to represent the American working people; AALL members dealt with workers at a distance and usually without any personal knowledge of the conditions that workers wanted urgently to reform.[7] Insurance companies did have considerable contact with the working population. In 1917, there were 37.5 million industrial policies in force in 22 companies. It should be recalled, however, that industrial policies were largely for loss of wages due to illness and not for indemnification of health services costs. When health insurance became a dead issue, the partisan activities of private insurance companies ceased.

PHARMACEUTICAL COMPANIES

Pharmaceutical companies were another group whose opposition was not anticipated by the proponents of health insurance. One of the companies' first actions was a resolution against government-sponsored health insurance passed in May 1917 by the Detroit branch of the American Pharmaceutical Association (APA).[8] In August 1917, the entire APA passed a similar resolution at its annual convention.[9] In August 1918, the APA's Committee on Compulsory Health Insurance reported at the annual meeting that Germany was attempting to export compulsory health insurance in order to raise production costs in the United States so that Germany could compete favorably in the international market.[10] Eventually other pharmaceutical interests joined in: the National Association of Retail Druggists and the American Drug Manufacturers' Association.

Pharmaceutical manufacturers presumably feared government as a monopoly buyer. The retail pharmacists feared that hospitals would establish their own pharmaceutical outlets under a government health insurance system.[11]

BUSINESS AND INDUSTRY

American business and industry are hardly a monolith regarding health and welfare policy, but the opinions of the Chamber of Commerce and the National Association of Manufacturers do carry some weight. These two organizations, initially at least, favored health insurance. In a short time, however, particularly in New York State, business interests, including private insurance companies, joined the opposition.[12] Their preference was voluntary health insurance. In time, the opposition of business and industrial interests increased in intensity.

THE AMERICAN HOSPITAL ASSOCIATION

As both the "doctor's workshop" and the custodian of institutional resources, the general hospital, as represented by the AHA, faced an ambiguous situation. The general hospital had become a central health services institution, and it constantly needed money. Would compulsory health insurance covering hospital services improve its cash flow? Cash came mainly from private, paying patients, but so far they were not a problem. What did seem to be a problem for hospitals by 1916 was the influence of third-party reimbursement under worker compensation. Apparently, reimbursement for indigent patients may not yet have been regarded as a problem, since the tradition of charity care, as enshrined in the charters of voluntary hospitals, was still sufficiently strong and the indigent were sufficiently apathetic. Losses could be recovered from private patients, who were the majority of patients, from philanthropists, and from state and local governments. Worker compensation payments forced hospitals into cost negotiations, which, according to the hospitals, were not negotiations at all but take it or leave it propositions.

Resolutions presented at the 1916 and 1918 annual conventions of the AHA showed that, while leaders appeared to be neither wholly against nor wholly for health insurance, they regarded it as inevitable. In his presidential address in 1916, Winford H. Smith, superintendent of the Johns Hopkins Hospital, said:

> We have accustomed ourselves, or are doing so, to the Workmen's Compensation Acts, as they affect our hospitals' health insurance, and the effect of the same on hospitals is another problem which we shall be forced to consider. Health insurance is doubtless in the minds of both of us a thing to be desired. In any event, it will surely be with us before many years.[13]

Smith went on to say that the AHA should appoint a committee to study the subject in order to arrive at "sound conclusions" and "sound principles." A committee on health insurance was appointed, with Michael M. Davis and S. S. Goldwater among the members. Davis was Mr. Health Insurance in the United States for over five decades thereafter. There is no evidence that this committee made any recommendations, but another body, the Committee on Social Insurance chaired by Thomas Howell, superintendent of New York Hospital, backed the AHA's endorsement of health insurance in 1918. The actual recommendation was made by the Legislative Committee, at least partly on the following grounds:

> Too long, however, hospital people sat idly by and let state legislatures and workmen's compensation commissions make plans for the injured workmen without careful thought for the sufficiency of the care and with almost no regard for the cost to the hospital of the service rendered.[14]

Following the tradition of third party payments for indigent patients, hospitals were paid less than actual costs in worker compensation cases. One may infer from the recommendations adopted by the AHA in 1918 that hospital administrators hoped the custom of paying hospitals less than cost would be rectified if health insurance were adopted by the several states. The AHA offered to advise and cooperate with state health insurance commissions and state legislatures in incorporating proper payment principles into proposed legislation. Although hospitals were becoming big enterprises, as measured by the capital and operating income they needed, it was difficult for them to put over the image of a community institution with cash-flow problems. The AHA did not seem to be active in health insurance beyond these expressions of concern over their financial solvency. The hospitals also needed to be deferential toward physicians in determining how strong a stand to take on health insurance.

In that era, the AHA was made up only of individuals; institutional membership was adopted shortly thereafter. It should be remembered that in 1918 there were over 5,000 general hospitals and 500,000 beds, a sizable political constituency bound to the middle-class community leadership through boards of trustees and other connections. Nevertheless, the AHA was not yet cohesive enough nor accustomed enough to political action to speak with one voice in the same way that the AMA was beginning to speak for physicians. A resolution similar to the one adopted by the AMA in 1920 was inconceivable.

NURSING

The nursing profession spoke with greater emphasis than did the hospital representatives, not to mention the physicians. Most registered nurses at the time were engaged in private duty; they were not employed by the hospitals, but by private patients in the hospitals. In 1916, three organizations of nurses—the American Nurses' Association, the National League for Nursing Education, and the National Association of Public Health Nurses, established a Joint Committee on Health Insurance. This committee reported favorably on health insurance in principle and recommended that the subject be studied.[15] Mary Beard, in her presidential address at the annual convention of the National Organization for Public Health Nursing in 1917, admonished: "We must set our house in order against the day when nursing under health insurance Acts will be ours to administer."[16]

She counseled preparedness as much as endorsement. Thus, in contrast to physicians, hospital administrators, and pharmacists, nurses were quite forthright. Assuming self-interest on the part of all the contending groups, one may speculate why nurses took the stand they did. Perhaps a public image of selflessness was sufficient incentive in itself.

THE U.S. PUBLIC HEALTH SERVICE

By 1912 the PHS was a recognized entity for health affairs in the federal government and an emerging interest group in the governmental bureaucracy. Although the service had not yet worked out a cooperative federal-state program, it was undoubtedly conscious of the possibilities for expanding responsibility, influence, and power. Also, it seems reasonable to assume that top-level officers envisioned local, that is, county, health departments throughout the country (city health departments already existed). County departments were already being established in a number of local areas between 1915 and 1920.

Public health officers were confronted with the possibility of becoming the administrative agents for government-sponsored health insurance, although it seemed that no proposal had mentioned this possibility. Private insurance companies, on the other hand, had been suggested as possible administrators, with government agencies handling the finances. It seems unlikely that physicians in private practice would have accepted PHS administration had health insurance legislation passed. In any case, the top public health officer, Surgeon-General Rupert Blue, was reported to be in favor of government-sponsored health insurance; B. S. Warren, a surgeon in the PHS, was an active proponent. Warren saw the administrative potential for public health departments as early as 1915, when he suggested that physicians in government agencies (who were presumed to be neutral agents, in contrast to private practitioners involved with their own patients) should do the certifying for disability compensation. The concept was to link health officers with preventive and curative medicine.[17]

An official stand was taken in Washington, D.C., in May 1916 at a conference of the PHS and the health officers of the states and territories. Twenty-three states and territories were represented, and a resolution was passed unanimously adopting the report of the Committee on Health Insurance; this report supported the establishment of a government-sponsored scheme.[18]

OBSERVATIONS ON AN ABORTED MOVEMENT

The reasons that compulsory health insurance was not adopted between 1915 and 1920 are quite clear. For one thing, the AALL did not have a broad base of support from organized labor, the largest and most powerful interest group at that time. The members of the AALL seemed to believe that any social reform as logical as health insurance would succeed on its own merits. Selig Perlman, for example, a professor of labor economics at the University of Wisconsin during this period, felt that intellectual leaders of social reform frequently underestimated the strength of the opposition.[19]

The AALL had not anticipated the rancorous opposition of the state medical societies given the early and sympathetic interest of AMA leaders. Attacks from private insurance companies were ineffective, since they did not even sell health insurance at the time. The inclusion of funeral benefits may have been recognized as a tactical error because of the possible threat to industrial life insurance. Another unexpected assault came from Christian Scientists and related practitioners, who saw in health insurance an attempt on the part of medicine to eliminate other ways of thinking. But most disheartening of all was the general indifference of organized labor.

The need for health insurance was difficult to explain. The risk concept of health services costs was not generally understood. Probably there were not enough visible cases of families incurring high-cost medical episodes unless they were poor, but the middle class was having difficulties. It was felt sufficient that a family should be thrifty and save for the rainy day of medical costs; further, it was assumed that people had a large degree of control over their health—if they led prudent and moral lives.

There was confusion at that time, as there still is, about whether to regard health insurance as (1) a health service or a risk to be paid from a pooled fund or (2) as a way of forestalling poverty or raising the general level of health. During this early period there was no broad base of support or, for that matter, of opposition. The political fight was between individual giants, and the general public seemed to have little interest.

At a combined annual meeting of the AALL and the American Sociological Society in 1930, Rubinow tried to explain the failure to enact compulsory health insurance ten years earlier. He felt that extravagant promises had been made by the proponents and that exaggerated dire consequences had been predicted by opponents. He said wistfully:

> It might have been unnecessary to make those promises if it had been possible for each economic group clearly to formulate its own interest in legislation, and if the legislative process were a simple equation of definite, measurable, recognized group influences. In other words, these

things would have been possible if the process of legislation were only a process of social accounting and not colored by numerous psychologic attitudes and rationalizations.[20]

He recognized, belatedly, the nature of the American political process, where experts are on tap, not on top.

There may be some question as to how relevant this fairly detailed account of the first foray into government-sponsored health insurance is to the development of the American health services. The health services were allowed to evolve without let or hindrance; they were shaped by the providers and voluntary committee boards and were bought by the general public with no thought of influencing the nature or organization of them. The delivery system was accepted as a given, with the minor and uninfluential exception of Michael M. Davis and Andrew R. Warner, who advocated outpatient departments of hospitals and group practice clinics for the general public as well as the poor. Even when the concept of health insurance emerged, there was no intention of reorganizing the delivery system, but simply of devising a payment mechanism. The physicians saw it otherwise, largely intuitively. Third party payments could interfere with the prerogatives of physicians to diagnose and treat as they saw fit and to determine method and amount of payments. Physicians did not regard method, amount, or source of payments as a public affair. In this they were wrong, although they have been rather successful in lumping the two prerogatives together under the rubric of professionalism. To this day, hospitals and physicians are sparring with funding sources in order to maintain maximum autonomy.

NOTES

1. American Association for Labor Legislation, "Report of Work, 1919," *American Labor Legislation Review* 10 (March 1920):74.
2. American Federation of Labor, *Proceedings of the 28th Annual Convention*, St. Paul, Minn., June 10–20, 1918, pp. 282–83. Washington, D.C.
3. American Federation of Labor, *Proceedings of the 29th Annual Convention*, Atlantic City, N.J., June 9–23, 1919, pp. 378–79. Washington, D.C.
4. William G. Curtis, "Social Insurance," address before the Convention of National Association of Casualty and Surety Agents, White Sulphur Springs, W.V., September 20, 1916, *Insurance Economics Society of America*, Bulletin No. 1 (1916):14.
5. *Insurance Economics Society of America*, Bulletin No. 2 (1916):9.
6. Frederick L. Hoffman, *Facts and Fallacies of Compulsory Health Insurance* (Newark, N.J.: Prudential Insurance Company of America, 1917),p.50.

7. ———, "Health Insurance and the Public," *Pennsylvania Medical Journal* 22 (July 1919):664.
8. *Journal of the American Pharmaceutical Association* 6 (June 1917):569.
9. *Journal of the American Pharmaceutical Association* 6 (December 1917):1081.
10. *Journal of the American Pharmaceutical Association* 7 (October 1918):900.
11. J. H. Beal, "Concerning Proposed Compulsory Health Insurance Legislation," *Journal of the American Pharmaceutical Association* 6 (August 1917):701–11; Harry B. Mason, "What Compulsory Health Insurance Would Mean to the Druggist," *Journal of the American Pharmaceutical Association* 6 (October 1917):881–90; Editorial, *National Association of Retail Druggists Journal* 25 (March 21, 1918):1018.
12. *American Labor Legislation Review* 7 (March 1917):11 and 7 (December 1917):644.
13. Report of the 18th Annual Conference, Philadelphia, September 26–30, *Transactions of the American Hospital Association* 18 (1916):32.
14. Report of the Legislative Committee, 20th Annual Conference, Atlantic City, N.J., September 24–28, *Transactions of the American Hospital Association* 20 (1918):50.
15. Report of the Twentieth Annual Convention of the American Nurses' Association, Philadelphia, April 26–May 2, *American Journal of Nursing* 17 (July 1917):864–66.
16. *Public Health Nurse Quarterly* 19 (July 1917):213.
17. *American Labor Legislation Review* 6 (March 1916):28–31.
18. *Journal of the American Medical Association* 67 (9 September 1916):321.
19. Selig Perlman, *A Theory of the Labor Movement* (New York: Macmillan, 1928), pp. 151, 179.
20. I. M. Rubinow, "Public and Private Interests in Social Insurance," *American Labor Legislation Review* 21 (June 1931):184.

8

The Persistent Idea
of Health Insurance

The 1920s and early 1930s were quiet as far as action on compulsory health insurance was concerned. The unequivocal resolution adopted by the House of Delegates of the AMA and the apparent apathy of organized labor certainly settled the issue for the time being. The country was also moving into a period of unprecedented prosperity following World War I. The presidencies of Harding and Coolidge symbolized "back to normalcy," and major health and welfare innovations were given little consideration in either the public or the private sector. Still, the idea of health insurance would not go away.

A seemingly innocuous bill for a public health program was introduced in Congress in 1921. Called the Sheppard-Towner bill, it would provide grants-in-aid to state health departments for maternal and child health programs. Except for the short-lived Chamberlain-Kahn Act in 1918[1] for control of venereal disease, this bill set a precedent in the field of public health. According to the bill, the Children's Bureau, a federal agency, would administer grants to the states for programs that were normally the state's responsibility. The bill aroused a great deal of controversy because of federal-state division of responsibility for health and welfare matters, and many physicians opposed it. They claimed that there would be undue interference in state affairs and regimentation of medical practice. Although the bill scarcely proposed government-sponsored health insurance, some believed it had unfavorable implications for private practice. Nevertheless, the Sheppard-Towner Act was passed in 1922, with strong support from citizens' groups and women's clubs. To be against it was like being against mothers and infants. The act was officially disapproved by the AMA House of Delegates at its annual meeting in 1922.[2]

The Sheppard-Towner Act was discontinued in 1929, but not because of any particular action by the AMA. Congress was not in the
mood to continue appropriations, and without them the federal government was unable to stimulate programs in state health departments.

Perhaps the twenties and early thirties can be regarded as the
period during which health care reformers expressed their faith in facts
to support policy formulation. Many AALL members were prominent
in the massive studies of the American health services conducted by the
Committee on the Cost of Medical Care between 1928 and 1931. Research and fact finding may be conducted with little political controversy; it is not until actual public policy recommendations are made on
the basis of research findings that controversy arises. Shortly after 1920,
morbidity studies were conducted by the Public Health Service. In order
to contribute to "a picture of the public-health situation as a whole,
drawn in proper perspective and painted in true colors," the PHS
launched a series of observations on the incidence of illness in a representative sample of the general population in Hagerstown, Maryland.[3]
A series of studies showed the rates of illness according to age, sex, and
family income.[4]

The actions leading to studies of social and economic aspects of
health care were discussed on several occasions in 1925 and 1926 by
leading physicians, public health professionals, and economists.[5] In
April 1926, an informal conference was held in Washington, D.C. At
this meeting a committee of five was appointed to plan a series of
studies on the economic and social aspects of health services.*

The activities of this committee culminated in a conference held
simultaneously with the annual meeting of the AMA in Washington,
D.C. in May 1927. The conference was attended by 60 people, a large
group at that time for so specialized and technical a subject. It indicated
that there was a critical mass of highly placed and technically competent
people in health services research. These people had connections with
private foundations and academic centers. The result was the creation
of the Committee on the Cost of Medical Care (CCMC), which consisted
of 42 persons: 14 private practitioners of medicine, 6 public health professionals, 8 persons from institutions and organizations involved with
medicine (such as hospitals, the AMA, and insurance companies), 5
economists, and 9 persons representing the public at large. The chair-

---

*The affiliations of the committee members reveal the faith put in studies to help
formulate policy: Winford H. Smith, director, Johns Hopkins Hospital, chairman; Michael
M. Davis, medical sociologist and economist, former director of the Boston Dispensary;
Walter H. Hamilton, professor of public health, Yale University; Lewellys F. Barker, private practitioner; and Henry H. Moore, economist, Chicago, secretary.

man of the committee was Ray Lyman Wilbur, a physician and president of Stanford University. The membership read like a who's who in health services public policy.

The CCMC laid out several areas for intensive study: (1) incidence of disease and disability in the population, (2) existing facilities, (3) family expenditures for services, (4) incomes of providers of service, and (5) plans for health services for particular groups of the population. Other agencies, such as the American Dental Association, the AMA, the Metropolitan Life Insurance Co., the National Bureau of Economic Research, and the National Tuberculosis Association, contributed studies in related areas in cooperation with the CCMC.

Six foundations contributed heavily to the CCMC endeavor, making it a completely private undertaking. These foundations were the Carnegie Corporation, the Josiah Macy, Jr., Foundation, the Milbank Memorial Fund, the Russell Sage Foundation, the Twentieth Century Fund, and the Julius Rosenwald Fund. Although philanthropic foundations had played an influential role in the health field up to this time, from contributing capital funds to hospitals to funding demonstrations in public health practice, their support of the CCMC endeavor represented a significant departure in philanthropic activity. First, it was financed jointly and second, it was explicitly concerned with the consumer's problem in paying for personal health services. No other country appeared to be as interested in the details of the public's problems as the United States was. The health services edifice had been raised, and now there was a desire to learn what needs it should serve, how much it cost (as measured by consumer expenditures), and how it was to be paid for on a daily basis. Capital expenditures were apparently not yet considered a problem. Hospitals were capitalized by various forms of philanthropy, and physicians financed their own offices and worked in hospitals with no direct cost to themselves.

The foundations contributed about $1 million for research. Such a sum was rare enough for research in medicine in those days, let alone for novel and generally untried social and economic research in health care payment and delivery. Virtually everyone of note in the health field and the social sciences participated. The CCMC mustered the resources of a nation. A full-time staff of 75 technical experts in research and statistics was engaged to work under Harry H. Moore, a career PHS economist appointed director of this enterprise. Some members of the research staff remained active in the financing and delivery aspects of the health services for years thereafter.*

---

*For example, C. Rufus Rorem, an economist, became a prime mover in the establishment of the Blue Cross Plan; I. S. Falk, a bacteriologist turned medical economist, became

In the twenties and early thirties, then, the country was in a trough between the attempts to introduce compulsory health insurance legislation and the beginnings of voluntary health insurance. During this hiatus, professionals in health and social research laid the basis for collecting and organizing data on health services, data that, it was hoped, would lead to the formulation of national policy. It seems that these reformers still did not relate their research to the exigencies of the political process, even after the experience of 1915 to 1920.

The intensive research years from 1928 to 1933 appeared to serve as a period of watchful waiting for the groups that had a direct interest in the findings. The AMA, for example, wrote on its editorial page:

> Most physicians and most economists and most social workers are willing to wait until the Committee on the Cost of Medical Care, a group with which the medical profession is cooperating whole heartedly, has brought into the situation data on which to base reasonable action for the future.[6]

In effect, the AMA was expressing the same opinion it had in 1916, when government-sponsored health insurance was being studied before possible legislation in 16 states.

Twenty-eight reports were published; the first 27 were field studies, and the last one, in 1932, contained the sweeping recommendations that were supposed to flow directly from the research results. In essence, the studies, particularly No. 26, showed that illness and expenditures for health services fall unevenly on families and that a small minority experience severe illnesses and large health care expenditures. Overall, 10 percent of the families incur 40 percent of the expenditures in a year. A few studies of health service organizations that employed physicians in group practice units attached to an industry or that operated as independent plans were carried out.

Reactions to the reports were immediate, showing the power of research results when parties at interest sense that the stakes are high. Recommendations based on CCMC research split the committee itself into factions. Majority and minority reports were prepared. In brief, those who supported the majority report (39 out of 50) recommended that:

> ... medical service, both preventive and therapeutic, should be furnished largely by organized groups of physicians, dentists, nurses, pharmacists

director of research and statistics of the U.S. Social Security Commission; Louis S. Reed, medical economist, joined the PHS; Margaret C. Klem, lawyer, occupied several important posts in federal health agencies; and Nathan Sinai, Professor of Public Health, returned to the school of public health at the University of Michigan and eventually established a training and research unit in health services. I became his first research staff member.

and the associated personnel. Such groups should be organized, prefer-
ably around a hospital, for rendering complete office and hospital care.
The form of organizations should encourage the maintenance of high
standards and the development or preservation of a personal relation
between patient and physician.

. . . the costs of medical care should be placed on a group payment
basis, through the use of insurance, through the use of taxation, or
through the use of both these methods. This is not meant to preclude the
continuation of medical service provided on an individual fee basis for
those who prefer the present method.[7]

Private insurance companies were proscribed from being administrators or carriers for health insurance benefits, contrary to the model
bill of 1916. It was believed that they would tend to increase costs and
ignore quality considerations because there would be no physicians involved in the formulation of policies.[8] The CCMC was drawing here on
the European experience with health insurance administered without
physician participation in the making of policy. The physician was presumably at the mercy of the third party payer.

The signers of the majority report were apparently quite self-con-
scious about allegations of impersonal care in group practice arrangements, allegations that continue to this day: "Group practice in no way
inhibits the patient from giving his confidence to different physicians.
The business relation between physician and patient is not considered
a necessary part of the personal relation. . . ."[9]

The majority report, then, recommended virtual reorganization of
fee-for-service and solo medical practice, as well as group prepayment
for services and the application of the insurance principle. Such a plan
could be financed from either private or government sources, or both.
Drawing again on European experience, the signers of the majority
report felt that physicians could best guard their professional prerogatives as groups negotiating with insurance agencies of various kinds.
Solo practitioners were considered vulnerable and unable to bargain
effectively.

In retrospect, it is difficult to conceive that those who signed the
majority report actually believed it would be practical to carry out their
major recommendations on any large scale. They apparently did not
believe, however, that it was possible to attach the insurance mechanism to the prevailing fee-for-service structure of physicians' services.
They surely felt that fee-for-service payment was undesirable and
should be eliminated as soon as possible because it discouraged the
formation of group practice units. As usual, there was no strategy for
change: research findings were supposed to be self-evident and logical
in their application.

The response of the signers of the minority report was anything but vague: it was as clear and unequivocal as it was vigorous. It is unlikely that supporters of the majority report fully expected the well-articulated response of supporters of the minority report.

The minority report attacked the recommendation for group practice units based in or adjacent to hospitals. Insurance was cautiously accepted in principle. Selected quotes from the minority report reveal the members' perceptions of the medical organization milieu they found themselves in:

> The medical center plan is the adoption by medicine of the technique of big business, that is, mass production. It seems almost impossible for those who are not engaged in the practice of medicine to understand that the profession of medicine is a personal service and cannot adopt mass production methods without changing its character. . . . It is the belief of the minority group that the majority report has presented this entire question in a distorted manner. The evils of contract practice are widespread and pernicious. The studies published by the committee show only the favorable aspects. They were selected because they were considered the most favorable examples of this type of practice in the United States. For each of these plans, a score of the opposite can be found.[10]

These counterrecommendations are worth describing at length because they explicitly stated for the first time organized medicine's position on public policy (other than its specific stand on government health insurance in 1920). Then proper role of government was presented as follows:

> The minority recommends that government competition in the practice of medicine be discontinued and that its activities be restricted (a) to the care of the indigent and of those patients with diseases which can be cared for only in governmental institutions; (b) to the promotion of public health; (c) to the support of the medical departments of the Army and Navy, Coast and Geologic Survey, and other government services which cannot because of their nature or location be served by the general medical profession; and (d) to the care of veterans suffering from bona fide service-connected disabilities and diseases, except in the case of tuberculosis and nervous and mental diseases.[11]

Everything else was to be monopolized by private practice.

The minority report recommended that the general practitioner be restored to a central place in medical practice. The minority believed that the creation of group practice units would simply accelerate the trend toward specialization, thus blaming group practice for specialization rather than specialization for group practice. It was estimated that

85 percent of all illness and injury could be treated "efficiently by any general practitioner with very simple equipment."[12] That figure persists as conventional wisdom to this day.

Supporters of the minority report said that they were not opposed to insurance within the framework of private practice, as they were alleged to be; they were only opposed to abuses, which in their minds had usually accompanied insurance for medical care. Accordingly, the minority recommended that state or county medical societies initiate plans for medical care embodying the following "safeguards":

1. The plan must be under the control of the medical profession
2. It must guarantee not only nominal but actual free choice of physicians
3. It must include all, or a large majority, of the members of the county medical society
4. Funds must be administered on a nonprofit basis
5. The plan should provide for direct payment by the patient of a certain minimum amount, the common fund providing only that portion beyond the patient's means
6. It should make adequate provision for community care of the indigent
7. It must be entirely separate from any plan providing cash benefits (such as disability)
8. It must not require certification of disability by the physician treating the disease or disability (so as to avoid divided loyalty)

Such plans should be initiated by county medical societies with the approval and supervision of the state and national medical societies.

The CCMC majority recommendations apparently moved representatives of organized medicine to spell out how physicians' services should be organized and how the insurance principle should be applied. The policy established by the AMA in 1920 dealt exclusively with source of payment, that is, government and compulsory enrollment. The proponents of government-sponsored health insurance had accepted the existing form of medical practice with no particular thought being given to its characteristics. In 1932, however, organization of services became the primary issue; the insurance method of pooling funds was a subsidiary, although highly important, issue. The medical profession's response to the CCMC majority report was to attach the insurance method to the existing structure of medical practice and to put it under the control of the medical societies, a medical guild concept. The minority report's reaffirmation of the proper role of government and its interpretation of the role of insurance was an accurate statement of the medical profession's outlook.

The minority report paid no attention to one of the majority report's recommendations, possibly because it was more or less incidental: that is, that general hospital insurance be provided on a voluntary basis. Individuals or groups in the community could pay agreed-on annual sums to cover the costs of hospital services when needed. The staff of the CCMC had reported on the beginnings of such plans at Baylor University Hospital in Dallas, Texas, and Community Hospital in Grinnell, Iowa. The Judicial Council of the AMA had alluded to these plans in a report to the House of Delegates in 1931. The report did not oppose them, possibly because they did not concern physicians' services directly, but it did say that the plans were not charging high enough premiums to meet their obligations.

The voluntary insurance of 1932 was not the same as the voluntary insurance of today. The term was loosely applied to some types of contract and corporate practices. Moreover, voluntary health insurance, the AMA pointed out, would inevitably lead to government-sponsored health insurance, a prediction hardly without foundation. The medical profession was in a dilemma no matter what action it recommended. Logically and inevitably, then, it built its defenses in the form of medical society-sponsored and medically controlled insurance based on the criteria set forth in the minority report.

In an editorial in the December 3, 1932, issue of the *Journal of the American Medical Association*, the AMA wished to make it clear that the minority report was not to be interpreted as being:

> opposed to any individual carrying insurance against the occurrence of a major illness or operation so that he might receive at such time funds sufficient to pay the hospital and physician he might select. No doubt, insurance companies could sell such policies most reasonably if a sufficient number of persons could be induced to insure themselves and their families in this manner. Such a procedure is foresighted, American, economical. It preserves personal relationships and the free choice of physician and hospital; moreover, it makes the patient responsible to the physician and places squarely on the physician the responsibility for the care of the patient.[13]

In other words, the physician is completely free of a contractual relationship with the insurance agencies. In this same editorial, however, there appeared an attack on the majority report of the CCMC which has become a classic:

The alignment is clear—on the one side the forces representing the great foundations, public health officials and social theory—even socialism and communism—inciting to revolution; on the other side, the organized medical profession of this country urging an orderly evaluation guided by controlled experimentation which will observe principles that have been found through the centuries to be necessary to the sound practice of medicine.[14]

The CCMC majority report was also criticized from the left by none other than the AALL, which was active in promoting compulsory health insurance in a number of states. The AALL accused the CCMC of pussyfooting and compromising.[15]

It can be said that, in the early 1930s, the issues of compulsory and voluntary health insurance were being clarified, the positions of the major providers could be seen, and a factual basis for rational discussion of the problems of health services and the delivery system was available. To the extent that controversy was based on lack of facts, the range of controversy surrounding the incidence of illness and the problems families had in paying for health services should have narrowed. The principle of insurance was accepted, but implementation of the principle was, and has remained, a political issue. The supply of hospitals and physicians, pharmacists, nurses, and so on was in place. A delivery system with voluntary hospitals (plus public hospitals) and autonomous private practitioners charging fees was in place, and any changes in the source of payment would have to deal with it. The group practice, prepayment type of arrangement visualized in the CCMC majority report took a long time to become an effective reference point. We now enter the second stage in the development of the American health services: the era of the third party payer.

NOTES

1. See Odin W. Anderson, *Syphilis and Society—Problems of Control in the United States, 1912–1964*, Research Series No. 22 (Chicago: Center for Health Administration Studies, Graduate School of Business, University of Chicago, 1965).
2. *Journal of the American Medical Association* 78 (3 June 1922):1709.
3. Edgar Sydenstricker, "The Incidence of Illness in a General Population Group," *Public Health Reports* 60 (13 February 1925):279–91.
4. Selwyn D. Collins, *Economic Status and Health*, U.S. Public Health Service Bulletin No. 165 (Washington, D.C.: Government Printing Office, 1927).
5. Committee on the Cost of Medical Care, *Five-Year Program*, adopted February 13, 1928 (Washington, D.C.: Committee on the Cost of Medical Care, 1928).

6. Editorial, *Journal of the American Medical Association* 92 (10 August 1929):459.
7. Committee on the Cost of Medical Care, No. 28. *Final Report,* adopted October 21, 1932 (Chicago: The University of Chicago Press, 1933), p. 120.
8. Ibid., pp. 50–51.
9. Ibid., p. 39.
10. Ibid., pp. 154, 158.
11. Ibid., p. 174.
12. Ibid.
13. *Journal of the American Medical Association* 99 (3 December 1932):1951.
14. Ibid., p. 1952. The editor of the *Journal of the American Medical Association* at that time, Morris Fishbein, M.D., loved words and was a good phrase maker. It is thus possible that this colorful paragraph, although serious in intent, was written tongue in cheek. Dr. Fishbein said in an interview with me, however, that the political situation at that time was so volatile—with impending nationalization of the economy as the Depression worsened—that strong words were needed. He permitted me to quote him.
15. *American Labor Legislation Review* 22 (December 1932):162.

PART III

The Era of the Third Party Payer, 1930–1965

9

The Issue of Equity Revived: Government Health Insurance

INTRODUCTION

By the early thirties, a tremendous and imposing health services delivery infrastructure was in place. It was second to none in the industrial nations of the world in its variety, capability, and magnitude. It naturally reflected the mass production, mass consumption, and entrepreneurial characteristics of the economy; in its very large private sector, it reflected the hands-off nature of the political system.

The sheer numbers of facilities, personnel, educational facilities, and expenditures at this time are revealing (see Table 9.1).

The number of medical schools and students dropped between 1905 and 1930 because of the upgrading of medical schools as they became affiliated with universities. Consequently, the ratio of physicians to population also dropped somewhat, from 146 per 100,000 to 125 in 1930. It would seem reasonable to assume that by and large, physicians in 1930 were better trained than those in 1910. The number of dental schools decreased for the same reason, but the ratio of dentists to population increased. The spectacular increases, of course, were in general hospital beds, nurses, pharmacists, and various technical personnel associated with laboratories, surgery, and radiology.

Specialization among physicians had already begun, particularly in surgery. Rosemary Stevens observes that the specialties were normally recognized as such between 1900 and 1930 and that they came of

TABLE 9.1   Hospital Facilities, Personnel, and
Educational Facilities in 1930

Personnel, Facility	Number	Ratio (per 100,000 Population)
Hospitals	6,719	
Beds	955,869	690
Physicians	153,803	125
Nurses	214,300	174
Pharmacists	84,000	6.8
Dentists	71,105	58
School		
Medical	76	NA
Students	21,597	
Graduates	4,565	
Nursing	1,885*	NA
Students	78,770	
Graduates	23,810	
Dental	38	NA
Students	7,813	
Graduates	1,561	
Pharmacy	77	NA

*Figures for 1929.

age from 1930 to 1950. She classifies them in Table 9.2. In 1929, there were 14 recognized specialties among the full-time specialty groupings in table 9.2. Still, fully 83 percent of physicians regarded themselves as being engaged in primary practice, in whole or in part. Even some of the full time specialists, such as pediatricians, obstetrician-gynecologists, and internists, regarded themselves as first-contact physicians.

It is useful to classify hospitals and beds by ownership and type of patient served. Ownership implies control and reveals the degree of pluralism in the system in regard to ownership and source of funding. Table 9.3 shows the distribution of hospitals and beds by ownership in 1930.

Around one-quarter of the hospitals were supported by government, particularly local government, and three-quarters were private hospitals, mainly nonprofit hospitals. These had only one-third of the beds, but they provided care for the bulk of the short-term patients. Government hospitals were generally responsible for long-term care for mental and tuberculosis patients, as well as for relatively long-term care for veterans. The full complement of hospital beds amounted to 6.9 per 1,000 population, 3 of them being general hospital beds.

TABLE 9.2 Medical Specialists in 1931

Specialist		Number	Percent
Part-time specialists		120,399	82.9
and general practitioners			
Full-time specialists		24,826	17.1
Medical	6,674		4.6
Surgical	14,450		10.0
Psychiatry,			
neurology	1,401		1.0
Other	2,301		1.6
Total		145,225	100.0

Source: Rosemary Stevens, *American Medicine and the Public Interest* (New Haven, Conn.: Yale University Press, 1971), p. 181. Reprinted with permission of the publisher, copyright 1971.

TABLE 9.3 Distribution of Hospitals and Beds by Ownership, 1930

Hospital Ownership	Hospitals		Beds	
	Number	Percent	Number	Percent
Government	1,812	27	619,726	65
Federal	288	4	63,581	
State	581	9	405,309	
Local	943	14	150,836	
Private	4,907	73	336,143	35
Church	1,017	15	116,846	
Nonprofit	2,090	30	159,297	
Proprietary*	1,800	18	60,000	
Total	6,719	100	955,869	100

*Proprietary hospitals are categorized as "other" (that is nonchurch) in 1930 data, but one can estimate the numbers from data before and after 1930.

The distribution of hospitals and beds by type of hospital (and, therefore, by type of patient) for 1930 is noted in Table 9.4. General and mental hospital beds are divided evenly. Around 116,000 general hospital beds were owned by government, probably local government, and 336,143 were owned privately. One-fourth of the general hospital beds were owned by government, mostly county and municipal government, for the indigent population. In addition, an undetermined number of beds in the voluntary hospital were for indigent patients. Hospital care was based on a two-class system as far as site of care and overlapping with the private sector were concerned. The public general hospital provided space for spillover indigent patients from the voluntary hospitals and a buttress against the mainstream of hospital services.

TABLE 9.4   Distribution of Hospitals and Beds by Type of Hospital, 1930

Type of Hospital	Hospitals		Beds	
	Number	Percent	Number	Percent
General	5,643	84	452,010	47
Mental	561	8	437,919	46
Tuberculosis	515	8	65,940	7
Total	6,719	100	955,869	100

Indeed, a two-class hospital system based on ability to pay was necessary because there was no voluntary health insurance to speak of and voluntary hospitals could afford to provide only a modicum of free care. Government subsidy was niggardly at best and below the actual cost of the voluntary hospital's daily expenses. Public general hospitals, then, became a relatively self-contained system. Conventional wisdom has it that the technical quality of care was equal in both systems, but that amenities were not.

Systematic data on use and expenditures were being collected during this period, but they were not published until 1946. In effect, this imposing health services delivery infrastructure had been erected without any knowledge of how much it would cost, how much it would be used, or how much it would be needed. Not until after it had come into being were there any data, or any interest in data, on how it was performing. Simply knowing that it was performing at all was sufficient evidence·that it was useful and wanted.

The federal government began to produce systematic data on expenditures by service component and source of funding annually in 1946, retrospective to 1929. The total expenditures are broken down in Table 9.5.

Spending was at its height at the end of the twenties; by 1933, as the Depression deepened, it had dropped off considerably, by about one-third. Expenditures reached a low of just under $2 billion in 1933, picking up thereafter. At the same time, total health expenditures as a percent of the GNP increased about 15 percent, indicating a shrinking economy but not proportionately shrinking health services. Private expenditures decreased somewhat, relative to public expenditures. In fact, public expenditures increased absolutely. Apparently, government had to pick up the slack left by the weakening private sector.

During the late twenties and early thirties, according to CCMC studies, 40 percent of the population saw a physician at least once during a year, and 7 percent underwent surgery. The rate of admission to hospitals was 59 per 1,000 population; the number of days per 1,000

TABLE 9.5   Expenditures on Health Care, 1929 and 1935

Expenditures	1929	1935
Total	$3.6 billion	$2.8 billion
Per capita	$29.16	$22.04
Private	87%	81%
Public	13%	19%
As percent of GNP	3.5%	4.1%

was about 1,300. Forty-four percent of maternity cases were hospitalized. Twenty-six percent of the population consulted a dentist. These data are essentially pre-Depression figures; data on national utilization were not available again until 1952. Visits to physicians most likely dropped, as did hospital admissions.

These data show that personal health services had become a tremendous private and public enterprise, already consuming 3 to 4 percent of the GNP and 3 percent of the average family income. As for equity, there was an expected and large disparity among income groups: the lower the income, the lower the use of physicians' services. Hospital use was higher among groups making less than $1,200 a year than among those immediately above them, particularly in cities. The disparity between low and high incomes was greater for dentists' services than for any other component of health care.

HEALTH INSURANCE REVIVED

The problem of increasingly expensive episodes of illness would not go away, but it was submerged as a potential political issue by unemployment and increasing destitution. The extent to which interest in health insurance was rekindled by the Great Depression is, therefore, a moot question. Undoubtedly, deep concern with the problem of income security in general led to emphasis on unemployment compensation, old-age insurance, old-age assistance (relief), and many other measures to protect a family's earning power. Costs of personal health services could also threaten family solvency. State and local governments were deeply involved in seeking to relieve the distress of the unemployed through cash relief and work relief. By 1932, however, state and local governments turned to the federal government for assistance; they were going bankrupt. Thus, early appropriations for the alleviation of economic distress were viewed as short-term remedies, although there was a growing realization that some deficiencies were inherent in the economic system. Booms and depressions were among them, but their effects could at least be moderated by income maintenance programs. Such were the considerations that laid the groundwork for long-range legislation to cushion loss of jobs and income.

In 1934, President Franklin D. Roosevelt appointed the Committee on Economic Security to investigate income security and recommend legislation for a program "against misfortunes which cannot be wholly eliminated in this man-made world of ours." One of the issues to be considered by the committee was the problem of personal health services. The committee was composed of selected members of the President's official family.*

Numerous other sections were established to advise the Committee on Economic Security. Throughout these sections were scattered many of the persons who had been involved with the majority and minority reports of the CCMC. Particularly important was the Medical Advisory Committee, which was charged with considering health insurance. Edwin E. Witte, professor of economics at the University of Wisconsin, Madison, was appointed director of the technical staff reporting to the Committee on Economic Security. Witte reported that there was a great deal of pulling and hauling in setting up the Medical Advisory Committee so that it would represent various opinions, interest groups, and geographic areas.[1] Other important advisory committees concerned with health, although not necessarily directly with health insurance, were drawn from the fields of public health, hospitals, dentistry, and nursing.

The technical staff concerned with health insurance was drawn logically enough from the staff of the CCMC which had finished its mission only two years before.† Other staff members were involved in unemployment compensation, old-age pensions, unemployment relief, and related problems. Two staff members of the health insurance section, Edgar Sydenstricker and I. S. Falk, figured prominently in the deliberations to come.

Sydenstricker was the scientific director of the Milbank Memorial Fund, New York City, and had been active in health insurance since

---

*Frances Perkins, Secretary of Labor, chair; Henry Morgenthau, Jr., Secretary of the Treasury; Henry A. Wallace, Secretary of Agriculture; Homer Cummings, Attorney General; and Harry L. Hopkins, Federal Emergency Relief Administration.

†The health insurance staff had as consultants W. Frank Walker, director, Division of Health Studies, Commonwealth Fund, New York City; Ira V. Hiscock, professor of public health, School of Medicine, Yale University; Michael M. Davis, Director of Medical Services, Julius Rosenwald Fund, Chicago (a former member of CCMC); R. G. Leland, and A. M. Simons, Bureau of Medical Economics, AMA; George St. J. Perrot, U.S. Public Health Service; Maurice Leven, Brookings Institution, Washington, D.C. (on the technical staff of CCMC).

1916. Before joining Milbank, he had been in the Public Health Service and had pioneered in studies of morbidity in the population and the use of health services and expenditures. He had been a member of the CCMC and submitted a statement as an individual protesting the shortcomings of all recommendations. I. S. Falk, Sydenstricker's associate at the Milbank Memorial Fund, had been associate director of the study for the CCMC and was senior author of report No. 26, the household survey.

The investigation of policy problems regarding health insurance did not get far. Witte reported that President Roosevelt was not interested in health insurance at that time, being more concerned with income transfer programs such as unemployment compensation and old-age pensions. Further, the members of the section on Insurance gave health insurance a low priority. Public health measures dealing with maternal and child health programs, aid to the blind, and aid to crippled children were given higher priority. They were noncontroversial and were supported by many groups, including the AMA. Such health programs became Title V of the Social Security Act. The maternal and child health program was actually a reactivation of the Sheppard-Turner Act, which had been in effect from 1922 to 1929.

Witte reported that the mention of health insurance in the Social Security Bill was meant only as a recommendation that the problem be studied. No legislation was proposed. Health insurance received only brief mention in the report of the Committee on Economic Security, even though the committee had had to devote a great deal of attention to the controversial subject. The *Journal of the American Medical Association* indicated in an editorial the considerable concern felt in medical circles:

> The headquarters office of the American Medical Association has been besieged with telephone calls, telegrams, and letters on this subject. . . . Some physicians are apparently opposed to all change and feel that the American Medical Association should officially make itself felt in opposition to the entire program of the government.[2]

It became evident, however, that health insurance would not be part of the Social Security Act. The Committee on Economic Security in its report to the President on January 15, 1935, wrote:

> We are not prepared at this time to make recommendations for a system of health insurance. We have enlisted the cooperation of advising groups representing the medical and dental professions and hospital management in the development of a plan for health insurance which will be beneficial alike to the public and the professions concerned. We have

asked these groups to complete their work by March 1, 1935, and expect to make a further report on this subject at that time or shortly thereafter.[3]

This bland statement belies Witte's revelation later that health insurance was so controversial that even research on it could not be proposed, much less legislation. The purpose of research is to enlighten in the hope of leading to rational recommendations for policy. The question is, Whose rationality? The CCMC's findings were assumed to flow from research, and they resulted in controversial and conflicting recommendations. Political solutions rely more on consensus than on facts— consensus on the nature of the solutions, rather than the self-evident nature of the facts. Witte remarked:

> When in 1934 the Committee on Economic Security announced that it was studying health insurance, it was at once subject to misrepresentation and vilification. In the original social security bill there was one line to the effect that the Social Security Board should study the problem and make a report therein to Congress. That little line was responsible for so many telegrams to the Members of Congress that the entire Ways and Means Committee unanimously struck it out of the bill.[4]

In February 1935, the AMA held a special session to discuss the future of government health insurance in the context of the emerging Social Security Act. At this meeting, the AMA's stand in opposition to government-sponsored health insurance was reaffirmed. There was just enough suspicion of the Committee on Economic Security to question its good faith that health insurance legislation was not actively being considered. The AMA pointed to the committee's preliminary report to Congress on January 17, 1935, in which 11 principles were regarded by the AMA as laying the basis for a plan for government-sponsored health insurance.[5]

In any case, the Social Security Act was passed in August 1935 with no reference to health insurance. The health measures it did embody supported noncontroversial public health programs, particularly maternal and infant welfare. Nevertheless, health insurance as an issue would not go away. Many regarded it as the missing spoke in the wheel of social insurance. As a subject for continued study, health insurance fell under the Social Security Board's charge to study and recommend:

> ... the most effective methods of finding economic security through social insurance, and as legislation and matters of administrative policy concerning old age pensions, unemployment compensation, accident compensation and related subjects.[6]

Originally, the last three words "and related subjects" had been preceded by "health insurance." As an example of the incremental nature of policy making in this country, the board established the Bureau of Research and Statistics to study these many social insurance subjects. I. S. Falk, whose major interests were health insurance, became assistant director and later director, and Margaret C. Klem was given charge of a division of medical economics within the bureau. Both Falk and Klem had been on the technical staff of the CCMC studies. As a result, the Bureau of Research and Statistics conducted many studies in the "related subject" of health services and health insurance, and the subject continued to be controversial, even for study.

The formulation and passage in 1935 of the Social Security Act, and the social insurance framework it established for continued political discussion of income transfer problems, pointed to health insurance as unfinished business. Also, the CCMC report had achieved wide publicity, particularly among provider interest groups and government, and had established a climate of debate on health insurance alternatives—voluntary or compulsory. Proposed legislation for some form of compulsory health insurance was not long in coming. The interest in further research on illness and use of services continued after the CCMC recommendations had been published, indicating Americans' insatiable appetite for information and facts whether they result in action or not.

During the winter of 1935–36, for example, the PHS launched a large household survey of the incidence of illness and related social and economic factors. Known as the National Health Survey, it gathered data in interviews with more than 700,000 householders in urban areas and 37,000 householders in rural areas.[7] It was widely supposed that the National Health Survey was prompted in part to give unemployed white collar workers jobs as part of the Works Progress Administration (WPA). Whatever the reason for it, it was the most extensive morbidity survey ever made up to that time. In fact, the combined results of the CCMC studies and the National Health Survey of 1935–36 provided the basic data on health and medical care in the United States until the early 1950s. They were used to justify the need for health insurance by showing that the use of services fell far short of the need, as revealed by sick persons not attended by physicians.

After the passage of the Social Security Act, the President appointed an Interdepartmental Committee to Coordinate Health and Welfare activities. This committee was composed of experts in various aspects of health and welfare in the federal government and was set up to assure that the provisions of the Social Security Act were being carried out and to suggest improvements. The Technical Committee on Medical Care, consisting chiefly of personnel from federal agencies concerned with health problems, was created in 1937.* The Social Security Act and the New Deal had created civil service jobs for people who were experts in health insurance, medical care, and public health; many of them, particularly Falk, were sympathetic to expanding the act to include health insurance. The Technical Committee was charged with reviewing the health service activities of the federal government and recommending actions toward a national health program.

As the deliberations of the Technical Committee progressed, its members became increasingly bold about two aspects of the national health picture:

> First, that existing services for the conservation of national health are inadequate to secure to the citizens of the United States such health of body and mind as they should have; and second, that nothing less than a national comprehensive health program can lay the basis for action adequate to the nation's need.[8]

The relationship between the health of the citizens and a comprehensive health program was assumed to be reasonable and direct at that time.

The Technical Committee submitted early in 1938 very broad recommendations for expanding the public health services dealing with specific diseases and maternal and child health, which had essentially been mandated already by Title V of the Social Security Act. It further recommended that hospital facilities be expanded through government subsidy; that experiments be made in health service programs for the needy; that insurance be provided against the loss of wages because of illness; and that, as part of this total package, "a general program of medical care" be established.

Thereupon, the President instructed the chair of the Interdepartmental Committee to consider the desirability of inviting representatives of the public and the health professions to discuss ways of dealing with the recommendations presented by the Technical Committee. The result was the first National Health Conference held in this country, in Washington, D.C., July 18–20, 1938. A review of the roster reveals that the 176 people who attended the conference figured prominently in health and welfare activities and represented the full range of opinion and expert knowledge in this country. The conferees were not expected

---

*The members were Martha M. Eliot, Children's Bureau, chair; I. S. Falk, Social Security Board; and Joseph W. Mountin, George St. J. Perrott, and Clifford E. Waller, all of the Public Health Service.

to endorse the recommendations of the Technical Committee; their function was to clarify issues and stimulate criticism, presumably constructive criticism. Clearly, the federal bureaucracy was taking the lead in promoting discussion of a national health program.

Considering the political composition of the Congress and the euphoria surrounding the New Deal, it probably was no coincidence that in 1939, the year after the National Health Conference, the first of a seemingly endless string of health insurance bills was introduced in Congress. The first, which aroused a great deal of interest, was proposed by Senator Robert F. Wagner of New York (S. 1920). It was followed by the Capper bill in 1941 (S. 489), the Eliot bill in 1942 (H.R. 7354), and the Wagner-Murray-Dingell bill in 1945 (S. 1606). There were no substantive differences among these bills; they were all to be federally initiated with state participation. The intent was to take the burden of high-cost illness off the backs of the people. No direct reorganization of the existing delivery system was envisioned. The major issue at that time was a profoundly ideological one—the appropriateness of the government's using payroll deductions or taxation, or both, to pay for health services for everyone versus voluntary enrollment in health insurance plans.

Two related bills were introduced in 1945: the Pepper bill (S. 1318), to expand maternal and child health programs, and the Hill-Burton bill, to assist in the federal financing of hospital and medical facilities in the states. The Hill-Burton bill, officially known as the Hospital Survey and Construction Act, was passed in 1946 with broad support and endorsement of the AMA. It represented public policy adapted to traditional social and political values, and was the first instance of planning for hospital facilities.[9] The hospitals, particularly the voluntary hospitals, were running short of capital funds as the traditional sources of philanthropy and community fund drives were drying up. Also, people who lived in rural areas were clamoring for more hospitals. The act was designed to be a one-shot subsidy for hospital expansion and renovation based on state-by-state inventory of existing facilities. The subsidy was to be matched by the hospitals and the states. No operating expenses were permitted. Thus, government involvement was temporary and salutary; the subsidy stimulated the flow of matching funds so that, on average, the federal government contributed only one-quarter of all capital expenditures over the years.

To illustrate the incremental approach of the American political system, Wilbur Cohen (who later helped draft Medicare and became Secretary of HEW under President Lyndon Johnson) relates that when he was a young staff person in Washington in 1943 he and Falk helped to draft the Wagner-Murray-Dingell bill of 1943:

I delivered the omnibus measure to Senator Robert F. Wagner, with the draft of what I thought was a brilliant speech for his introduction of the bill to the Senate. I had enthusiastically and wholeheartedly devoted hours to participating in the social policy incorporated into this monumental and historic leviathan of public policy—a bold and innovative combination of creative ideals which came second only to Thomas Jefferson's imaginative proposals incorporated in the Declaration of Independence.

Then Senator Wagner and I sat around his office discussing trivialities for about an hour. When in my youthful impatience I asked the Senator if he was going to look at the bill or draft statement or if he wished to discuss any policy options with me he said, "No, it would take a number of years before the bill would even be enacted—it would be redrafted innumerable times, and his role was to introduce it so that future members of Congress could carry it forward to realization long after he was gone."[10]

By far the most vociferous and visible opponent of the string of health insurance bills introduced between 1939 and 1949 was the AMA. Its methods of opposition went beyond rhetoric and stretched the bounds of good taste and credibility. After the Wagner Act of 1939 was introduced, an agency called the National Physicians' Committee for the Extension of Medical Services was set up. The AMA denied any official connection with it, but it was headed by a physician. This organization distributed 25 million propaganda leaflets, some featuring a copy of the classic painting of a devoted physician sitting at the bedside of a sick child with the caption: "Do you want the Government in this picture?" The National Physicians' Committee was superseded in 1949 by the California public relations firm of Whitaker and Baxter, which had waged a successful attack on Governor Earl Warren's health insurance bill. Physicians were asked to contribute $25 each toward a war chest of $3.5 million. The propaganda excesses continued, but only for a short time after Truman left office; Eisenhower's presidency created a calmer political atmosphere.[11] The government, through the proposed health insurance legislation, was then attempting to reduce the cost of health services to nothing in order to stimulate the supply of hospitals and beds and to improve geographic access to beds.

In 1947, three health-related bills were in the congressional hopper. One, sponsored by Senator Robert A. Taft, would assist states in providing medical care for the indigent (S. 545). A second, introduced by Senators Robert F. Wagner and James E. Murray (and others as the concept gained in political popularity), spelled out a comprehensive health insurance system for the general population (S. 1320), and the third (S. 1714) dealt with maternal and child health. Hearings were held on only two of the health insurance bills, the Wagner bill of 1939 (S.

1620) and the Wagner-Murray-Dingell bill of 1945 (S. 1606). Many and varied witnesses testified for or against the bills.

Their views were usually predictable, depending on whom they represented—organized labor, organized medicine, business and industry, other providers, or citizens' groups.

Recommendations for a national health program were made by both Presidents Roosevelt and Truman. The White House, the PHS, and the Social Security Administration showed intensifying interest in a broad national health program. In 1939, President Roosevelt recommended to Congress that the report of the Interdepartmental Committee and the Technical Committee be studied carefully. In his message to Congress in 1941 he said, "We should widen the opportunities for adequate medical care."

In 1942, as an incremental gesture, the President recommended that permanent and temporary disability payments and payments for hospitalization be established as an expansion of the Social Security Act. The Social Security Act was regarded as the basic vehicle for national health insurance in the United States largely because of its tremendous taxing potential through payroll deductions. In his message in 1943, President Roosevelt repeated his previous recommendations for adequate medical care and protection from the "economic fears of old age, sickness, accident, and unemployment."

The next presidential pronouncement on this subject came in 1946 from Harry Truman, who forcefully, as was his style, recommended compulsory health insurance and ways in which to carry it out. This was the first instance in the history of the United States of a chief executive's making such a recommendation. President Truman repeated this recommendation until the end of his term in 1952. In fact, he felt that his inability to establish a compulsory health insurance program was one of his unfinished tasks as President.[12] It should be noted that not one of the national health insurance proposals reached the floor of Congress for debate. After 1935, activity for government-sponsored health insurance on the federal level became dominant over action on the state level. By 1940, action had moved to the national level, with the Social Security Act as the framework. There was consensus by then that the federal government should take the lead in health and welfare matters, in cooperation with the states. This leadership took the form of grants-in-aid to the states and was carried out with a high degree of refinement. The Supreme Court declaration that the general intent of the Social Security Act was constitutional provided legitimacy for this shift to the federal government.

The federal government, because of its enormous taxing power, was in a position to return money to the states—if the states met certain minimum standards. States were not compelled to join in unemployment insurance or the categorical assistance programs, such as the grants-in-aid for special public health activities, but if they did not, they would not recover money paid by their citizens in federal taxes. The Old Age, Survivors, and Disability Insurance program (OASDI), however, was and is completely administered by the federal government through the Social Security Administration and its regional offices. Old-age insurance was considered a national problem because of the mobility of the population. Other programs came under federal influence in order to narrow the gap between low- and high-income states and to establish a national health and welfare policy.

Although the main action was taking place in Washington, there was some activity on the state level. From 1939 to about 1950, government-sponsored health insurance bills were introduced in 12 states concurrently with federal legislation.[13] In California, such legislation had the personal support of Governor Warren, and the battle was an extremely bitter one. Warren had had the bill drawn up by Nathan Sinai, professor of public health at the University of Michigan and a former member of the CCMC technical staff. None of the state bills ever reached the floors of the legislatures for debate, not to mention passage.

While universal health insurance was being debated, the federal government was being forced into providing health services for special groups who had suffered unduly from the unemployment and destitution caused by the Great Depression. In 1933, when state and local governments were no longer able to carry the mounting relief load, the federal government, at the risk of bankruptcy, established the Federal Emergency Relief Administration (FERA) to assist the states with unemployment relief through grants-in-aid. In June 1933, the program was expanded to provide at least minimal health services for those receiving unemployment relief.

Rules and Regulations No. 7[14] of FERA was unprecedented in that under it the federal government helped states pay for physicians' services for persons receiving public assistance. Hospitals were supposed to carry out their traditional charitable functions without federal assistance. The rules were expressed in general terms in order to permit states to formulate policies appropriate for local conditions, and they varied considerably, both between and within states. Representatives of the AMA participated in the formulation of rules and regulations. Official state and local relief agencies entered into agreements with medical societies and individual physicians for services to persons receiving unemployment relief. One of the rules was that patients had free choice of physicians. Physicians were now receiving federal money for treating low-income patients.

The FERA program was short-lived, coming to an end in late 1935, the year in which the emergency relief program was changed to a permanent public assistance program as part of the Social Security Act. Although the FERA program did not last long, one observer felt that it had a long-term influence:

> Probably the most valuable contribution . . . was the public awareness which it created of health needs and of the inadequacy of existing facilities, especially in rural areas. The scarcity of physicians in sparsely settled regions, the absence of clinics, of hospitals, of sanitariums and of facilities for convalescent care became matters of general knowledge and concern.[15]

Another medical program that was a direct result of the Depression was the one designed for low-income farmers by the Farm Security Administration (FSA) in the Department of Agriculture. Prominent in its administration were Frederick Mott and Milton Roemer, both career physicians in the Public Health Service. Mott and Roemer were part of the corps of PHS physicians anticipating and supporting some form of national health insurance. Although no such insurance was enacted, these physicians contributed greatly to the development of prepaid group practices. Mott played a tremendous role in the implementation of the universal hospital insurance plan established in the Province of Saskatchewan in 1947.

The FSA's medical program is reported to have originated because many low-income farmers had defaulted on their FSA loans. Many such defaults were blamed on the low health status of the economically marginal farmers, whose poor health was believed to have decreased their productivity. By 1944, the medical program was operating in about 1,000 counties in 39 states. The program came to an end in July 1946, when Congress refused to continue appropriations.

Another special program inaugurated during World War II served the wives and dependents of men in the armed forces. It was called the Emergency Maternity and Infant Care program (EMIC). It was administered by the Children's Bureau through state health departments and was financed entirely by the federal government through special appropriations from Congress. The wives of men in the lowest pay grades were provided antepartum, obstetrical, and postpartum care by the physicians and hospitals of their choice. By the time its total commitments had been fulfilled, the EMIC program had paid for the care of over 1.2 million maternity patients, an expenditure of about $130 million. The program was abolished on July 1, 1947, having served its wartime purpose.[16] The EMIC program highlighted the difficulty of determining appropriate methods and amounts of payment for physicians and hospitals under contract to a government agency. This is a seemingly mundane problem, but it continues to be a major technical one between providers and third party payers.

Still another program connected with the military is the provision of hospital and physicians' services for veterans with service-related disabilities. Hospital care for veterans came into being shortly after World War I. At first the federal government contracted for services with voluntary hospitals, but in time over 175 hospitals exclusively for veterans were built and maintained throughout the country by the Veterans Administration (VA). Although up to 1950 the VA hospitals accounted for only 5 percent of total expenditures for health services, they nevertheless have been a visible portion of total federal expenditures for health services.

From early on, the VA program has been untouchable politically. It has been controversial among physicians, however, not because of its intent, but because of its administration. The original and continuing intent of Congress was to provide medical care for veterans whose illness or disability resulted from military service. Frequently, of course, it is difficult to differentiate between service-related and nonservice-related disabilities: a person's medical history cannot be split up that easily. Consequently whenever there is reasonable doubt, decisions tend to be made in favor of the veteran. The difficulty of administration is compounded by the proviso that, even if a disability is not service-related, the veteran can receive free care by declaring his inability to pay for care elsewhere. There was no stigma attached to receiving VA care, but it was very demeaning to declare oneself indigent.

NOTES

1. Edwin E. Witte, *The Development of the Social Security Act* (Madison: University of Wisconsin Press, 1962).
2. Editorial, *Journal of the American Medical Association* 103 (24 November 1934):1627.
3. Committee on Economic Security, *Report to the President* (Washington, D.C.: Government Printing Office, 1935), p. 6.
4. Interdepartmental Committee to Coordinate Health and Welfare Activities, *The Nation's Health* (Washington, D.C.: Government Printing Office, 1939), p. 103.
5. *Journal of the American Medical Association* 104 (2 March 1935):751.
6. Social Security Act, Title XII, Sec. 702.
7. George St. J. Perrott and Clark Tibbitts, "The National Health Survey," *Public Health Reports* 54 (15 September 1939):1663.
8. Interdepartmental Committee, *Nation's Health*, p. 12.
9. See the sympathetic evaluation by Judith R. Lave and Lester B. Lave, *The*

Hospital Construction Act: An Evaluation of the Hill-Burton Program, 1948–1973 (Washington, D.C.: American Enterprise Institute for Public Policy Research, 1974).

10. Wilbur Cohen, "From Medicare to National Health Insurance," *Toward New Human Rights: The Social Policies of the Kennedy and Johnson Administrations,* ed. David C. Warner (Austin, Texas: Lyndon B. Johnson School of Public Affairs, 1977), p. 144. See also Daniel T. Hirshfield, *The Lost Reform: The Campaign for Compulsory Health Insurance in the U.S. from 1932 to 1943* (Cambridge, Mass.: Harvard University Press, 1970).

11. See details in "The American Medical Association: Power, Purpose and Politics in Organized Medicine," *Yale Law Journal* 63 (May 1954):938–1022, particularly pp. 1077–78.

12. "The Truman Memoirs," *Life* 40 (23 January 1956):104. See also Monte M. Poen, *Harry S. Truman Versus the Medical Lobby: The Genesis of Medicare* (Columbia: University of Missouri Press, 1979).

13. Adela Stucke, "Note on Compulsory Sickness Insurance Legislation in the States, 1939–1944," *Public Health Reports* 60 (28 December 1945):1551–64; "Compulsory Health Insurance Laws Introduced in Various States," *Tic,* 1 June 1944, pp. 2–7 (published by Ticonium Laboratory, Albany, N.Y.).

14. U.S. Federal Emergency Relief Administration, Rules and Regulations No. 7, *Government Medical Care Provided in the Home to Recipients of Unemployment Relief* (Washington, D.C.: Government Printing Office, 1933).

15. Josephine C. Brown, *Public Relief, 1929–1939* (New York: Holt, 1940), p. 257.

16. A full description of the origin and operation of the EMIC program is found in Nathan Sinai and Odin W. Anderson, *E.M.I.C., A Study of Administrative Experience,* Bureau of Health Economics Research Series No.3 (Ann Arbor: School of Public Health, University of Michigan, 1948).

10

The Rise of Voluntary Health Insurance: The Self-Help Answer to the Issue of Equity

The Blue Cross hospital plans and the Blue Shield medical plans emerged in the thirties. Early Blue Cross plans were initiated a few years before compulsory national health insurance legislation was being promoted in Congress. Blue Shield plans, sponsored by some state and county medical societies, were set up in response to both the Blue Cross plans, in order to forestall being absorbed by hospital insurance, and compulsory health insurance.

The first major Blue Cross plans were established to help both the self-reliant patient who had little money and the hospitals, whose incomes were falling drastically. J. Douglas Colman, a reliable and interested observer and a prime mover in the Blue Cross plan in Baltimore, had this to say 30 years later:

> One of the canards I'd like to demolish, if I could, is that the people who brought Blue Cross into being did it to keep hospitals out of the red. Those who were involved in the early days were concerned with the ability of people to avail themselves of hospital service. As a matter of fact, the boards of trustees of hospitals worried about the liabilities they might be incurring for their hospitals in Blue Cross, because in almost every state the hospitals had to guarantee the delivery of service. The concern of the trustees was not to solve the financial problems of the hospitals, but whether or not they dare take on that additional problem.[1]

As for Blue Shield plans, it is doubtful that they were established to alleviate physicians' cash flow problems or patients' problems in

125

paying for service. For voluntary hospitals and physicians alike, the establishment of hospitals and medical prepayment plans manifested their desire to maintain control over their own destinies as providers, a characteristic desire of all institutions. It also filled a clear public need, as revealed by the CCMC studies, for some form of insurance to help pay for the unpredictable and occasionally high costs of personal health services. The hospital prepayment plans were promoted aggressively by hospital sponsors and administrators and were sanctioned by the AHA. The medical plans, however, were simply offered to the public rather than aggressively promoted, and they were never officially sanctioned by the AMA. Physicians' activities were mainly on the level of the state and county medical societies.

If the voluntary, nonprofit community hospital had not been the backbone of the hospital delivery system in the United States, Blue Cross would not have been invented. Further, if the private practice of medicine, linked to the voluntary hospitals, had not been the backbone of the medical delivery system, Blue Shield would not have followed. The sequence was inevitable. American hospitals and physicians have an entrepreneurial ethos that reflects the prevailing business ethos, and the social and political environments support it. The Blue Cross and Blue Shield pioneers were part and parcel of a lively middle-class entrepreneurial culture.[2] As observed by Wiebe:

> In part, the new middle class was a class only by courtesy of the historians' afterthought. Covering too wide a range to form a tightly knit group, it divided into two main categories. One included those with strong professional aspirations in such fields as medicine, law, economics, administration, social work, and architecture. The second comprised specialists in business, labor, and in agriculture awakening both to their distinctiveness and to their ties with similar people in the same occupation. In fact, consciousness of unique skills and functions, an awareness that came to mold much of their lives, characterized all members of the class. They demonstrated it by a proud identification as lawyers or teachers, by a determination to improve the contents of medicine or the procedures of a particular business, and by an eagerness to join others like themselves in a craft union, professional organization, trade association or agricultural cooperative.[3]

In the late 1920s and early 1930s, a man in Essex County, New Jersey, one in Chicago, one in St. Paul, and still another in Cleveland were independently pondering some form of prepayment for hospital care that would involve all the hospitals in the community. The man in New Jersey, son of a feed and grain dealer, was Frank Van Dyke, a promoter-salesman with a high school education. The man in Chicago, C. Rufus Rorem, son of a small-town merchant and farm owner in Iowa, was a certified public accountant with a Ph.D. in economics from the University of Chicago. Rorem was a scholar and theorist with a drive for application. The man in St. Paul, E. A. Van Steenwyk, son of a harness- and shoemaker, also came from a small town in Iowa. He had a teacher's certificate from Mankato State Teachers College in Minnesota and had attended the University of Minnesota for one year. Van Steenwyk was a practical dreamer. John Mannix, from Cleveland, was born into an Irish immigrant family that had experienced a great deal of illness. He had a high school education and was a self-taught hospital accountant with a flair for large-scale action. The fusion of these men, with their variety of talents and similar aims, resulted in a movement.

At the beginning of the thirties, these men were between 30 and 36 years of age. They embodied the virtues of hard work, enlightened self-interest, enthusiasm, pragmatism, and, in their view, dedication to the public interest. They were clearly products of the stratum of society described by Wiebe. They were basically Calvinist in outlook, even though Mannix was a Roman Catholic and Rorem a Quaker.

When Rorem became an assistant professor of accounting in the School of Business at the University of Chicago in 1928, he met Michael M. Davis, previously mentioned in connection with CCMC studies, who had a long-time interest in health insurance. Davis was Rorem's senior by 15 years and was then on the staff of the Julius Rosenwald Fund, a Chicago-based foundation established by Rosenwald of Sears, Roebuck, and Company. The Fund was designed to support activities that would help people to help themselves, for example by giving grants for higher education for blacks. Davis was in charge of the Fund's Division of Medical Economics and was looking for someone to study capital investment in hospitals. He was also active at the time in getting the CCMC started. Rorem accepted the assignment because, as he said some 40 years later, "From my point of view, we had picked the key point where all the conflicts and the changes were going to come."[4] The study of capital investments in hospitals sponsored by the CCMC became a landmark study.[5]

By the end of 1935, 15 Blue Cross plans had been established in 11 states, and by 1936, six more had been started. At the same time, there was a move to create a coordinating agency to give the now rapidly growing movement a national focus and a broad base. As luck would have it, the Rosenwald Fund had decided to eliminate its Division of Medical Economics, partly because, according to Rorem, it had become too controversial. Davis had known Julius Rosenwald since 1915, and had become a friend of his son Lessing. A settlement was made in 1936 between Davis and Rorem on the one hand and Lessing Rosenwald on the other. Davis and Rorem were each given custody of a substantial amount of money for those days, $175,000 and $100,000, respectively, for four years. Rorem later received an extension for a year and an additional $25,000. The conditions were that the money be spent in the field of medical care and that a nonprofit agency be found to which the Rosenwald Fund could legally grant the money. Davis set up his own agency, known as the Committee for Research in Medical Economics, which was concerned with research into and promotion of national health insurance. Rorem took the voluntary, nonprofit route and sought an agency through which he could promote hospital prepayment and uniform accounting as a tool of hospital administration. Davis and Rorem were not necessarily at odds regarding the future sponsorship of health insurance in the United States: Davis saw voluntary health insurance as a stage leading to some form of national health insurance; Rorem, however, was willing to give the private, nonprofit sector a try, hoping it would succeed.[6] It is in the best tradition of philanthropic foundations to fund two people with similar objectives but divergent means of obtaining them.

After consulting with two agencies that might qualify to administer his nest egg, Rorem sought the help of the AHA. He reports that AHA officers quickly accepted his proposal. A body known as the Committee on Hospital Service was created; although established under AHA auspices, the committee operated independently of it. The AHA was a very small, struggling organization at that time, and the Blue Cross movement started outside it. Likewise, Blue Shield was started outside the AMA by maverick physicians. Apparently, professional associations find it difficult to initiate new developments because they might change the status quo.

As for the role of government, Rorem said: "Governments tend to emphasize equity, not efficiency; certainty, not originality. They do not provide the basis for much experiment or innovation, which are natural fields for private enterprise, whether nonprofit or not."[7]

The hospital plans became known as Blue Cross plans shortly after they changed from single- to multihospital systems. Eventually, most of them operated statewide. By 1946, there were Blue Cross plans in 43 states serving 20 million members. From the beginning, the Blue Cross plans were sanctioned in principle by the AHA. In 1937, the AHA established a clearinghouse for the plans in its Chicago office. Known as the Blue Cross Commission, it superseded the Committee on Hospital Services. The commission acted as a central agency for the accumulation of cost and utilization data from member plans. It established standards with which plans complied, and it served as a consultant to the plans.

Blue Cross plans assumed certain characteristics early on in order to blend with the traditions of voluntary hospitals and to differentiate themselves from private insurance companies.

1. They were incorporated as nonprofit organizations and there-fore had no stockholders or profits for individuals.
2. Their boards of directors represented hospitals, physicians, and the general public and were self-perpetuating.
3. They were usually supervised by state insurance commissions.
4. As nonprofit corporations, they held low cash reserves (hospitals were assumed to guarantee a reserve of service instead of cash).
5. They emphasized hospital benefits in the form of service rather than in cash indemnity.
6. They placed all employees on salary and offered no commission to sales personnel.

Thus, Blue Cross plans declared that they were not commercial organizations competing in the open market, but organizations attempting to provide a service to the public at cost and to generate a surplus sufficient to cover their cost of operation. Blue Cross drew over itself the service mantle of the voluntary hospital. This was not an easy task, since hospital insurance can be sold only to those who are willing and able to buy it, whereas hospital care is traditionally provided to all who have need of it.

Action comparable to that of the state hospital associations was also taken by state medical societies and a few of the larger county medical societies. As early as 1932, the Michigan State Medical Society initiated a series of studies on medical care.[8] A report was prepared by Nathan Sinai, then on the technical staff of the CCMC and in the School of Public Health at the University of Michigan. The California, Michigan, and Pennsylvania medical societies established the first state medical society-sponsored plans in 1939. There was, however, another plan already underway in Tacoma, Washington, under the sponsorship of the Pierce County Medical Society; its purpose was to counteract the growth of contract medical practice for employed groups under the aegis of various industries, particularly the lumber industry. Eventually, 23 county societies in Washington established such plans, offering free choice of physician, fee-for-service payment, and physicians' services in and out of the hospital. They set up a surveillance mechanism to flush out unusual practices. These plans went curiously and unjustifiably ignored by the physician-sponsored plans that emerged later, because they offered home and office calls. The later plans limited their benefits mainly to in-hospital physician services. The state of Washington showed that out-of-hospital physicians' services could be insured, but medical societies in other states could not believe the evidence.

By the end of the 1950s, medical society-sponsored plans, which became known as Blue Shield plans to show their relationship to Blue Cross, were in operation in all states and accounted for almost one-half of the coverage of physicians' services. The chief characteristics of the medical society-sponsored plans were:

1. They were incorporated as nonprofit corporations.

2. Their boards of directors were comprised mostly of physicians.

3. They offered benefits either in the form of services or cash indemnity. The service benefit was usually limited to persons under certain incomes.

4. They favored cash reserves but assumed that participating physicians would be a service reserve analogous to the Blue Cross concept for hospitals.

5. They offered free choice of physician and assumed that the great majority of physicians would participate.

In 1946, the Blue Shield plans established a national federation similar to the original Blue Cross Commission called the Associated Medical Care Plans, Inc. (It was later superseded by the National Association of Blue Shield Plans.) Revealing ambivalence about setting up their own plans and encouraging adherence to a standard fee schedule, some state medical societies cooperated with private insurance companies to underwrite and administer health insurance. Physicians did not have contracts with the insurance companies, thus their traditional financial relationship with patients remained intact.

Incorporating Blue Cross and Blue Shield plans as nonprofit entities posed problems. Were the plans insurance? If so, were they required to incorporate under state insurance laws dealing with stock and mutual insurance companies and to be supervised by the state departments of insurance? Were they to be defined as a special type of insurance and supervised by the departments of insurance? Or were they to be incorporated under state laws relating to nonprofit corporations and to be supervised by a state agency other than the department of insurance?[9]

To resolve these questions, the hospital and medical associations asked the state legislatures for special legislation that would enable them to be supervised by state departments of insurance. The state legislatures complied rapidly, revealing their support of the concept.

Classified as a special type of insurance exempt from the usual financial criteria for private insurance companies, the voluntary plans were thus relieved of the obligation to maintain substantial cash reserves and were exempt from taxes. By 1950, almost all the states had passed such enabling legislation.

The enabling legislation gave providers special privileges because of the value of voluntarism. They were legally out of the marketplace, yet they had to "sell" insurance contracts. Hospitals and physicians were permitted to control their financing and organization on the guild pattern; at the same time the public was provided an easier way of paying for services. According to law, then, the hospital and medical society plans were not in the insurance business: they were prepayment agencies, budgeting agencies, yet in effect still insurance agencies because they were involved in pooling risks.

The new legislation also facilitated an extension of the voluntary hospital board concept to hospital insurance plans. The medical profession was drawn into the same orbit in its medical plans and became familiar with the daily operations of insurance. An attempt by the medical societies to control the incorporation and operation of medical care plans was successful in 20 states; laypersons could not set up a plan unless physicians controlled the board of directors. This proscription made it difficult for certain types of group or prepayment plans to get started.

The existence of a voluntary, nonprofit sector in a country so seemingly committed to private and profit-making enterprise is fascinating. One would imagine that there need be only two types of enterprises: the purely profit-making and the purely governmental. Few social scientists have attempted to formulate theories for the existence of the nonprofit sector. In a larger context, Dahl and Lindblom have attempted to do so. In 1953, they set forth a continuum showing the choices available in the United States between government ownership and private enterprise in areas ranging from education to power production.[10]

Specifically, Weisbrod has made the intriguing observation that the nonprofit sector results from both market failure and failure of government to conduct enterprises that are not held strictly accountable to the bottom line or to administrative and financial legalities.[11] He presents a scheme of the great range of enterprises classified as voluntary and nonprofit, from social clubs to Blue Cross plans. Private insurance companies resent the tax-exempt status of Blue Cross and Blue Shield plans because it can constitute a competitive advantage. Nevertheless, the fact that the status has been granted shows the special regard that elected representatives have for the health services.

THE EMERGENCE OF DELIVERY
ALTERNATIVES

The United States is the only country (except, perhaps, for Australia) in which alternative forms of personal health delivery have thrived. Unlike physicians in any other country, American physicians reflect the prevailing culture of entrepreneurship. They can organize, and they are venturesome. As specialization began to occur, physicians in the solo-practice fee-for-service mainstream adjusted by establishing informal referral networks and concentrating their offices in medical arts buildings in the cities. Other physicians created private group practice. These formalized the relationships among participating doctors, incorporating them in order to hire support staff and set up joint financing and accounting. Private clinics charged fees, as did solo practitioners, but the income was divided in a variety of ways among the partners.

An unintended offshoot of private group practice was group practice prepayment, in which a known population is enrolled and participating physicians are salaried. From the standpoint of the mainstream, this mode of delivery was revolutionary. It struck at the heart of solo-practice fee-for-service delivery and to some degree at the free choice of physician. It put a group of physicians in competition with individual physicians, even though the latter participated in Blue Shield plans, which enrolled a known population.

The conflicts and debates about methods of organizing physicians' services took place outside the controversies over government-sponsored health insurance. The group practice recommendations of the CCMC in 1933 were made more or less independently of any endorsement of the insurance principle or sponsorship of particular types of health insurance.

According to Stevens, "after 1918 the idea of group practice began to flower."[12] By 1930, there were about 150 group practices in the United States, involving 1,500 to 2,000 physicians (out of 154,000) and concentrated mainly in the West and Midwest. The typical group practice had up to ten full-time physicians and included at least internal medicine, surgery, and eye, ear, nose, and throat. Only a few included general practitioners, and doctors in the typical group obtained hospital affiliations to admit their patients.

Several private medical groups were established before 1930, possibly overshadowing the small group practice clinics. Their names are household words: May Clinic in Rochester, Minnesota; Crile Clinic in Cleveland, Ohio; Lahey Clinic in Boston; and Ochsner Clinic in New Orleans. Although many medical centers were established in association with medical schools and teaching hospitals, these clinics became training centers in their own right. Their establishment was frequently greeted with hostility from local physicians, who feared competition. Yet this initial hostility apparently had little effect on the success of the clinics, since they became nationally and internationally famous. Private group practice clinics became increasingly a part of the system for delivering physicians' services.

The real conflict between medical societies and innovative physicians came when prepayment was added to group practice. An early and geographically remote battleground that nonetheless received national attention was the clinic and prepayment plan established in 1929 by farmers in Elk City, Oklahoma, under the medical leadership of Michael Shadid. Shadid was a Syrian immigrant who had earned his M.D. at Washington University in St. Louis. Shadid was convinced that the contemporary method of practice was not serving the people adequately, and he made it his mission to have it do so.[13]

Shadid's good intentions and idealism were direct and ingenuous; he was a man who believed that something ought to succeed on its merits. His medical competence seems never to have been questioned, but, when group practice and prepayment were combined, the issues were joined as far as the local medical society was concerned. When Shadid led the establishment of the Community Hospital in Elk City, the hostility he encountered from local physicians was awesome. It is unlikely that this hostility would have been any less intense had he worked quietly, but Shadid's wrath was biblical and aimed at what he considered to be not only medical commercialism, but also poor quality medical care given by local physicians. As a result, he gained much publicity and the sympathy of the governor of Oklahoma when the medical society attempted to deprive him of his license to practice. After years of struggle and near bankruptcy, and with considerable difficulty in hiring staff, Shadid's Elk City Cooperative finally stabilized at a workable level, and the turbulence subsided. In time, physicians on the staff of the cooperative became members in good standing of the county medical society.

A similar situation arose in Los Angeles in the 1930s with the creation of the Ross-Loos clinic, a group practice prepayment plan that was physician-owned and -controlled. Drs. Ross and Loos fought the opposition of the California Medical Association and eventually won without court action. They confined themselves to the adjudication machinery of the state medical society and the AMA.[14]

In 1937, another fight with organized medicine loomed, this time in Washington, D.C., with even more national publicity. The plaintiff was a cooperative group practice plan organized by government employees, the Group Health Association. Members were articulate and educated civil servants who enlisted the services of the U.S. Attorney General versus the medical society of the District of Columbia and the AMA. The medical society and the AMA were indicted under the antitrust act for restraint of trade because staff physicians had been prevented by the local medical society from obtaining admitting privileges in the city's hospitals. The Attorney General ruled that the medical society was restraining trade, although he did not necessarily call the practice of medicine a trade. Naturally, the medical association argued that the antitrust laws were being inappropriately applied to medical practice, which was indisputably a profession. The defendants lost, suffering a small fine, and physicians in the Group Health Association eventually obtained admitting privileges in the city.[15]

With only slight variations, the litigation in Washington, D.C., was repeated in Seattle, San Diego, and elsewhere. The actions in Seattle took place in 1949, when the Group Health Cooperative of Puget Sound brought suit against the King County Medical Bureau, the local medical prepayment plan sponsored and operated by the King County Medical Society. The plan was sued for being party to the exclusion of Group Health physicians from appointments to local hospitals.[16] The King County Medical Bureau lost. In the San Diego case, and for similar reasons, the San Diego Medical Society lost to the Complete Service Bureau.[17]

Probably the most significant confrontation between organized medicine and group practice prepayment plans took place between the Health Insurance Plan of Greater New York (HIP) and the New York County Medical Society. HIP was established in New York City in 1946 with great flourish by Mayor Fiorello La Guardia, who promised this newest and largest group practice prepayment plan contracts for over 250,000 employees, with the city paying one-half of the premium. The plan was run by a prestigious community board, and a philanthropic foundation provided its startup costs. Over 30 group practice units were set up throughout the city's boroughs.

Organized medicine was hostile to HIP: the 1,000 or so physicians practicing in HIP units found it difficult to obtain hospital appointments. The columns of newspapers and local medical journals were soon full of charges and countercharges. The stakes for organized medicine were felt to be exceedingly high, as were the stakes for group practice prepayment plans. HIP had the support of the eminent citizens on its board of directors, and its medical leadership was in the hands of a physician with impeccable clinical credentials, George Baehr.

The complaints of the HIP physicians, spearheaded by physicians in Queens, reached the Judicial Council of the AMA in 1954. The council refused to consider the case on the grounds that it involved alleged unethical conduct—namely, professional participation in a group plan. This refusal was tantamount to the AMA's saying that the Medical Society of Queens did not have a case.[18] As far as the AMA was concerned, the fight with HIP was a local medical society matter, and the prestige of the national organization could not be involved in the adjudication.

Such were the agonies of bringing forth a new method for delivering physicians' services in a country that prides itself on competition and medical associations that espouse initiative and free enterprise.

A major group practice prepayment plan that somehow escaped direct confrontation with medical societies was the Kaiser-Permanente plan, originated by Dr. Sidney Garfield. Kaiser-Permanente may have escaped trouble because it was established during World War II for shipyard workers, who were removed from adequate health services, and it was backed by a big industry, the Kaiser Family Enterprises. The plan also built its own hospitals, thus avoiding the problem of admitting privileges for its physicians. After the war, and with considerable organizational know-how, the Kaiser plan began to expand up and down the West Coast, becoming a significant influence on the medical establishment. Rather than attempting to destroy the Kaiser plans, medical societies began to compete with them, a salutory development more in line with American thought than the previous, fruitless confrontations.

In general, organized medicine does not understand free enterprise and competition. The group practice plans emerged in the private sector of an open economy and used government when necessary to keep the system open, a classic of government function in a liberal-democratic political system. By 1950, the United States had achieved, because of its economic system, delivery alternatives that did not exist anywhere else in the world.

NOTES

1. Report of an interview with J. Douglas Colman when he received the Kimball Award from the American Hospital Association for meritorious service to hospital affairs, *Hospitals*, 39 (16 April, 1965), no. 8, p. 46.
2. A detailed treatment of the development of the Blue Cross plans can be found in Odin W. Anderson, *Blue Cross Since 1929: Accountability and the Public Trust* (Cambridge, Mass.: Ballinger, 1975). A much less sympathetic book is Sylvia A. Law's *Blue Cross: What Went Wrong?* 2d. ed. (New Haven, Conn.: Yale University Press, 1976). Law loved the original idea and its idealism but was disappointed that Blue Cross had not attained what she saw as its social objectives.

3. Robert H. Wiebe, *The Search for Order, 1877–1920* (New York: Hill and Wang, 1967), p. 112.
4. Interview with Rorem, New York City, December 17, 1970.
5. C. Rufus Rorem, *The Public's Investment in Hospitals* (Chicago: University of Chicago Press, 1930).
6. Interview with Michael M. Davis, Chevy Chase, Md., February 7, 1971.
7. Rorem, interview.
8. Michigan State Medical Society, Committee on Survey of Medical Service and Health Agencies, Nathan Sinai, Director, *Report to the House of Delegates* (Lansing: Michigan State Medical Society, 1933).
9. For background, see Odin W. Anderson, *State Enabling Legislation for Non-Profit Hospital and Medical Plans, 1944*, Research Series No. 1 (Ann Arbor: Michigan Public Health Economics, School of Public Health, University of Michigan, 1944).
10. Robert A. Dahl and Charles E. Lindblom, *Politics, Economics, and Welfare* (New York: Harper, 1953), p. 10.
11. Burton A. Weisbrod, *The Voluntary Nonprofit Sector: An Economic Analysis* (Toronto: Heath, 1977) and "The Private Nonprofit Sector—What Is It?" Institute for Research on Poverty Discussion Paper No. 416–77, University of Wisconsin, Madison, May 1977.
12. Rosemary Stevens, *American Medicine and the Public Interest* (New Haven, Conn.: Yale University Press, 1971), p. 141.
13. Michael A. Shadid, *A Doctor for the People* (New York: Vanguard, 1939).
14. Mary Ross, "The Case of the Ross-Loos Clinic," *Survey Graphic* 24 (June 1935):300–304.
15. Michael M. Davis, "The AMA Case," *Survey Graphic* 32 (April 1943): 117–19, 143–44, and Wendell Berge, "Justice and the Future of Medicine," *Public Health Reports* 60 (5 January, 1945):1–16. See also Edward D. Berkowitz and Wendy Wolff, *Group Health Association: A Portrait of a Health Maintenance Organization* (Philadelphia: Temple University Press, 1988).
16. Group Health Cooperative of Puget Sound vs King County Medical Society et al. 39 Wash. (2d)(1951) p. 586.
17. Complete Service Bureau vs San Diego Medical Society, 43 Calif. (2d)(1954) p. 201.
18. "Appeal of Dr. Ben E. Landess to the Judicial Council of the American Medical Association," *Journal of the American Medical Association* 157 (26 February, 1955):753.

11

Voluntary Versus Compulsory Insurance: The Emergence of a Compromise

Whether to share the cost of health services through compulsory insurance from the government or voluntary insurance from private companies was the primary issue up to 1948. Although the growth of voluntary health insurance was rapid, proponents of government health insurance saw it as inadequate to cover the entire population with the necessary range of services. It would not cover the poor or self-employed, and its financing mechanism was regressive. Still, the proponents of government insurance did not have a coalition in Congress. The several bills introduced had been supported by maverick members. The voluntary plans seemed, however, to see these bills as a real threat to their future, so they continued to expand their coverage in order to make government-sponsored health insurance irrelevant.

In this political atmosphere, President Truman called another federal conference on the state of the nation's health and its health services. The National Health Assembly, held in May 1948, was sponsored by the Federal Security Agency (a precursor of the DHEW and DHHS). Oscar Ewing, then secretary of the agency, was an outspoken supporter of government-sponsored health insurance. The administration wished to call together experts, special interests, and representatives of the public for a reappraisal of the status of health services, financing and health of the population.

Revealing the popularity of conferences on issues that will not be settled by facts alone, the 1948 conference was attended by 800 people, far more than attended the 1938 conference. The ability of Americans to sit and listen to the obvious for several days is astonishing, but it seems to be the price one must pay for the testing and creating of consensus.

Ewing tried to set the stage by stating overall objectives with which no one would disagree in principle, but with which many would disagree vigorously regarding implementation. The report on the meeting set forth in detail the supply of hospitals, physicians, nurses, dentists, and all other health resources and judged the numbers inadequate. Detailed data were presented on income groups, mortality and morbidity, and deaths attributable to inadequate facilities and financing. The primary data continued to be the 1928–1931 studies of the CCMC and the National Health Survey of 1935–1936. Additional information in 1948 was the extent of enrollment in voluntary health insurance.

There was too much dependence on the private market, in Ewing's view, to assure an adequate supply of health services, since the ability of people to pay would not equal their need for services. He said, "Plainly ... if we are to move toward an ultimate goal, we cannot continue to use the purchasing-power demand as our exclusive criterion of the adequacy of supply."[1] It seems curious that Ewing did not recognize that the issue was in practice settled, in that the "principle of contributory health insurance should be the basic method of financing medical care for the large majority of the American people." There was no agreement, however, on the question of government-sponsored health insurance. Ewing emphasized that such a program "must be clearly understood as in no way expressing the views of the assembly. It took no position one way or another on this issue."[2]

Ewing made the interesting prediction, given current knowledge, that voluntary health insurance would probably never be able to cover more than one-half of the population.[3] Candid proponents of voluntary insurance would probably not have gone much above this figure. In the early forties, proponents were somewhat startled by the rapid growth of voluntary plans and began to ride the tide. They seemed to believe that, if the government would take care of the poor and persons living in hard-to-reach areas, voluntary health insurance would take care of self-supporting persons who wanted health insurance. In 1948, 40 percent of the population was covered by hospital insurance, 23 percent by surgical insurance, and 9 percent by insurance for physicians' services outside the hospital. In 1940, hospital insurance covered 9 percent of the population. It seems that the chief reason for Ewing's pessimistic prediction was his observation that voluntary health insurance premiums were not, and probably legally could not be, graduated according to family income, as government-sponsored health insurance premiums could be.

While Congress sat on pending health insurance legislation, voluntary health insurance became the backbone of health services funding. Congress did agree to increase and distribute more equitably general hospital beds, through the Hospital Survey and Construction Act of 1946. The report of the National Health Assembly stressed an impending shortage of physicians, nurses, and dentists, based on contemporary personnel-population ratios. At that time, however, there was no consensus that this was a serious problem.

The National Health Assembly was seemingly ineffective in influencing public policy, but President Truman was undaunted. Three years later, he set up the President's Commission on the Health Needs of the Nation by means of a congressional appropriation entitled Emergency Fund for the President, National Defense (Public Law 137). The president was authorized to establish such a commission under the umbrella of national preparedness, and his doing so reflected his concern with national health problems. Truman took great pains to assure that the commission had complete freedom in making public policy recommendations concerning the health services, regardless of the known policy of his administration. Government commissions in this country can rarely, if ever, be instructed to deliver a certain recommendation: to do so would not only wreck their credibility, it would prevent them from being established altogether, because no one would want to serve on them. In order to assure objectivity and a range of interests and opinions, Truman appointed members representing the public, labor, medicine, dentistry, nursing, and hospitals. Presumably the appointees were to speak in the public interest rather than in their own.

Gunnar Gundersen, a member of the AMA Board of Trustees, was named to represent medical practice. However, the president of the AMA at that time, John W. Cline, claimed in the *Journal of the American Medical Association* that Truman had named Gundersen without Gundersen's approval. Gundersen turned down the offer, giving as his reasons:

> I believe I am correct in assuming that the commission is designed, both in its majority membership and its objectives, as an instrument of practical politics to relieve President Truman from an embarrassing position as an unsuccessful advocate of compulsory health insurance. I certainly cannot subscribe to such a masquerade, and today have requested that my name be removed from consideration as a commission member.[4]

Cline observed:

This is a stacked committee, but among its membership are to be found sincere and able men who have accepted the appointment with the finest intentions. However, in such an obviously political framework and in the short space of time that the Commission has been allowed for its work, they will be ineffectual.[5]

As an expression of the AMA's pique, no representative was named by the AMA to replace Gundersen. The commission went ahead and assembled staff, collected and organized existing data and litera-ture, conducted extensive hearings all over the country for those who wished to be heard—and it seems that everyone was heard—and is-sued a report with recommendations in 12 months. Cline's complaint that too short a time was allowed seems to have been justified, but for the wrong reasons.

The chairman of the commission was Paul B. Magnuson, Professor Emeritus, Northwestern University Medical School. Chester I. Barnard, appointed vice-chairman, was at that time director of the National Sci-ence Foundation. In a short time, a competent technical staff was re-cruited under the direction of Lester Breslow, then of the California State Health Department, an able epidemiologist who was knowledge-able about the health services situation in the United States.

The staff collected and organized virtually all relevant information on the status of the health field up to 1950, providing a single, volumi-nous, organized source of information for the health field as of that time.[6] It proved to be a benchmark, both as technical information and as a mirror of emerging public policy regarding the proper role of gov-ernment and private efforts in health services. The amount of material assembled in so short a time is incredible. It is likely that new ground was broken on policy. Recommendations were not clear-cut, to be sure, yet the stalemate reached by the National Assembly four years earlier was absent. It would seem, moreover, that the AMA could take less exception to this report than to any previous public document on the subject.

In his letter of transmittal to President Truman, Magnuson clari-fied the role of government as it had never been clarified before:

The building up of our health resources in terms of training more health personnel and providing more physical facilities must start from the ground up. We have recommended federal grants-in-aid to these and other necessary activities because we believe that the role of the federal government is to stimulate them, not to control them. Government must take the leadership in the promotion of good health, its major energies should go here rather than in extensive direct operation of the health services.[7]

In other words, government should set the stage and establish a climate for the nation's health services, as it traditionally does for the economy in general. The government should poke and prod here and there, providing information on cost and needs and assisting in financing, but it should not control or operate these services. Reality, of course, is sometimes different in that government itself can become an interest group.

In addition to clarifying the role of government, the commission's report set forth principles that had not been made explicit before, including the responsibility of the individual. Coupled with a declaration that "attainment and preservation of health is a basic human right," came another declaration equally straightforward: "the effort of the individual himself is a vitally important factor in attaining and maintaining health." And to set the stage, the report stated unequivocally that:

> . . . a society must assure its citizens access to professional services, education concerning personal health practices, and a reasonably safe physical environment. Only then can individual responsibility for health exercised through personal action reach its full potential.[8]

Left to social and political determination, perforce, was the definition of adequate facilities, adequate access, and individual responsibility. Twenty years later these were to become live topics, including life style, a new term in the context of health.

The lack of consensus about means and sources of financing persisted, but for the first time it seemed that voluntary health insurance might be the means. The commission's recommendations regarding source of control and financing are ambiguous, but the ambiguity stems from an unwillingness, or more likely an inability, to suggest anything else and a desire to give voluntary alternatives a fair trial. Proponents of voluntary health insurance had been asking for a chance for years. The committee's recommendations were a policy breakthrough that few recognized, a typical characteristic of incremental policy developments as described by Lindblom.[9] Belief in the principle of health insurance was reaffirmed, and it was recommended that:

> the present prepayment plans be expanded to provide as much health service to as many people as they can; be judged by the criteria mentioned earlier in this chapter; and be aided by government by allowing payroll deductions for government employees (as in industry), removing the restrictions on organization of prepayment plans, and promoting research on health service administration.[10]

This last is of interest because professional administrators of hospitals and health service plans were being produced by programs in health services administration in universities across the country.

As a seeming counterweight to the foregoing recommendations, the commission also recommended that:

> funds collected through the Old-age and Survivors Insurance mechanism be utilized to purchase personal health service benefits on a prepayment basis for beneficiaries of that insurance program, under a plan which meets federal standards and which does not involve a means test.[11]

This recommendation presaged the Medicare Act of 1965. Further, a general recommendation was made that "federal grants-in-aid be made from general tax revenues for the purpose of assisting the states in making personal health services available to the general population."[12] This recommendation apparently was to give the states an incentive for starting their own health insurance schemes in place of a compulsory national plan. These two recommendations were clearly so general as to be innocuous, but they kept the flame of national health insurance burning.

It would seem that, with 58 percent of the population having some type of voluntary health insurance, these recommendations may have reflected the relative power positions of proponents of private and public financing. Alternatives of private or public financing were to be given a try. Ironically, whereas it was the "conservatives" who signed the CCMC minority report in 1933, objecting to group practice prepayment and allusions to government health insurance, it was the "liberal" members of the commission who signed a minority report in 1952, objecting to the recommendations because they did not go far enough. They felt that the states should not be given the choice of entering or not entering a federal-state health insurance system, because the federal government "must through law assure equality of services in the states." The signers of this minority report were A. J. Hayes, International Association of Machinists; Walter P. Reuther, United Auto Workers-Congress of Industrial Organizations; and Elizabeth S. Magee, National Consumers' League.

Publication of the report of the president's commission coincided with a change in administration in Washington; the country elected its first Republican president in 30 years, Dwight D. Eisenhower. Although the Truman administration was friendly to government-sponsored health insurance and not necessarily unfriendly to voluntary health insurance, Truman himself was never able to induce Congress to bring any of the compulsory health insurance bills to the floor. They never got beyond the hearings; Congress as a whole had been singularly reluctant to commit itself on this issue. The AMA has traditionally been given the credit, or the blame, as the case may be, for Congress' failure to enact a compulsory health insurance law; its skillful lobbying and the influence of personal physicians on members of Congress are cited as the reasons. A more realistic assessment is that the AMA won by default, because public support was not strong enough. This interpretation seems particularly plausible because Congress paid little attention to the AMA's equally fierce opposition to the Medicare Act.

NOTES

1. U.S. Federal Security Agency, *The National Health, A Ten-Year Program: A Report to the President* (Washington, D.C.: Federal Security Agency, 1948), p. 7.
2. Ibid., p. 10.
3. Ibid., p. 87.
4. John W. Cline, "The President's Page," *Journal of the American Medical Association* 148 (19 January 1952):208–9.
5. Ibid.
6. The President's Commission on the Health Needs of the Nation, *Building America's Health*: vol. 1, *Findings and Recommendations*; vol. 2, *America's Health Status: Needs and Resources*; vol. 3, *A Statistical Appendix*; vol. 4, *Financing a Health Program for America*; vol. 5, *The People Speak: Excerpts from Regional Public Hearings on Health* (Washington, D.C.: Government Printing Office, 1952).
7. Ibid., vol. 1, p. vii.
8. Ibid., vol. 1, p. 2.
9. Charles E. Lindblom, "The Science of Muddling Through," *American Political Science Review* 19 (Spring 1959):79–88.
10. The President's Commission, *Building*, vol. I, pp. 47–48.
11. Ibid., vol. I, pp. 47–48.
12. Ibid., vol. I, pp. 47–48.

12

Ferment Within
the Compromise

By the beginning of the Eisenhower administration, a compromise had been reached regarding the primary source of payment for personal health services*—the private sector. This compromise, reached by default, not by outright political bargaining, marked the culmination of many years of activity and debate regarding the fundamental characteristics of the health services in the United States. The undebated decision was to allow the private sector of the health services economy—primarily through voluntary health insurance—to be the chief source of funds for services to individuals. With few exceptions, such as the VA hospitals, the government, when mandated to do so, would buy services from the private sector. Reactions to government support for the training of personnel and for capital funds for voluntary hospitals (as expressed through the Hospital Construction Act in 1946) seem ambivalent, as do reactions to employers' deducting as a business expense their contributions to employees' health insurance.

Having gone through a fearful depression and an even more fearful world war, Americans were tired. The Eisenhower administration provided a desired calm. In addition, the country had begun an unprecedented boom, which made health and welfare problems seem relatively unimportant. Still, the middle and upper classes worried about

---

*In contrast to my thinking in *The Uneasy Equilibrium* (1968), I prefer the term "compromise" to "consensus." A compromise implies continuing tension held together by a consensus. A consensus implies general agreement so that public policy is quite easily formulated; there is little tension. The period from the 1950s to 1965 represents a series of cumulative compromises.

145

costly health care episodes. Voluntary health insurance entered this breach while a benign government looked on.

The federal government, particularly after 1950, began to finance medical research generously. It funded research in its own agencies—for example, the National Institutes of Health—and in universities, through research grants. The Eisenhower administration helped to set and expand these precedents.

Finally, an extremely important development was the emergence during World War II of collective bargaining as the main arena in which union members could obtain increased health insurance benefits. This development removed the issue of health insurance from the political sphere. Labor unions were still paying lip service to the desirability of some type of government-sponsored health insurance, but after their constant successes at the bargaining table, their insistence on national health insurance became muted. Nevertheless, as late as 1952, the last year of the Truman administration, William Green, the aging and long-time president of the AFL, said:

> Facts and logic are on the side of national health insurance. Sooner or later the time-worn, threadbare arguments against it will give way to the irresistible force of the American people's good common sense. Sooner or later the program for which labor pleads will be enacted.[1]

Early in 1953, George Meany, Green's successor, disagreed with the majority report of the President's Commission on the Health Needs of the Nation and supported Green's statement.[2]

When the Eisenhower administration came into power in 1952, the personal health services enterprise was robust. By 1950, voluntary health insurance had begun to have a visible impact as a source of funding for families: 57 percent had at least hospital insurance, up from 8.9 percent in 1940 and 24 percent in 1945. Voluntary health insurance was paying for 17.5 percent of hospital expenditures by 1950 and 10 percent of expenditures on physicians' services; the public sector was paying 48 percent and 5 percent, respectively. The rest was out-of-pocket or direct pay. There was very little coverage of other types of goods and services.

The use of services also increased considerably, from 40 percent of the population seeing a physician at least once a year in the early thirties to 65 percent doing so by the early fifties. Similarly, hospital use climbed from 59 admissions to 120 admissions per 1,000 population. The percentage of the population seeking dental services increased from 21 in the early thirties to 34 in the early fifties. Twenty percent of the low-income pregnant women who had live births saw a physician during the first trimester of their pregnancies in the early thirties, compared with 59 percent of the high-income women (dividing family incomes roughly into thirds). By 1953, these percentages had increased to 42 and 89 percent, respectively. It is obvious that there was greater use of services, as was exhorted and intended. Discrepancies between income groups and geographic areas remained, of course, but the trend was clearly in the direction intended.

The chief issue was the pace of improvement in use and expenditures covered by insurance. The Eisenhower administration had inherited a very rapid momentum, for by 1955 voluntary health insurance was paying 27 percent of all hospital bills and 22 percent of all physicians' bills, an increase of 17 percent and 5 percent, respectively. The public sector stabilized around 20 percent of all expenditures for all services until after the Medicare Act of 1965.

Beginning in the 1950s, subsidies for medical research also began to increase rapidly, particularly subsidies from the federal government; these went up from $73 million in 1950 to $139 million in 1955 to $471 million in 1960. Private funding increased from $37 million in 1900 to $55 million in 1955 to $121 million in 1960. The health services enterprise was obviously taking off, even without a boost from national health insurance. Another element described earlier, and one peculiar to the American scene, was the prepaid group practice plan, which was outside the mainstream Blue Cross-Blue Shield plans and private insurance companies.

PREPAID GROUP PRACTICE PLANS

Prepaid group practice plans were here to stay, notwithstanding the slow initial growth in their enrollments. It took corporate structures like the Kaiser-Permanente plans to provide the needed capital, organizational prowess, and marketing skills. Smaller plans usually had many financial difficulties, not all of them resulting from the opposition of the medical societies. They learned, to give a simple example, that it was essential that there be an explicit contract between participating physicians and the plan![3]

In 1954, the Council on Medical Service of the AMA, chaired by Leonard Larson, a moderate on the question of group practice prepayment, cooperated with a special committee of physicians to survey the various forms of group practice plans in the United States. Larson and his group were charged with examining the quality of medical care, the matter of free choice of physicians, working conditions of physicians, and related matters. A detailed and well-reasoned report was published in 1959 commending the general level of quality of the group practice units but recommending an amendment to the principle of free choice of physicians. The amendment would have the AMA consider the advisability of officially approving the free choice of group plan physicians or solo-practice physicians.[4] The AMA House of Delegates adopted this recommendation.

The AMA was apparently endorsing free choice of delivery systems, a refinement of the free choice of physicians, as health services began to take on corporate characteristics. Thus, it seemed that, with the publication of the Larson report and the ensuing recommendations, the issue of group practice prepayment versus solo practice and prepayment was settled on the national level. It was certainly settled in principle, and the hostile atmosphere dissipated enough that physicians who wished to participate in group practice plans would not be pilloried by their medical society colleagues for doing so. Local skirmishes continued, however: for example, in some areas served by the United Mine Workers, the union attempted to set up plans. The relatively autonomous nature of local and state medical societies, which were not yet tuned in to the main trends, resulted in some unhappy repetitions of experience. It seems that, as far as social innovations are concerned, no one believes that in similar circumstances a given experience will be repeated elsewhere.

All forms of practice began to exist side by side in the early fifties. Still, it should be realized that private solo practice (with increasing specialization and informal referral networks) was the backbone of the delivery system for physicians' services.

REINSURANCE

Even during the Eisenhower era the issue of government health insurance would not go away. In his State of the Union Message in January 1954, Eisenhower said: "I am flatly opposed to the socialization of medicine. The great need for hospital and medical services can best be met by the initiation of private plans."[5] He had mentioned this in his campaign speeches. He said that the proper role of government in medical care was to support medical research and to see that the poor receive care, the classic American philosophy. But Eisenhower also attempted to reformulate government's role in accordance with the new conditions created by voluntary health insurance.[6]

The problem at that time, and still a problem, was the high-cost episode of illness, which voluntary health insurance was not designed to meet and was afraid to meet for fear of bankrupting the insurance agencies. Instead of recommending some sort of government coverage,

Eisenhower suggested that the federal government partially back up the insurance industry, in somewhat the same way that the Federal Deposit Insurance Corporation backs up the banks. This was the concept of reinsurance, one already in use by the insurance companies. Under reinsurance, when one company does not dare to cover a possible contingency such as tornadoes by itself, it spreads the risks and profits by agreement over several companies. Reinsurance as it applies to voluntary health insurance has been given little attention in the historical literature, possibly because it got nowhere with the insurance agencies. I believe it is worthwhile to describe the concept and the situation because they illustrate America's desire to put the private sector on the front line, with government staying in the background.

The Eisenhower administration reasoned that the federal government, with its great resources, could back up insurance agencies, thereby enabling high-risk and low-income groups to buy insurance.* Presumably, the insuring of persons in low-income groups would also help prevent them from resorting to public assistance and private charity.

Reinsurance was intended to increase the proportion of people covered by voluntary health insurance and to improve their ability to pay for catastrophic illnesses.

In 1954, the administration held unpublicized meetings with representatives of the insurance companies and the Blue Cross and Blue Shield plans to discuss the probability of reinsurance. Rumor has it that the insurance agencies were cool to the idea. AMA president David B. Allman called it the familiar "opening wedge" and said with due consistency that the federal government should stay out of health insurance completely.[7] The view was reaffirmed by the Board of Trustees of the AMA at its annual meeting in June 1954: "It is apparent that this program involves subsidization of voluntary health insurance and federal regulation and control."[8] It would seem that the voluntary health insurance sector now felt secure enough about the administration's stand on compulsory health insurance to feel no need to compromise at all.

Opposition also came from labor. The AFL's director of social security, Nelson Cruikshank, a long-time supporter of government-sponsored health insurance, opposed reinsurance for other reasons. He

---

*This recommendation was embodied in the Wolverton bill (H.R. 6944). The premium charge for reinsurance of any health service contract of any approved association would be 2 percent per year of the gross payments received by the association on all health contracts. A Health Service Reinsurance Corporation would be set up, with a hospital service reinsurance fund of $2.5 million. The federal government would pay two-thirds of any hospital bill in excess of $1,000 a year for any individual. The premiums would be scaled according to income (*New York Times*, 11 January 1954, sect. C, p.10).

stated that, if government were to buttress voluntary health insurance at all, it should do so through direct subsidy. That way the relationship between voluntary health insurance and federal administrative agency would be direct rather than indirect, as it would be under a program of reinsurance.[9] Accountability to the public would be blurred under reinsurance.

Even in the face of opposition from those with whom the government would have to deal were the reinsurance bill to be enacted, the administration pushed the bill to a vote on the House floor in July 1954. The bill suffered a decisive defeat, with a vote of 238 against and 134 for it. A post-mortem in the *New York Times* speculated on the reasons for the defeat of this seemingly innocuous measure:

> It appeared that the bill simply had got caught in a crossfire by the conservative wings of both parties from one direction and by New Deal and Fair Deal Democrats from the other. . . . The Conservatives believed that the plan had socialistic tendencies. Others held that it fell short of meeting the average family's needs for health protection. Opponents also argued that the bill had been too hastily considered in Committee and presented to the House without adequate explanation.[10]

Its primary advocate, Oveta Hobby, the Secretary of HEW, urged the AMA House of Delegates in November 1954 to consider supporting the concept. She felt impelled to reemphasize that, although the administration favored reinsurance, it opposed compulsory national health insurance. She observed that experience over the last six years had shown a widening gap between health care costs covered by voluntary health insurance and the total costs of care. Her clincher was:

> In order to help voluntary health insurance to close the gaps in coverage and benefits, we have urged a voluntary reinsurance system. It is, we believe, the only proposal that is clearly consistent with the principle of self-help.[11]

In his annual message to the nation in January 1955, President Eisenhower repeated his recommendation for some type of reinsurance.[12] Again the AMA opposed the concept; this time it offered details of the reasons for its opposition: (1) extensive private funds are available within the insurance industry for such purposes; (2) reinsurance does not make insurable what otherwise would be an uninsurable risk; (3) reinsurance will not fulfill its intended purpose and might even inhibit the satisfactory progress made to date by voluntary plans; and (4) it is a potential subsidy.[13] The most important reason for the AMA's opposition was doubtless the last. As a subsidy, reinsurance would interfere with the operation of voluntary health insurance. The AMA's fears of a potential subsidy were not groundless. It is doubtful, however, that the AMA's argument about uninsurable risks could be sustained, at least not in relation to the costs that the administration wished to help insurance agencies meet.

In the summer of 1955, Oveta Hobby was succeeded as Secretary of HEW by Marion Folsom of Eastman Kodak, chairman of the Folsom report. Although a supporter of the reinsurance concept, calling it the "keystone of the Eisenhower health program," Folsom was not hopeful that it would be accepted by the incoming Congress. He was quoted in a *New York Times* interview as acknowledging that the insurance companies were not keen on it. They engaged in HEW discussions out of courtesy to an administration of which they generally approved. Folsom also said that "the people who want compulsory Federal health insurance say it won't do the job, that it won't reach the lower-income people, and that it is inadequate.... [T]he doctors shy away and don't want the Federal Government to do anything." His reasonable conclusion, given the circumstances, was that "a workable program had not been found."[14]

In his message to Congress in January 1956, President Eisenhower made his last reference to reinsurance in an annual message. He still hoped Congress would consider the concept favorably, but he sounded discouraged:

> Last year and the year before I urged enactment of a proposal for Federal insurance to encourage increased protection against the cost of medical care through voluntary prepayment plans. Since legislation was introduced, private insurance organizations have developed new types of policies and prepayment plans and have extended coverage to groups formerly unprotected. There are now indications that the organizations writing health prepayment plans might progress more rapidly by joining together—sharing or pooling risks to offer broad benefits and expanded coverage on reasonable terms in fields of special needs.... the administration is considering legislative proposals which would permit such pooling. But, if practical and useful methods cannot be developed along these lines, then I will again urge enactment of the proposal made last year.[15]

In the meantime, the Prudential Life Insurance Company had indeed invented and begun to market another form of health insurance: major medical insurance. Perversely, payment for the total medical bill from the first-dollar was expanding, but, because they feared open-ended, very high cost episodes without some dollar limitation, insurance agencies were cautious.

The issue, but not the problem, faded away in June 1956, when the administration urged Congress to enact legislation allowing *small* companies to pool their resources without running afoul of antitrust laws. The original reinsurance proposal had been watered down considerably, and Secretary Folsom described the latest proposal as "simply a step in helping obtain adequate financial protection for more Americans against long hospitalization and costly illnesses."[16]

Subsequently, reinsurance was replaced by expanded support of medical research, grants-in-aid for facilities and training of health personnel, and grants-in-aid for medical care for recipients of public assistance. The policy of no, or at most limited, government intervention in health insurance for the general public remained intact, but not for long. It was threatened again in the early 1960s, when medical care for the elderly became a political issue. It was becoming evident that voluntary health insurance could not provide complete coverage for the elderly and still remain solvent.

ENDEAVORS FOR SPECIAL GROUPS

After the demise of the reinsurance concept, the Eisenhower administration focused on the expansion of programs for special groups. It was a comfortable policy, continuing what was already in being, and it was well within the accepted bounds of government and private activities. These less controversial problems had bipartisan support as well as support from various interest groups in the country. They encountered only occasional opposition from the AMA, whenever it felt that basic principles of voluntary health insurance and private medical practice were being threatened. One successful bipartisan endeavor, the Hill-Burton Act, has been described as "one of the most successful and popular health programs ever initiated by the federal government."[17]

The special groups that received continuing attention from the federal government represented a mixed bag of ad hoc problems. No priorities had been set, and no overall policy tied them together. The groups and problems included veterans, persons unemployed because of permanent, total disability, wives and dependents of men in the military service, recipients of old-age assistance in the states, continuation and expansion of the Hospital Survey and Construction Act, legislation to assist in grants to educational institutions for the training of health personnel, and a tremendous increase in federal grants for medical research. In the American context, these were and are accepted responsibilities of government—they are not concerned with payment for health services by self-supporting segments of the population. The Eisenhower administration let voluntary health insurance have its head: the reinsurance proposal was simply a means of helping it along.

The AMA as Continuing Watchdog

The AMA took exception to two issues. The first of these was the expansion of the Old Age, Survivors, and Disability Insurance (OASDI) portion of the Social Security Act to include payments to persons under the age of 65 years (but not younger than 50) who were unemployed because of permanent, total disability. This measure failed of enactment at the close of the Truman administration; it was revived under Eisenhower with apparently bipartisan support. This issue might be regarded as peripheral to health insurance and health services delivery because it does not involve services, but opponents feared it would spread to include services as well. Worker compensation had demonstrated that possibility.

As early as 1954, premiums had been waived for OASDI recipients at age 65; thus their pension rights were continued just as if their employment and payroll deductions had not ceased. Four years later, the waiver was expanded (as H.R. 7225) to include beneficiaries between ages 50 and 65 who had to leave employment because of permanent, total disability. Little public attention was paid to this measure, but the AMA opposed it strenuously. Its reasons were stated by its Board of Trustees:

> Because of the piecemeal approach to the socialization of medicine of which this proposal is the keystone, the medical profession and the nation as a whole have not been as alert to the dangers as they were during the 1949–1950 campaign against the Truman-sponsored compulsory health insurance bills. The present danger, in fact, is greater. If this bill is adopted, it can be confidently predicted that the cash disability benefits will be extended to the temporarily disabled and that eventually the federal government will initiate a system of compulsory health insurance as a necessary counterpart to the cash benefits program.[18]

The disability issue could be an opening wedge, but hardly a keystone. It is doubtful that Congress and the bureaucracy were as premeditated as the AMA made them out to be, but the AMA's worries were not unfounded.

The second issue was whether to provide some form of health services for the wives and dependents of men in the armed forces. Precedents for this had been established during World War II, with the Emergency Maternity and Infant Care program. The program had been discontinued after the war, but, as the United States moved into a cold war and began maintaining a large standing army and occupation forces throughout the world, congressional interest in the welfare of military dependents was revived.

In 1953, Senator James E. Murray (D-Mont.) introduced a bill (S.1459) that would provide for the medical care of the wives and dependents of men in military service. The AMA opposed the bill, although it was careful to point out that it was not opposed in principle to the government's providing medical care to wives and dependents "if it is determined by Congress to be a proper emolument of military service."[19] The AMA was mainly concerned with the manner of implementation; it approved the mechanism of payment—premiums paid voluntarily by service personnel to private insurance agencies to cover the cost of physician and hospital care. Persons in the military were to be regarded, in effect, as employees.

The following year, Senator Leverett Saltonstall (R-Mass.) introduced S.3363 (which became Public Law 569 in October 1956), the Dependents' Medical Care Program, or Medicare. (This bill was no ancestor of the 1965 Medicare Act for the aged.) This program made possible a variety of approaches, depending on the accessibility of military medical facilities and the dependents' preference for civilian facilities. The Department of Defense could contract with state and local medical societies and their Blue Shield plans for specified services on a prepaid basis. The latter resulted in extensive negotiations on fee schedules between the representatives of the state medical societies and the Department of Defense. The first annual report of the Office for Dependents' Medical Care in the Department of Defense reveals the traditional public policy underlying governmental and private relations when government is mandated to provide health services for a special segment of the population. "It was the policy of the Office for Dependents' Medical Care from the beginning of the program to preserve the customary practice of medicine for the dependents of the military whenever possible."[20]

In the main, this program operated quite smoothly. The policy of utilizing the private health service system is probably due as much to the desires of the dependents as to the AMA and its constituent societies. Every so often there was some fuss over negotiated fee schedules versus cash indemnity, the latter method entailing no contract between the physician and the insurance agency.

The one great exception to the government's general policy of buying medical and hospital care from the private sector was (and is) the VA hospitals. The health services system developed by the VA, with the solicitude and generosity of Congress, has been supported by the AMA in principle, although attacked by it frequently in practice. The AMA's unhappiness has stemmed almost entirely from the VA policy (sustained by Congress) of admitting veterans with nonservice-related disabilities, reported to be 60 percent of all VA patients. This practice is counter to the AMA's policy of no free care for persons who can afford to pay through insurance or otherwise, a view consistent with the general outlook of the public. With regard to veterans, however, public sentiment seems to support a more liberal policy and to accept the veteran's own definition of inability to pay. This is due in no small part to the vigorous activity of the American Legion in supporting VA hospitals and mobilizing the veterans' voting power.

A public fight took place in the 1950s between the AMA and the American Legion over the issue of free treatment for veterans with nonservice-related conditions who the AMA felt could afford to pay for care. It is relevant because it points up the inconsistencies of interest groups in supporting one policy or another, thereby revealing the ad hoc nature of policy positions. To observers of the political scene, the VA-AMA fight was amusing because the contenders are usually conservative politically. The American Legion bitterly attacked the AMA's allegations that many self-supporting veterans were receiving free care at VA hospitals for nonservice-related disabilities. Legion commander A. J. Connell opened fire on the AMA early in 1954 and followed with an article in the *American Legion Magazine* denying the abuses alleged by the AMA. He wrote:

> It is possible that this most powerful and monopolistic medical guild, The American Medical Association, having virtual control and guidance of the nation's health program costing $11 billion annually and with its autocratic direction of the doctor from the time he is a medical student until he finishes his years of practice, will come out flatly and say no veteran should have care not approved by the AMA.[21]

As the controversy continued into the summer of 1954, the president of the AMA, Walter B. Martin, and its secretary and general manager, George F. Lull, felt impelled to issue public statements in reply to the American Legion commander. Lull stated: "Leaders of certain veterans' organizations unwittingly are planting the seeds of socialization when they continue to foster free care for veterans with non-service connected disabilities." Martin asserted:

> It would be unfortunate, indeed, if, in our efforts to reward patriotism, we were responsible for the creation of a system of Government medicine, against the will of the majority, with its inevitable deterioration in the quality of medical care for veterans and non-veterans alike.[22]

A year later, Martin, as retiring AMA president, was still speaking out on the problem of medical care for veterans, but on a different basis. He urged that the federal government contract with existing voluntary hospitals for the care of veterans in order to sustain the system and to avoid duplication of facilities. He observed on the president's page of the AMA *Journal:* "The present policy is producing a centrifugal force that is drawing more and more patients and more physicians and other health personnel into the federal vortex."[23]

In the meantime, the VA was expanding its full-time medical staff, developing medical research opportunities and facilities, and, in some places, becoming affiliated with medical schools. Martin's prediction, although reasonable at the time, did not come to pass. Government-owned and -operated health services are still held in such low regard that VA hospitals are seldom held up as models.

Always the Poor

Another accepted government responsibility that continues to be a chronic political issue is medical care for the poor. In 1957, Congress enacted amendments to the Social Security Act permitting states to use part of their federal grant-in-aid funds to pay the providers of health services for persons on public assistance in various categories. Until that time, federal regulations had not permitted the matching of state funds to pay providers of services; grants-in-aid for public assistance had been intended solely as cash payments to the recipients of assistance. The states were free, of course, to set up any health services program they desired, but federal funds could not be used. In 1957, therefore, the federal government entered directly into the payment of health services providers.

More far-reaching from a public policy standpoint, however, was the enactment of what is popularly known as the Kerr-Mills bill (or Medical Assistance Act), which went into effect on October 1, 1960, as Public Law 86–778. For the first time, the federal government recognized the concept of medical indigency. Many people 65 years of age and over who were not receiving old-age assistance (at that time about 15 percent of the age group) and who were, therefore, not eligible for health services provided by the state welfare programs could not afford to pay for health services even though they were self-supporting in other respects. The Medical Assistance Act, permitting grants to the states from the federal government, was to serve as a financial stimulant to the states to expand their medical care programs for low-income aged persons who did not qualify for old-age assistance.

The Kerr-Mills bill went through Congress with little controversy and with the support of the AMA. The Medical Assistance Act fulfilled the AMA's requirement that government assistance be given only to persons below certain income levels and that payments be made to the private sector of the health services economy. Most states entered into this grants-in-aid agreement.

THE GOVERNMENT AS EMPLOYER

Another act of Congress authorized payment of about one-half of the health insurance premiums of 3 million or so federal employees and their dependents.[24] No public policy precedents were set thereby, because the program was not a tax-supported government health services venture for self-supporting Americans. The federal government was simply emulating, belatedly, long-standing precedents set by employers in private industry and unions acting in their capacity as employers and contributing to health insurance as a wage supplement or fringe benefit. The health insurance industry had been urging the federal government to take such a step for years; when it finally did so, the insurance agencies set up various types of national contracts. Competition among the insurance carriers was stiff but orderly, and 7 million or more stable, desirable new members were added to the voluntary health insurance enrollment.

Medical Research

At the same time, federal grants for medical research were expanded: by 1965, the federal government had become the major source of research funds. The Hill-Burton Act was revived, with significant amendments, at five-year intervals. The amendments related to diagnostic facilities, nursing homes, and extensive renovations of existing hospitals that did not necessarily increase the number of beds.

Need for Personnel

One notable aspect of federal support in the health field during this period was the increasing assistance for training various types of health personnel.[25] There was generally bipartisan support for this kind of assistance, in order to assure a supply of health facilities and the personnel to staff them. President Eisenhower enunciated this policy in his budget message of January 1957. He urged Congress to enact legislation allowing the federal government to assist medical and dental schools with their teaching facilities as well as their research. Thus by 1957, the administration had accepted the consensus of the experts that there was a pending shortage of health personnel. Eisenhower justified his plea for federal assistance "to prevent the already acute shortage of trained manpower from becoming critical."[26]

Bipartisan interest in this problem became fully evident when Senator Lester Hill (D-Ala.) and 12 other senators introduced S.1323 on March 4, 1955. The bill was a five-year plan for federal aid for medical and dental school construction. The bill was accepted by many deans of the schools, but it was rejected by the AMA. The rejection was based on fear of federal intervention in medical schools.[27]

In 1958, however, the AMA endorsed legislation for federal grants to help build and equip medical and dental schools, advising Congress that it opposed any financial incentive to increase enrollment that might tempt schools to accept more students than they could train properly. A statement from F. J. L. Blasingame, executive secretary of the AMA, outlined the AMA's requirements in endorsing the legislation:

> Generally, the American Medical Association is opposed to federal aid in those areas where the private citizens and local communities are capable of providing for themselves. We believe federal aid to be a dangerous device because of the degree of control and regulation which must necessarily accompany federal funds. We believe, however, that there is sufficient need for assistance in the expansion, construction, and remodeling of the physical facilities of medical schools to justify a one-time expenditure of federal funds, on a matching basis, provided, of course, that maximum freedom of the schools from federal control is assured.[28]

The Health Professions Education Assistance Act of 1963 for the construction and expansion of medical schools is notable. These schools were the last of the training facilities for health personnel to be recipients of federal support. This legislation provided loans to medical students to help finance their education, whereas the original bill in 1955 (S.1323) had provided scholarships: medical education was apparently regarded as a worthwhile investment, not a gift. Federal scholarships for the training of other types of health personnel were the rule, and eventually the differentiation between them and medical students was abandoned. Following the pattern set by the Hill-Burton Act, grants for medical school facilities were to be one-time grants for capital construction. It is worth noting that, regarding the start-up grants provided to hospitals, no one criticized the government for "federal interference."

Thus federal legislation relating to health during this period was relatively noncontroversial—grants for research, facilities, and training of personnel in order to make health services more effective and more accessible, leaving the financing and the structure of the delivery system intact. The poor got the Kerr-Mills Act; the better-off were being increasingly covered by voluntary health insurance. The admitted deficiencies in voluntary health insurance—little or no coverage for the self-employed, inadequate coverage of high-cost episodes—were tolerated politically. There was no outcry leading to political action, with one exceedingly important exception—the aged. The agitation for a federal program for the aged and its eventual success demonstrated the pragmatic nature of American politics. The ideological arguments of the forties and early fifties involving individual rights and volition versus compulsion vanished. The aged became a special case.

NOTES

1. William Green, "A National Health Program for a Stronger America," *American Federalist* 59 (February 1952):6.
2. "AFL Backs National Health Plan," *Michigan CIO News* 15 (1 January 1953):2.
3. William A. MacColl, *Group Practice and Prepayment of Medical Care* (Washington, D.C.: Public Affairs Press, 1966).
4. American Medical Association, "Report of the Commission in Medical Care Plan," *Journal of the American Medical Association,* special edition, 17 January 1959.
5. *Christian Science Monitor,* 7 January 1954, p. 6.
6. Ibid.
7. "Reinsurance Fought by AMA," *New York Times,* 6 April 1965, sect. C, p. 31.
8. American Medical Association, *Digest of Official Actions,* 1946–1958 (Chicago: American Medical Association, 1959), p. 343.
9. *Washington Post and Times-Herald,* 6 April 1954, p. 3.
10. John D. Morris, "Eisenhower Plan for Health Funds Rejected in House," *New York Times,* 14 July 1954, p. 1.
11. "AMA Asked to Back Reinsurance Plans," *Washington Post and Times-Herald,* 30 November 1954, p. 8.
12. William H. Lawrence, "President Revives Wide Health Plan with Reinsurance," *New York Times,* 1 February 1955, p. 1.
13. "AMA Policy on Reinsurance," *AMA Washington Letter,* 5 April 1955.
14. Bess Furman, "Folsom May Drop Hobby Health Plan," *New York Times,* 17 January 1956, sect. C, p. 10.
15. Text of Eisenhower's Message to Congress on Health, *New York Times,* 17 January 1956, sect. C, p. 10.
16. *AMA Washington News Letter,* 5 February 1956.
17. Ibid.
18. "Special Message from the Board of Trustees—National Compulsory Disability Benefits," *Journal of the American Medical Association* 158 (23 July 1958):1032.
19. American Medical Association, *Digest,* p. 95.
20. U.S. Department of Defense, Office for Dependents' Medical Care, *First Annual Report* (Washington, D.C.: Government Printing Office, 1958).
21. *Washington Report in the Medical Sciences,* 1 February 1954.

22. Nate Haseltine, "AMA Claims Legion Aids Socialization," *Washington Post and Times-Herald*, 31 August 1954, p. 1.
23. Walter B. Martin, "The President's Pages," *Journal of the American Medical Association* 157 (26 March 1955):1128.
24. For more details, see Odin W. Anderson and J. Joel May, *The Federal Employees' Health Benefits Program, 1961–1968: A Model for National Health Insurance*, Health Administration Perspective No. A9 (Chicago: Center for Health Administration Studies, Graduate School of Business, University of Chicago, 1971).
25. See Elmer L. Hill and Lucy M. Kramer, "Training for Service and Leadership in the Health Professions," *U.S. Health, Education, and Welfare Indicators*, August 1964, pp. xxiii–xxvii.
26. Ibid.
27. Ibid.
28. "AMA Endorses 'Bricks and Mortar' Aid to Medical Schools," *AMA Washington Letter*, 18 April 1958.

13

The Aged: A Policy Breakthrough and Reformulation of the Compromise

THE EISENHOWER ADMINISTRATION, 1952–1960

With the report of the President's Commission on the Health Needs of the Nation in 1953, an unofficial consensus regarding the respective roles of government and the private sector materialized. Voluntary health insurance was given its head, and government supported medical research, construction of health facilities, and training of health personnel.

The problem of health services for the aged, however, threatened this consensus. Persons aged 65 and over—65 being the criterion set for receiving OASDI pensions—comprised about 10 percent of the population, but they incurred a disproportionately large share of the expenditures for health services. The elderly do not fit neatly into traditional classifications of special groups or special problems, for they have so many problems simultaneously that they cut across such boundaries. This creates great confusion whenever attempts are made to justify governmental concern on the basis of precedents. The aged are on the cutting edge of public policy changes.

It has been documented beyond all doubt that the aged have more illnesses, use more health services, and have an average lower income than the younger segments of the population. They also have less health insurance coverage. But not all of the aged fall below the poverty line, they are not all ill or disabled, and they do not all suffer from disease, even diseases peculiar to their age group. Moreover, health insurance coverage among the elderly is increasing. Consequently, the aged have been assisted by government if they are poor, if they have special disabilities ordinarily cared for by government, such as blindness or psychosis, or if they are veterans. That is, assistance has been based on criteria other than just age.

Proponents of a federal health service program for all the aged, regardless of income or special condition, prefer to regard the aged as a special group defined mainly by age. To them, multiple problems among the aged, whether directly related to aging or compounded by it, warrant preferential handling. Opponents argue that such a program would constitute a change in public policy. An entire age group would come under a government program, regardless of need. The main point at issue is whether or not income should be eliminated as a criterion for a government-sponsored health services program.

Unquestionably, any federal health service program for the aged not based on income would be a public policy breakthrough. Even so, future expansion of that program would be debated on its merits rather than on an ideological position such as freedom versus compulsion. The process is what Skidmore aptly refers to as the American process of rhetorical reconciliation. This practice, according to him, "helps explain how American society escapes many of the strains that might be expected when its professed ideals conflict with many of its accepted practices."[1]

Developments in the Public Sector

From 1952 on, many bills were introduced in Congress proposing health services for OASDI beneficiaries. During Eisenhower's first term, 1952–1956, several such bills were introduced in Congress, separately or jointly by Representative John D. Dingell (D-Mich.), Senator James E. Murray (D-Mont.), Senator Hubert Humphrey (D-Minn.), Representative Emanuel Celler (D-N.Y.), and Senator Herbert H. Lehman (D-N.Y.), all New Deal-style Democrats. Two of them, Dingell and Murray, had been associated with previous universal health insurance bills. It would seem that these bills were introduced mainly to keep the issue of government health insurance alive. Government-sponsored health insurance for the entire population was not a viable political issue any more, but insurance for the aged might be.

In 1953, 31 percent of persons aged 65 and over had some type of hospital insurance, compared with 57 percent of the general population. Five years later, the respective percentages were 43 and 65, indicating a faster rate of growth in coverage for the aged. Presumably, however, the rate of growth was not fast enough to prevent insurance for the aged from becoming a political issue.[2] Furthermore, benefits for the aged were not as broad as those for the rest of the population.

Many national conferences on the aged were held between 1950 and 1960. Most of them, along with the proposed legislation for the aged, were extensively documented and widely disseminated.[3]

During Eisenhower's second term, 1956 to 1960, Congress' interest in health care legislation for the aged quickened considerably, on both sides of the aisle. The bill destined to receive prominence and publicity was that introduced by Representative Aime J. Forand (D-R.I.) in 1957 (H.R. 9467). Parallel bills were sponsored by congressmen Kenneth A. Roberts (D-Ala.); John J. Allen (R-Calif.); and John D. Dingell (D-Mich.). Forand's name remained in the political limelight as a result of his introduction of another bill in 1959 (H.R. 4700). These bills included hospital care and physician's services in the hospital, particularly surgical services. Arthur S. Flemming, Secretary of DHEW, testified forcefully against the second Forand bill in July 1959. The bill was contrary to the administration's stand against compulsory health insurance in any form.

Unequivocal opposition was to be expected from the AMA. The AHA was not able to assume such a position. Although it remained opposed in principle to the Forand type of legislation, the AHA hedged its opposition somewhat, thereby increasing the AMA's anxiety. The AHA was not opposed in principle to some type of federal subsidy. As institutions, the voluntary hospitals, the bulk of the AHA's constituency, were products of the charitable and community traditions; physicians, on the other hand, drew primarily on their professional conscience, with little corporate commitment. The fears of the AMA were expressed by its executive secretary, F. J. L. Blasingame, in a speech before the Mid-Year Conference for Presidents and Secretaries of Allied Hospital Associations. He appealed to the hospital representatives not to become "the soft spot in the dike of voluntary financing mechanisms. It would be tragic if the designers of state medicine are permitted to divide and conquer."[4]

On December 6, 1959, the AHA and AMA issued a joint resolution stating that they would mobilize their "full resources" to accelerate the development of adequately financed health care programs for needy persons, especially the aged needy. The gist of their opposition to the 1959 Forand bill was that it was not designed especially for the needy and that it would apply to all Social Security beneficiaries, thereby excluding most needy persons who were not yet eligible for Social Security benefits.[5]

Early in 1960, the AHA issued a strong statement opposing any

Forand-type bill. It believed that any federal mechanism for financing hospital care for so large a segment of the population carried with it inherent dangers. The following is a paraphrase:[6]

1. The federal government, as a major purchaser of hospital care, would become concerned with hospital costs and then be involved in the administration and operation of hospitals, with possible ill effects on the quality of service and interference with the care of patients.

2. The provision of prepaid hospital benefits unaccompanied by appropriate long-term facilities and benefits might lead to very high utilization of general hospitals for services that could be better provided in other ways.

3. Financing health care for one group through the Social Security mechanism would lead to financing for other groups and ultimately to a compulsory system for the entire population.

These are standard arguments, and the predictions are reasonable enough, considering the viewpoint. Early proponents of Medicare did have as their long-term strategy the spread of government health insurance from the elderly to the general population. The result would obviously have been more government surveillance over hospital accounting and reimbursement methods.

Senator Jacob Javitz (R-N.Y.) and seven other "liberal " Republican senators introduced S.3350 in April 1960, a plan for voluntary health insurance for the aged. The services to be covered were broader than in any bill introduced heretofore. Anyone would be eligible at age 65, and premiums would be based on ability to pay. Premiums would range from 50 cents to $13 dollars a month, with total costs to be shared by federal and state governments and, whatever extent possible, the individual insured.[7] On May 4, 1960, the administration proposed a "Medicare Program for the Aged," calling for the establishment of "Medicare" systems by the states under federal standards. Insurance would be available free to elderly persons receiving public assistance; other eligible persons would pay an annual fee of $24 dollars each. It was estimated that this proposal would cover all but 3.5 million of the 15.6 million people age 65 and over.[8] The president of the AMA, Louis Orr, opposed the proposal, saying that it was "based on the false premise that almost all persons over 65 need health care and cannot afford it."[9]

Not to be outdone by the Republicans, and to further the endeavors of their Democratic colleagues, Forand and Senators Pat McNamara of Michigan and Clinton P. Anderson of New Mexico placed proposals for a health program for the aged in the legislative hopper in May and June 1960.

As the bills for health care for the aged accumulated, they became increasingly hedged by limitations, restrictions, deductibles, and other forms of control, indicating a great fear of unexpected costs, despite all the estimates made from the abundant data. An overestimate of 10 percent, not to mention 25 percent, might be regarded as disastrous to plans for financing. Moreover, institutional aspects of care were emphasized almost exclusively; physicians' services—whether in or out of the hospital—were left out altogether. This was probably a tactic to avoid a head-on encounter with the AMA. This tactic was also used in Canada, which started universal health insurance with the hospital.

The exclusion of physicians' services may also have resulted from the cost-consciousness of Congress and the administration. HEW Secretary Flemming mentioned the fear of costs in his testimony opposing Anderson's proposed legislation. He raised the possibility of a "tax revolt" if Congress kept on adding new Social Security payroll deductions. Adding health insurance benefits, he said, "could very well bring the payroll tax up to somewhere between 15 and 20 percent." He added pointedly, "[W]e believe it is unsound to assume that revenue possibilities from a payroll tax are limitless."[10] Anderson's counterclaim was that it would be easier to finance health benefits through a payroll tax than through "another burden on the already overburdened states and on the income tax system of the United States." Tying methods and sources of funding to benefits had the advantage of keeping them clearly in sight and, presumably, bringing more discipline to funding. The administration's proposal was embodied in what eventually would become known as the Kerr-Mills bill, or the Medical Assistance Act. On June 23, 1960, the house voted overwhelmingly, 380 to 23, for this federal-state program of medical care for the needy; President Eisenhower signed the bill into law in September of that year. Both Senator Robert S. Kerr of Oklahoma and Representative Wilbur Mills of Arkansas were Democrats, but neither was partial to the Forand-McNamara-Anderson proposals to use the OASDI section of the Social Security Act as the vehicle for federal health care for the aged.

In the meantime, McNamara headed a new subcommittee of the Senate Labor and Public Welfare Committee created in 1959 to conduct a year-long study of the aged population. The subcommittee gathered mountains of data on the aged and conducted hearings in many cities through the country. Health care for the elderly was undoubtedly the most thoroughly aired social problem in the history of the country, but it is often difficult to determine what effect facts had on specific legislation. Opponents of Medicare for the aged felt that care should be provided for the needy aged, but they paid no attention to the fact that, as measured by standard poverty levels, two thirds of the aged were needy. It might be more expedient to include all the aged rather than try to classify them. Social surveys showed clearly, however, that the aged incurred a disproportionate share of expenditures for health services, thus taxing severely their already limited financial resources. This fact was the stimulus for Medicare.

In the summer and fall of 1960, preparations for national and state elections were underway. As might be expected, the issue of health services for the aged was in the forefront. At the State Governors' Conference in June, the governors went on record 30 to 13 in favor of using the Social Security system to finance health services for the aged. The states wanted to get out from under the tax burden of the aged as much as possible. This vote was a victory for Governors Nelson Rockefeller of New York, a liberal Republican, and G. Mennen Williams of Michigan, a Democrat.[11]

At their political conventions in July, both the Republican and Democratic parties endorsed in principle proposals for health care for the aged. The concept now had bipartisan support, but political issues of source and amount of funding, scope of benefits, need, and voluntary versus compulsory insurance were still unsettled. The Republican platform proposed that OASDI beneficiaries be given the option of purchasing private health insurance policies. The platform promised a federal health care program to those older citizens "needing it."[12]

Developments in the Private Sector

As early as June 1955, the Board of Trustees of the AHA recommended that responsibility for the care of the aged should be divided equally among the federal government, the state governments, the voluntary plans, and the beneficiaries themselves. In keeping with precedent, the trustees said that federal legislation should provide grants-in-aid to the states on a variable matching basis, depending on the state's economic health.[13]

In medical circles, a parallel proposal was submitted by the Commission on Geriatrics of the Pennsylvania Medical Society to the AMA House of Delegates in November 1956. The commission proposed a system of voluntary health insurance administratively connected with the OASDI program. The House of Delegates, however, did not accept the proposal, because it combined voluntary health insurance with a compulsory social insurance program. Further, the house wanted to wait and see whether voluntary health insurance could increase the enrollment of the elderly.[14]

In its attempts to avoid federal financing of health services for the aged, other than the traditional public assistance categories, the AMA House of Delegates adopted the following recommendations in December 1958:

> .... that the American Medical Association, the constituent and component medical societies, as well as physicians everywhere, expedite the development of an effective voluntary health insurance or prepayment program for the group 65 years of age and over with modest resources or low family income; that physicians agree to accept a level of compensation for medical services rendered to this group, which will permit the development of such insurance and prepayment plans at a reduced premium.[15]

The next step was to induce the constituent medical societies sponsoring or approving Blue Shield plans, as well as the plans themselves, to carry out AMA recommendations. Appeals were sent to the medical societies to give earnest consideration "to implementing special programs which would carry out the intent of the House of Delegates."[16] Officially, the AMA preferred to formalize the traditional sliding fee scale and embody it in a fee schedule rather than deal with a government agency that would pay for the care of the aged above a certain income level. The ostensible intent was to adapt the Robin Hood principle to the collective responsibility of physicians through a prepayment plan. The House of Delegates wanted physicians to act in a more concerted manner in regard to this vital policy issue.

On February 24, 1960, the House of Delegates of the California Medical Association approved the principle of federal subsidy to enable the needy to buy voluntary health insurance policies. This proposal was regarded by many as the medical profession's alternative to a bill linked to Social Security.[17] Nevertheless, the acceptance of a federal program continued to be limited to the concept of the "needy aged."

The expected line-up for and against some type of federal health care bill for the aged, in addition to the positions of the AHA and AMA, was the AFL-CIO, the American Nurses' Association, the National Council of Churches, and several leading newspapers for the idea and the American Dental Association, the National Association of Manufacturers, the U.S. Chamber of Commerce, the Farm Bureau, and private insurance companies against it. Early in 1961, the *New York Times* editorialized somewhat naively:

> Another great advantage of this setup would be its avoidance of anything that can be called socialized medicine. Every beneficiary would be free to

choose his own doctor and hospital, and there would be no government supervision or control of the practice of medicine.[18]

The case for the opposition is probably summed up equally naively in a statement from the Health Insurance Association of America: "The HIAA has pointed out to the American business community that if the Federal Government projects itself into the field of health insurance, the principle of competitive enterprise will be in peril."[19]

THE KENNEDY AND JOHNSON ADMINISTRATIONS, 1960–1965

With the election of John F. Kennedy in 1961, there was an air of expectation that there would be some successful federal action in health care for the aged, despite Kennedy's very narrow victory and a divided Congress. In short order, President Kennedy laid before Congress a broad program of federal insurance for the health care of the aged.[20] Immediately, Representative Cecil R. King (D-Calif.) and Senator Anderson, with the endorsement of other Democrats, introduced identical bills in their respective chambers (H.R. 4222 and S. 191). Javits and eight other Republicans introduced identical bills in their respective chambers (H.R. 4222 and S. 191). Seldom have so many names been listed on pending bills, and seldom have so many legislators wished simultaneously to get on record. The bandwagon was gathering passengers.

In January 1958, Representative John F. Fogarty (D-R.I.) had introduced a bill (H.R. 9822) to authorize the holding of a White House Conference on Aging before the end of that year. A skeptic might have questioned the value of another assembly, considering the great mass of data available and the complications and recommendations of several earlier conferences, but calling it a White House Conference gave it a special aura.

Fogarty was apparently conscious of the spate of data and proposals from other conferences when he said, "In spite of the many surveys, books, and conferences on aging, the greatest accomplishment to date has been the output of words."[21] After various delays to give the states time to collect information (with federal grants), arrange their own conferences, and formulate recommendations to the White House Conference, the date was set for January 1961.

From January 9 to 12, more than 2,500 delegates met in Washington, D.C. They represented 53 states and territories and more than 300 national voluntary organizations interested or active in aging. The delegates' "basic objectives were to define the circumstances, needs, and opportunities of America's older citizens, and to recommend actions by governmental and private groups that will enable all our people to achieve maximum satisfaction in their added years."[22] Within this blur of objectives, the most cogent issue was health care. The conference commended the efforts of voluntary health insurance and public assistance in one breath, but in the next breath it declared that such mechanisms "will continue to fall short of meeting the basic medical care needs of the aged as a whole. The majority of the delegates of Section 2 [by a vote of 170 to 99] believe that the Social Security Mechanism should be the basic means of financing health care for the aged."[23] Many informed citizens had spoken and helped to establish a "sense of the meeting," to which it was expected that Congress would pay attention. Yet Congress did not appear to be in a hurry, and the debate, studies, and wheeling and dealing continued.

With consummate timing, President Kennedy, in his State of the Union message, urged that OASDI be the mechanism for health services for the aged. "Private health insurance helps very few [of the aged], for its cost is high and its coverages limited," he said. "Public welfare cannot help those too afraid to seek relief but hard pressed to pay their own bills. Nor can their children or grandchildren always sacrifice their own health and family budgets to meet this constant drain."[24]

Liberal Republicans continued to press for a compromise bill using the OASDI mechanism, but providing various options to beneficiaries. These included institutional care or a major medical plan covering a wide range of services, thus enabling older persons eligible for health services to choose cash instead of service benefits if they already had adequate health insurance. Late in June 1962, a compromise proposal by five Republicans and 18 Democrats called for a government subsidy to provide Social Security health benefits to persons age 65 and over who were not entitled to regular retirement benefits. This was a fairly large minority and, for the sake of equity, one not to be ignored. The proposal would also have allowed Blue Cross or other private insurance agencies to administer the federal program.[25]

It is scarcely possible, and not even worthwhile, to distinguish among the bills introduced in Congress during this period. They represented the ad hoc policy making characteristic of the American political process. It is important to realize that the members of Congress who wished to consider a bill, and no one wanted to be left out, were in agreement that the Social Security mechanism and payroll deductions should be the basis of financing health services for the aged. Further, special attention should be paid to the low-income aged and those not eligible for Social Security pensions. Members of Congress differed on the extent to which private insurance agencies should be used as paying agencies by the government. The emphasis placed on the elderly "poor" as against emphasis on all aged regardless of income showed that members of Congress differed as to the acceptance of a means test for entitlement purposes. There were sharply different views regarding the restrictions placed on hospital days, the amount of deductibles, and similar limitations to control costs. In due course, however, the bill that emerged and passed was a work of art in political compromise, revealing that, once Congress achieves voting consensus, something will be passed. The administration's bill was the King-Anderson version, and it was on this bill that discussion and debate centered.

The relationship between HEW and the AMA was anything but cordial. Persons on the Social Security Administration staff were helping draft the bill. F. J. L. Blasingame, executive vice-president of the AMA, charged that Abraham A. Ribicoff, Secretary of HEW, was lobbying in favor of the King-Anderson bill by publishing with public money a booklet on health care for the aged; Ribicoff, he charged, had therefore broken the law. Ribicoff countered by citing his authority to do so under section 702 of the Social Security Act, which allowed him to recommend changes and publish facts showing need.[26] This seemingly innocuous action on Ribicoff's part illustrates the near impossibility of separating administration from politics when running a program like OASDI.[27] On May 21, 1962, the AMA paid for a national television hookup to blast at the proposal for medical care for the aged supported by the Kennedy administration, using an empty Madison Square Garden in New York as a setting. This telecast took place only a few days after President Kennedy had spoken to a packed Madison Square Garden to urge support for the administration's program. The audience was the White House Conference on Aging mentioned earlier.

During the same month, there were symptoms of unrest among rank and file physicians. A deluge of publicity followed a resolution originated by J. Bruce Henriksen, a physician from Point Pleasant, New Jersey, urging a medical boycott of President Kennedy's proposed health services program for the aged were it to be enacted. Reportedly, the resolution had the support of 200 physicians in five New Jersey hospitals. A furor was created in the state, and Blasingame himself was drawn in. He said, "the New Jersey physicians made it clear that they will continue to treat patients as they always have, and if the patients cannot afford to pay them, they will treat them free."[28] This was probably the first time that a sizable number of U.S. physicians had threatened to strike, although there were precedents in Canada and other countries with governmental health insurance systems.

There were immediate repercussions in the New Jersey State Assembly, which voted overwhelmingly on May 7 to condemn physicians who had declared they would not treat elderly patients under any program tied to Social Security. The voice vote came "after a long and emotional debate."[29] Meanwhile, a bill to penalize any physician who refused to treat a patient was introduced in the assembly and prepared for a final vote on May 14. The penalty was to be loss of license to practice, which, of course, meant the physician would be deprived of the usual source of livelihood. The bill was later withdrawn. The climax came when the state medical society disassociated itself from Henriksen's resolution but reaffirmed its opposition to President Kennedy's proposal.[30] Withholding of service obviously betrays the public trust and prerogatives society has accorded the medical profession.

Although written a year before the incident in New Jersey, an editorial in the *New England Journal of Medicine* accurately describes the manner in which American physicians react to proposed legislation in which they feel they have a high stake.

> Unfortunately for the side to which organized medicine cleaves, most spokesmen for the American Medical Association are, by virtue of their training, politically inexperienced. The Association, as a result, sometimes finds itself struggling to get out of an argument into which it naively wandered or was cleverly led. Its explanations, vexations and hair-trigger retorts, when silence might have been golden, have only tended to confuse the fundamental argument, delight its antagonists and embarrass member physicians. . . . And yet, the Association's stand on financing medical care of the aging—despite misinterpretation and misleading harangue and despite its honest bumbling in the political arena—is simple to understand. The House of Delegates has concluded that supplying medical and hospital services to a large segment of the population regardless of financial need, through a compulsory tax, as provided in the King-Anderson bill, is socialized medicine—an overworked term that can be variously defined but is generally interpreted as federally administered and controlled medical service. To be sure, it may be a small dose of socialized medicine, but according to the Association's definition it is socialized medicine nevertheless. The Association further believes, not without justification, that once Congress endorses the principles embodied in the bill, expansion of the program is inevitable.[31]

Physicians in the United States, unlike their counterparts in countries with government health insurance, appear to believe that the medical profession has the right to control both diagnosis and treatment and the methods, amounts, and sources of payment—in short, the delivery system itself. This does not seem to be reasonable, and it certainly is not practical.

Whereas the AMA's opposition to the King-Anderson bill was unequivocal, the AHA's position was not. In July 1962, the AHA released a policy statement opposing details of the King-Anderson bill but not the substance of it. The AHA accepted the Social Security Administration funding through payroll deductions, but it opposed having the program administered by the Social Security Administration. The AHA also wanted a test of financial need and believed that costs had been underestimated. The AHA policy read:

> We recognize that government assistance is necessary to enable many retired persons to obtain needed health care. We believe that such assistance should go to the individual to aid him or her in purchasing prepayment through the voluntary system. The Senate amendments permit the administration of the program by the Social Security Administration. We believe it does not belong there. The provision in the Senate amendments for purpose of coverage through Blue Cross or private insurance would make them mere fiscal agents for the government benefit program.[32]

On July 17, 1962, the Kennedy administration suffered a serious legislative defeat. The King-Anderson bill had been stalled in the House Ways and Means Committee, so Senate Democratic leaders decided to make an end run around it. They attached to a Senate bill already passed by the House an amendment that contained the essence of the King-Anderson bill—a health service program for the aged financed through Social Security—and forced a vote on it. The prevailing interpretation of this maneuver was that the Senate Democratic leaders were confident of Senate approval, and they hoped the Senate tally would demonstrate Congressional support for the program. Furthermore, according to the *Wall Street Journal*, "if the victory margin were big enough—[it] might even pry the bill loose from the Ways and Means Committee."[33]

The Senate, however, voted 52–48 against the amendment, following a motion by Kerr, the leading Democratic foe of the administration's health care plan for the aged, to table the proposal. Only five Republicans joined 43 Democrats in supporting the plan; it was opposed by 21 Democrats and 31 Republicans. The *Wall Street Journal* commented:

> The defeat was all the more humiliating for Mr. Kennedy because it was by no means necessary even to have a Senate vote on this issue this year. Even if the Senate's vote July 17 had gone the other way, there would have been no final congressional approval this year of the President's proposal. . . . [34]

The Senate vote did not kill the King-Anderson bill, but it raised doubts as to the Kennedy administration's ability to get such legislation through Congress.

The Senate action did not dampen interest in the King-Anderson bill, rather it foreshadowed greater compromises. In February 1963, Javitz reintroduced his bill; it included: (1) coverage for the estimated

2.5 million people age 65 and over not covered under the Social Security Act; (2) an option under which beneficiaries could choose to receive hospital care through approved private plans rather than the federal government; and (3) the establishment of a separate health insurance trust fund (that is, separate from other funds in OASDI) into which all health care funds would be deposited.[35]

The Javitz bill leaned toward the private sector:

> The provisions of our bill are essential if there is to be recognition that private enterprise is an important partner in the effort to meet the special needs of the aging and can help to limit Federal Government expansion in this field. If we are truly to prevent socialized medicine, the entire burden and responsibility for meeting the health needs of the aging should not fall entirely on the Federal Government.[36]

Somewhat in the same vein, a respected and prominent surgeon from Washington, D.C., Donald Stubbs, a medical moderate and chairman of the board of the District of Columbia Blue Shield plan introduced a resolution at the annual meeting of the National Association of Blue Shield Plans urging the development of a nonprofit national program for the aged. The program would provide uniform benefits covering two-thirds of the cost of medical and hospital care. The resolution recognized the relatively heavy expenses that would be involved, and it recommended support of legislation to provide federal aid for all of the aged who would choose to participate in a qualified voluntary prepayment program. It also recommended supplemental state or local assistance, with individual need determined locally. Opposition to Stubbs' resolution was led by Norman Welch, at that time chairman of the board of the Massachusetts Blue Shield Plan and speaker of the House of Delegates of the AMA. (A year later, Welch became president of the AMA.) Welch noted that the resolution was contrary to AMA policy because of its support in principle of a general federal subsidy for everyone in the aged population, irrespective of financial status. The opposition won.[37] AMA consistency on policy continued.

In November 1963, a group of national leaders who had founded an ad hoc committee called the National Committee on Health Care for the Aged sought to break the stalemate in Congress by proposing the use of both government and private insurance. They believed that a portion of the program could be financed through OASDI. Their proposal was not particularly new, but it aroused interest because the 12–member committee included three officials from the Eisenhower administration: Arthur S. Flemming and Marion B. Folsom, former secretaries of HEW, and Arthur Larson, former Undersecretary of Labor. Other members included representatives of private health insurance agencies, hospitals, medical schools, business, and educational groups. Folsom and Larson were already on record as favoring OASDI as a logical financing mechanism.[38]

The stalemate in Congress continued during 1964. Lyndon B. Johnson, then President, expressed continued support of health services for the aged through OASDI in his 1964 message to Congress. The stalemate was usually attributed to Wilbur Mills, who chaired the strategic House Ways and Means Committee. Mills was reported to be concerned about the financial integrity of the OASDI fund. Another cause of the delay was the proposal to increase the cash pension benefits under OASDI. An increase in benefits would necessitate an increase in payroll deductions from employers and employees; if a deduction for health care for the aged were added, the burden on the American payroll would be "intolerable." Proponents of health care for the aged were put in the uncomfortable position of having to oppose an increase in pensions if this were to jeopardize enactment of legislation for health care for the aged through OASDI. Health care for the aged was facing final, political trade-offs.

In September 1964, the Senate voted 60 to 28 to support a bill combining health insurance for the aged and increases in Social Security cash benefits.[39] On October 2, Senate and House conferees met to break the deadlock on the bill and failed, sending the entire Social Security bill down in defeat. Senate conferees voted 4 to 3 in favor of the bill and House conferees voted 3 to 2 against it. Aid to the elderly, either in the form of increased pension benefits or health insurance, was ruled out for the following year. The *New York Times* reported that this action, both a defeat and a victory for President Johnson, immediately made health care for the aged a dominant issue in the presidential campaign then underway. The element of victory lay in the fact that the administration had succeeded in warding off attempts to raise pensions without including health care for the aged.[40] Meanwhile, Republican presidential candidate Barry Goldwater called the health care bill "unnecessary," given the progress that had been made, and that was likely to continue, by the health insurance industry.[41]

The presidential election returned Johnson to the White House with an even greater majority of his party in control in both houses of Congress than before. The Democratic and Republican parties both had liberal and conservative wings in Congress, however, and passage of a health care bill for the aged was not necessarily assured. Certainly, the election results could reasonably be interpreted as conducive to health and welfare legislation, a fact of which the AMA was well aware. Shortly after Johnson's message to the nation, AMA president Donovan F. Ward proposed to a national conference on Kerr-Mills in Chicago that federal and state funds be used to help persons age 65 and over who had incomes below a certain level to purchase comprehensive health insurance benefits from voluntary health insurance agencies.[42] This AMA proposal became known as Eldercare, as distinguished from Medicare (which the AMA delighted in calling Fedicare, a humorous note in an otherwise humorless debate).

The Eldercare plan was notable for its comprehensiveness, as compared with the administration bill, which was limited to hospital and nursing home care.[43] The administration's omission of physicians' services was surely a tactical maneuver to avoid direct confrontation with the medical profession. In point of fact, if "means" had been defined generously—as, say, 20 percent of the population—Eldercare would have been a more equitable program for the aged than the administration bill. The AMA insisted, correctly, that the administration program was inadequate, given its narrow range of services. In doing so, however, the AMA walked directly into a trap set by Mills who accepted the AMA's criticism. He devised Part B, the provision for physicians' services in which the elderly could enroll voluntarily.

Wilbur Cohen casts some light on the hectic political environment in which policy was made, metaphorically shooting from the hip, after Lyndon B. Johnson became president following John F. Kennedy's assassination. Johnson readily accepted Part B plus $500 million for a federal subsidy to add to the premium to be charged the elderly. He accepted it in very unusual circumstances, even for the riotously pluralistic policy making system of the United States. Part B had to be put over quickly to catch the American Medical Association off-balance, as that organization could be counted on to oppose compulsory health insurance and to support a means test.

Cohen reports that, when he took the Part B idea to the president,

> The President did not bat an eye. He accepted the situation calmly, which I took for acceptance and clearance. It was a strange and unique way in which to make a major policy decision. There was no policy clearance with others in the Department [of HEW, of which Cohen was then the secretary] or in the Budget Bureau or White House. Mills had scored a coup. Johnson immediately realized it. I was the intermediary for a major expansion of our proposal and without any intervening details of the proposal as developed by the staff. In this case the Federal Government was moving into a major area of medical care with practically no review of alternatives, options, tradeoffs, or costs.[44]

As the passage of the Medicare bill became imminent, *Medical World News* reported an interesting theory among AMA leaders to explain their defeat on Medicare. They felt that their cause was doomed not by the merits of a bill whose time had come (the inexorable forces of history), but by a tragic event, the assassination of President Kennedy. The AMA officials believed that "Medicare could have been beaten—perhaps for all time—if John F. Kennedy's death had not suddenly and violently changed the whole political climate." According to them, the assassination started a chain reaction that greatly strengthened pro-Medicare forces and undermined their conservative opponents. It was pointed out that the late President had won by a very narrow margin in 1960 and that, despite a substantial Democratic majority in Congress, he was defeated on Medicare because of the coalition between Republicans and Southern Democrats. President Johnson, because of the new atmosphere, broke this coalition throwing the Republicans into a state of confusion. During the early months of 1964, Johnson worked to satisfy his consensus. After the House Ways and Means Committee shelved the King-Anderson bill, supporters of Medicare were reported to be in near despair. Johnson, however, decided to press for a Senate vote during the election campaign in order to put Goldwater on the spot. Although Johnson did not win congressional passage at the time, he succeeded in making Medicare an important issue during the 1964 election campaign. When the landslide for Johnson came, he felt he had a mandate. It was assumed that, if Kennedy had lived, he would have been reelected by another narrow margin and, therefore, without the mandate on which Johnson acted.

This is interesting historical speculation that may have been true for the short run, not for the long run. The aged would not have gone away, and their numbers were increasing.[45] Johnson's prescience did not extend to the shape and scope of the bill to be enacted. There was no understanding of how a particular bill would affect the delivery system or how it would set priorities of need. The strategy was to get passed a bill that would ostensibly meet catastrophic costs of acute illnesses and that would affect most of the aged and their families. Hard-core residuals like the chronically ill and those not covered by the bill would have to resort to welfare and Medicaid.

The AMA's Eldercare proposal was taken seriously by the House committee, probably to the AMA's surprise. Eldercare was added to, or, more aptly, grafted on to, the administration bill so that the aged could subscribe to physicians' services in and out of the hospital on a voluntary basis. Subscribers would pay $3 a month and the federal government $3 a month. This feature preserved the voluntary nature of the proposal as far as the AMA was concerned, although it did not respect the association's principle of low-income recipients; further, the revision violated the AMA's principles regarding the use of the OASDI for all the aged. Representative Mills was apparently ready to change his mind, but the stakes were high and he was not as inconsistent as many assumed at that time. The universal and compulsory hospital care portion of the bill became Part A, the voluntary physicians' care portion Part B.

How the bill that finally passed was put together is difficult to determine. It is unlikely that the chain of events and decisions could be reconstructed, even by the principals.[46] A 1974 conference sponsored by the Institute for Research on Poverty, University of Wisconsin–Madison, offered further insight into the "rationality" of the political process. Wilbur Cohen, present as a discussant of the papers being delivered, remarked,

> As I sat through these sessions, I got the feeling that people here [critical academics] assume there were a lot more alternatives to the decision makers in 1961, 1962, 1963, and 1964 than there really were. But when I look back on it, I cannot think of any basically different alternatives than the ones that were taken at that particular moment of time.[47]

In any case, the Medicare bill (H.R. 6675) was passed by the House in April 1965, by a resounding vote of 315 to 115. It exceeded in scope and cost anything envisioned by the Johnson administration, and it was called a "three-layer cake" (it might have been called more aptly a "marble cake"); a stunning symbol of the art of political compromise in this country. In H.R. 6675, social insurance, public assistance, a means test, private enterprise, and physicians' sensibilities and prerogatives converged. From some points of view, the program authorized by the bill was a medical and administrative monstrosity: "the outcome of 1965 was, to be sure, a model of unintended consequences. The final legislative package incorporated features which no one had fully foreseen, and aligned supporters and opponents in ways which surprised many of the leading actors."[48] Monstrosity or not, the Medicare Act expressed Americans' overriding concern about their ability to pay their medical bills. It was not a reorganization of the health care delivery system. Further, the bill accepted the premise that more money needed to be poured into hospital and physician services to relieve the financial pressure on a vulnerable segment of the population, to sustain the going system financially, and to take an onerous burden off the private insurance agencies, which had never been designed, or able, to underwrite exceedingly high-risk or low-income groups. In essence, H.R. 6675 satisfied everyone and no one. Still, it laid the groundwork for a politically tolerable resolution of a special problem.

A perceptive article about Wilbur Mills published in *Fortune* before the passage of H.R. 6675 contains some observations worth quoting:

In capitalizing on the inevitable, Mills sought to resolve three points of principle that had continually bothered him in the years when he was resisting Medicare.[49] Mills, according to *Fortune*, was determined, first and foremost, that any new program of medical assistance should not endanger the actuarial and financial integrity of the social security funds, which supply some 20 million persons with the minimum cash necessary for daily living.

Regarded as a conservative, Mills would seem to symbolize a solid acceptance of the Social Security Act as part of the American social fabric. The funded pension concept (despite criticisms that OASDI is not insurance) flows directly from a middle-class American value of produce and pay your own way. Mills' second point was that he sought to preserve the independence of the medical profession. He had no desire to set in motion forces that might lead, "along whatever path of good intentions, to government control of doctors and hospitals." Finally, Mills wanted "to avoid undermining the usefulness of the private health-insurance industry."[50]

The status quo of the health services establishment was upheld, although there was a public policy breakthrough in covering the aged and in using the Social Security mechanism to do so. Mills seems to have attempted to contain this breakthrough by building in features that would make expanding the bill to cover other segments of the population politically cumbersome, expensive, and discouraging. Mills overcame the limitations of the earlier King-Anderson bill by combining its basic features with the AMA's Eldercare plan and the essentially Republican proposal for a voluntary system of financing health services for the aged.

The AMA held its annual meeting in New York City in June 1965, faced with the imminent passage of H.R. 6675 by the Senate. Members of the House of Delegates from several states hoped to put the house on record as favoring a physician boycott of this legislation should it pass. Before the meeting, incoming president James F. Appel had expressed his opposition to any type of strike or boycott, but he was prepared to support any stand taken by the house. The delegates' decision opposing a boycott came after a reference committee hearing, at which more than 80 physicians testified.[51] The house rejected nine resolutions dealing with nonparticipation in Medicare, but "recommended that M.D.'s be reminded that it is each individual physician's obligation to decide for himself whether the conditions of a case for which he is about to accept responsibility permit him to provide his own highest quality of medical care."[52] Thus reason prevailed, but, in order not to antagonize physicians unduly, the Medicare Act enshrined the principle of usual, reasonable, and customary as a basis for determining fees.

Hospitals were also held in some awe by Congress, in that the reimbursement method was charges or costs, whichever was lower, and retrospective payment. The providers were given, in effect, an open-ended budget.

Perhaps this observation is conventional and plausible wisdom, but Wilbur Cohen, who was in the thick of it, observed that the principle of "reasonable cost" for both hospital and physician services was never seriously debated or opposed during the period from 1961 to 1965 as far as he could recall:

> No one criticized it during the legislative process as a "cost plus" principle. No one thought of it as a basis for inflationary price or cost rises. It was accepted not only because no other alternative was proposed, but because conventional wisdom at the time accepted *reasonable cost as a reasonable principle* [emphasis mine].[53]

The economy was both affluent and quite stable with respect to price. The rush of inflation came later, upsetting all cost projections.

The Medicare Act became Title 18 of the Social Security Act. Title 19, which became known as the Medicaid Act, was added at the same time. Medicare was a controversial measure and hence received more publicity than Medicaid, medical care for the poor being more or less traditional for government and private philanthropic institutions. There have been no studies on the politics of medical care for the poor leading to Medicaid, as there have been for Medicare, perhaps because there was little "politics" involved compared with Medicare.[54] The major political issues involved in Medicaid were scope of services, income level, and federal and state responsibilities. In the case of Medicaid, American society struggled with its conscience; in Medicare, American society struggled less with its conscience than with the problem of how to keep the nuclear family solvent by taking the aging parents and grandparents off its back. The aged were implicated in Medicaid, however, because many of them were poor and not connected with the labor market and thus not able to afford the deductibles and coinsurance required of Medicare recipients.

The Medicaid Act was a descendent of the Kerr-Mills bill (Medical Assistance Act) enacted in 1960. It recognized the existence of medical indigents, particularly among the aged, and was related to the federal-state categorical programs of public assistance (that is, programs giving income to the aged, blind, disabled, and families with dependent children).

In 1974, all categories except families with dependent children were federalized under Supplemental Security Income; Aid to Families with Dependent Children (AFDC) remained a joint federal-state program. Medicaid recognized a medically indigent category for federal subsidy, should a state wish it.

The Medicaid Act solidified further the concept of using federal matching funds for the states to pay physicians. It increased reliance on the private sector through contractual arrangements with providers and insurance agencies to bring the poor into the mainstream of the delivery system. Medicaid mandated a comprehensive range of services if the states were to be eligible for matching grants. The determination of recipients' eligibility was left to the states. There were strong financial incentives for the states to participate, although funds were matched differentially, depending on a formula based on the states' respective incomes. Finally, the federal commitment was open-ended as long as the foregoing requirements were met.

The combined federal financing engines of Medicare and Medicaid plus voluntary health insurance coverage of about 80 percent of the population, funded in large part by employers' contributions, resulted in an unprecedented flow of funds to the health services, funds that were tax-free to the employer and employee. Further, government stimulated the supply of hospital beds through the Hill-Burton Act and various loans and grants to train more health personnel. The federal government was providing massive support for medical research, which inevitably led to more effective and more expensive services. Thus, during the Johnson administration there was an outpouring of health legislation—and a resultant rise in expenditures.

NOTES

1. Max J. Skidmore, *Medicare and the Rhetoric of Reconciliation* (University, Ala.: University of Alabama Press, 1979). This book provides a worthwhile short history of the Social Security Act through the debate on Medicare for the elderly.
2. Odin W. Anderson, Patricia Collette, and Jacob J. Feldman, *Changes in Family Medical Care Expenditures and Voluntary Health Insurance, A Five-Year Resurvey* (Cambridge, Mass.: Harvard University Press, 1961), p. 3.
3. See, for example, U.S. Department of Health, Education, and Welfare, Special Staff on Aging, *The Nation and Its Older People: Report of the White House Conference on Aging* (Washington, D.C.: Government Printing Office, 1961).
4. *AMA News* (23 February 1959):2.
5. *Hospitals* 34 (1 January 1960):58.
6. "Health Care for the Retired Aged: Compulsory National Solutions or Voluntary Local Action?" *Hospitals* 34 (1 February 1960):48.
7. John D. Morris, "8 in GOP Offer Bill to Aid Aged," *New York Times*, 8 April 1960, p. 1.

8. ———, "1.2 Billion a Year Asked to Aid Aged," *New York Times*, 5 May 1960, p. 1.
9. Austin C. Wehrwein, "AMA Denounces Eisenhower Plan for the Care of the Aged," *New York Times*, 6 May 1960, p. 1.
10. Ibid.
11. "Governors Back Aged Care Plan," *New York Times*, 30 June 1960, Sect. C, p. 30.
12. "GOP View on Eldercare," *Washington Report on the Medical Sciences*, August 1960.
13. "Official Notes," *Hospitals* 30 (1 January 1956):80.
14. Official Proceedings of the House of Delegates, November 1956 and December 1957, in American Medical Association, *Digest of Official Actions, 1846–1958* (Chicago: American Medical Association, 1958), p. 348.
15. Ibid., p. 351.
16. *AMA News* 2 (9 February 1959):1.
17. "CMA Backs Aged Health Fund Plan," *San Francisco Chronicle*, 25 February 1960, p. 8.
18. "Health Goals for the Nation," *New York Times*, 10 February 1960, p. 8.
19. Robert R. Neal, "HIAA Girds Itself to Meet Challenge," *Eastern Underwriter* 60 (December 1959):58.
20. John D. Morris, "Kennedy Submits Aged Care Plan, Staff Fight Likely," *New York Times*, 10 February 1961, p. 1.
21. U.S. Department of Health, Education, and Welfare, *Nation*, p. 3.
22. Ibid., p. v.
23. Ibid., p. 129.
24. Text of John F. Kennedy's State of the Union Message, *New York Times*, 12 January 1962, sect. C, p. 12.
25. Marjorie Hunter, "23 Senators Give Compromise Plan on Medical Care," *New York Times*, 30 June 1962, p. 1.
26. "Ribicoff Accused of Lobbying Activity," *New York Times*, 10 May 1962, p. 27.
27. See Martha Derthick's well-documented study of politics and the management of Social Security funds, *Policy Making for Social Security* (Washington, D.C.: Brookings Institution, 1979).
28. Alfred E. Clark, "200 Jersey Doctors Back Move to Boycott Kennedy Health Plan," *New York Times*, 5 May 1962, p. 1.
29. George Cable Wright, "Jersey Assembly Attacks Doctors," *New York Times*, 5 May 1962, p. 1.
30. "New Jersey's Medical Society Divisions Threaten to Boycott Aged Care Measure," *Wall Street Journal*, 15 May 1962, p. 8.
31. "The Changing Order," *New England Journal of Medicine* 255 (20 July 1961):144.
32. American Hospital Association. Publicity release, July 1962.
33. "President's Plan for Medical Care Killed by Senate," *Wall Street Journal*, 18 July 1962, p. 2.
34. Ibid.

35. "Health Insurance Benefits Bill of 1963," *Congressional Record* 109 (19 February 1963):2367.
36. Ibid.
37. "Long-Sought Agreement Nears," *Medical World News*, 10 May 1963.
38. Marjorie Hunter, "New Plan Is Given on Medical Care," *New York Times*, 14 November 1963, sect. C, p. 5.
39. ———, "Aged Care Clears Senate, 60–28, House Delay Seen," *New York Times*, 4 September 1964, p. 1.
40. ———, "Administration Bill for Aid to Aged Through Social Security Dies as Congressional Conference Fails to Break Deadlock," *New York Times*, 3 October 1964.
41. Eve Edstrom, "Barry Calls Health Bill Unnecessary," *Washington Post and Times-Herald*, 21 July 1964, p. 2.
42. "AMA Program Offers Wide Health Coverage for Aging," *AMA News* 7 (18 January 1965):1.
43. "AMA Approves Last-Ditch Fight to Block 'Medicare,' Substitute Its Eldercare Plan," *Wall Street Journal*, 8 February 1965, p. 10.
44. Wilbur Cohen, "Medicare, Medicaid: 10 Lessons Learned," *Hospitals* 59 (August 1, 1985):6.
45. Michael J. O'Neil, "Capital Records," *Medical World News* (June 25, 1965):166.
46. The best account so far, in large part because of the authors' access to the principals, is Theodore R. Marmor and Jan S. Marmor, *The Politics of Medicare* (London: Routledge and Kegan Paul, 1970). See also James L. Sundquist, *Politics and Policy: The Eisenhower, Kennedy, and Johnson Years* (Washington, D.C.: Brookings Institution, 1968).
47. Reported in Robert H. Haveman, ed., *A Decade of Federal Antipoverty Programs: Achievements, Failures, and Lessons*, University of Wisconsin–Madison Institute for Research on Poverty, Poverty Policy Analysis Series (New York: Academic Press, 1977), p. 189.
48. Theodore R. Marmor and Jan S. Marmor, *The Politics of Medicare* (London: Routledge and Kegan Paul, 1970), p. 82.
49. Harold B. Meyers," Mr. Mills' Elder- Medi- Better Care," *Fortune* 71 (June 1965):166.
50. Ibid.
51. *AMA News* 8 (July 5, 1965):10.
52. Ibid.
53. Wilbur Cohen, "Medicare, Medicaid: 10 Lessons Learned." *Hospitals* 59 (August 1, 1985): 8.
54. The one that comes closest to the politics of medical care for the poor is Robert Stevens and Rosemary Stevens' *Welfare Medicine in America: A Case Study of Medicaid* (New York: Free Press, 1974). This book deals mainly with the experience rather than the legislative and political process of Medicaid, as do Steven M. Davidson, *Medicaid Decisions: A Systematic Analysis of the Cost Problem* (Cambridge, Mass.: Ballinger, 1980) and John Holahan, *Financing Medical Care for the Poor* (Lexington, Mass.: Lexington Books, 1975).

PART IV

The Era of Management and Control, 1965 to the Present

14

Attempts to Determine
Order and Direction

INTRODUCTION

The considerable increase in government funding of the health services, on top of private funding from voluntary health insurance, set the stage for the boom in the health services economy—or cost escalation, as it is popularly known.

Concepts of regulation, planning, management, and control of the health services enterprise began to be considered, albeit tentatively, in the latter fifties and early sixties, concurrent with the deliberations on Medicare and Medicaid. There was some doubt about the wisdom of increasing the supply of facilities and physicians, but there was great faith in promoting medical research. The latter would, of course, increase demand and costs. The sixties reveal this confusion of objectives, which became more explicit in the seventies.

It is difficult to set forth a coherent account retrospectively, since one cannot read into events a compelling logic and order that were not there. By the end of the fifties, Herman and Ann Somers had published a useful book on the status of the American health services; they pay particular attention to funding sources, especially voluntary health insurance. This book helped me to understand the welter of the period.[1]

It may be appropriate at this point to pause and take stock of the level of expenditures, use, and availability, in the aggregate, of personnel and facilities in 1965 (Table 14.1). There were the following hospital beds in 1965:

— 7,000 hospitals with 1,616 million beds
— 6,500 general hospitals with 1,069 million beds

TABLE 14.1   Health Care Expenditures in 1965*

Source and Destination of Funds	Percent
Sources of Funds	
Private (total)	78
Direct payment	51
Insurance	27
Public	
Federal	9
State and federal	12
Destination of Funds	
Hospital	
Private (total)	61
Direct payment	17
Insurance	44
Public	39
Physicians	
Private (total)	93
Direct payment	61
Insurance	32
Public	7
All other services	
Private (total)	87
Direct payment	82
Insurance	5
Public	13
Service Components' Share	
Hospital	37
Physician	23
Dentist	7
Drugs	15
Nursing home	6
Other	12

*Total expenditures on health care were $39 billion, or $198 per person, and constituted 5.9 percent of the gross national product.

— 4.2 general hospital beds per 1,000 population

— 3,676 nonprofit general hospitals with 552,000 beds

— 969 proprietary general hospitals with 54,100 beds

Approximately one-half of the general hospital beds were in nonprofit hospitals, but nonprofit hospitals continued to provide the bulk of the general hospital care. Church-owned beds accounted for around 25 percent of all general nonprofit hospital beds.

There were the following medical and dental personnel in 1965:

— 305,000 physicians, or 153 per 100,000 population

— 613,000 nurses, or 319 per 100,000 population

— 109,000 dentists, or 56 per 100,000 population

— 100,000 pharmacists, or 50 per 100,000 population

Insurance coverage was as follows:

— 71 percent of the population had hospital insurance

— 66 percent had surgical insurance

— 35 percent had major medical insurance (which overlaps hospital and surgical insurance)

— 20 percent of the population (age 65 and over) was covered by Medicare

— 5 percent was potentially covered by Medicaid

Utilization of services had been increasing every year, according to surveys. With an increasing proportion of services being covered by third party payers, there was no incentive on the part of patients or providers to contain costs. The cost per inpatient day for the voluntary hospitals stood at $45, up from $33 five years earlier. Hospital personnel per 100 patients stood at 252, up from 232 in 1960 (and up from 191 in 1950). Clearly, all indications were that cost increases would continue. What was not foreseen was the rising inflation, which exacerbated the problem.

In the late fifties and early sixties, the government and the country were beginning to try to specify problems more clearly and to impose more "system" on the health services enterprise. This meant coordination, integration, planning—all of the emerging buzz words. They were applied to specific services, in the case of mental health, and to global efforts as well.

One of the most intractable health problems is mental illness. National concern in the form of the Joint Commission on Mental Health and Illness preceded by a few years concern with other, somatic diseases, rising costs, and the organization of health services. In 1955, Congress passed the Mental Health Study Act. A series of excellent studies was completed covering needed personnel, social costs of mental illness, and concepts of mental health. This last was exceptionally good in that it examined the very concept of mental illness itself.[2] The studies culminated in a landmark report for the mental health field in 1961.[3] Although the recommendations of the commission were by no means startling, they were nevertheless necessary (for example, deemphasizing institutional care in favor of day care in community clinics).

The commission undoubtedly set the tone for subsequent, and salutary, developments in the mental health field that are now creating new problems, such as mental illness ghettos in the cities.

As for personnel, the U.S. Public Health Service prepared reports in consultation with relevant interest groups on the need for more nurses.[4] A voluntary group called the National Commission on Community Health Services was set up by the American Public Health Association and the National Health Council (NHC)—APHA being a group of public health professionals and NHC being a federation of voluntary health agencies. This commission was financed by several philanthropic foundations. In a highly systematic manner, it organized its activities into three projects. In one, six task forces were set up to deal with a wide range of health problems, from the effect of the environment on health to personal health services delivery systems. In another, 21 "successful" community programs throughout the country were evaluated. The third project dealt with the dissemination of health information. The commission's recommendations were quite general and rather self-evident: the desirability of health service areas, a general physician for everyone, comprehensive services, effective use of health personnel, and so on.[5] Although the voluntary sector of the health services was stressed, it was suggested that official public health agencies should be the major vehicles for carrying out these recommendations.

The global nature of the commission's recommendations is typical. Lacking a strategy, even a general one, most such commissions issue their recommendations as challenges and exhortations in a cloud of moralisms. An exception among the dozen or so reports published by the APHA-NHC commission was one by a political scientist who applied some social-system power-structure concepts to the analysis of five community programs that were deemed experimental and "successful." His observations were directed chiefly to the feasibility of planning at all in the American social and political context. He concludes, in colorful style:

> Nowhere in this free-wheeling, pluralistic, local autonomy will planners (health or otherwise) ever achieve the ideal state of affairs in which unadulterated schemes of technicians become the holy script of political leaders and policy implementers. In any event, sophisticated planners no longer see a comprehensive plan as the end of planning; they now visualize a planning process in which plans are formulated in broad contexts, offered to policy leaders as guidelines, and subjected to continuing restudy in an interplay between planners and policy leaders.[6]

Nowhere in the APHA-NHC commission's reports was there any recognition of the politics of health care. The bland statement that follows is an example of the lowest common denominator characteristic of committee reports generally:

> The responsible participation and involvement of all sectors of the community, coordination of efforts, and development of cooperative working arrangements are fundamental to effective action-planning. Health service objectives can be met through processes which provide opportunity for citizens to work together to understand . . . [etc., etc.][7]

The sixties, however, did see the establishment of a planning philosophy, such as it was, and a series of mechanisms to work toward a more visible system of interrelated health services. The conventional wisdom was that what was not set up formally could not possibly be a system. It was not generally recognized that there exists an informal network without which no formal system could operate.

The Hospital Survey and Construction Act of 1946 is regarded as the beginning of systems thinking, because the states had to inventory all their hospitals, draw up a general plan of adequate supply and undersupply, particularly for rural areas, and avoid duplication.[8] Some 15 years later, the report of a joint committee of the AHA and the PHS *Areawide Planning for Hospitals and Related Facilities,* was published.[9] This report represented a joint attempt by the public and private sectors to establish planning as an ongoing process, particularly in metropolitan areas. It was a partnership between the hospitals, through the AHA, and the federal government, through the PHS. Both sectors represented the public interest, the hospitals as community-oriented institutions and the PHS as an institution accountable to the Congress through HEW.

The committee was building on the hospital planning councils already in place in the major cities, such as Philadelphia, New York, and Chicago. These planning councils enabled hospital administrators in a given area to confer with one another and acted as clearinghouses for hospital operation information. As reported by the joint committee, however, few of the planning councils were genuinely representative of the community.[10] Only 12 or 13 of the 26 staffed councils were engaged in long-range planning. Financing varied widely, with hospital membership dues supporting from 10 to 75 percent of the costs of the councils; other funds came from Blue Cross plans, foundations, United Funds or community chests, and fees for special services. Voluntary planning associations were also funded by contributions from industry and membership organizations.

The Community Health Services and Facilities Act of 1961 was intended to stimulate and coordinate community health planning. The federal government, which had supported the joint committee and published its report, began to provide relatively large sums of money for development grants and operating funds for areawide planning agencies throughout the country. The number of such voluntary agencies increased from 14, when the report was published, to 25 in 1962, to 80 in 1966. In addition, the PHS, beginning in 1963, sponsored a number of annual institutes for the staffs of the planning agencies. It is reported that these institutes were well attended.

The first grant made under the act was in June 1961. In 1964, the Hill-Harris amendments to the Hill-Burton Act augmented the funds for planning and made it possible to provide matching funds to establish planning agencies in areas where there were none. By 1967, more than one-half of the 80 agencies in existence were receiving grants totalling $13 million.

In September 1963, the PHS prepared a manual to amplify the recommendations made in the report of the joint committee. The staffs attending the various institutes discussed the manual. From these discussions there emanated a list of 22 purposes and goals that the planning agencies should set for themselves, such as maintaining and improving the quality of care as economically as possible; discouraging duplication of facilities, developing more effective integration of facilities; determining and projecting needs for services, facilities, and personnel; maintaining flexibility in planning; maintaining a central storehouse of information for the area; and so on. In other words, the planning agencies were to do everything. A feasible task was to act as a central source of information on the health services and community characteristics.

This description may seem a little churlish, but the joint committee and the PHS had an intuitive sense of what was possible in the American context. Their intention seems to have been to establish a climate of planning, or at least of reasoning together, in a situation where a central authority was clearly unacceptable. As observed by May: "the only way such decisions [as the proper distribution of hospital beds] can be reached 'correctly' is with the participation of all interested parties in a setting where the horizons are broad enough to include the entire establishment."[11] When the horizons are broad enough, the result is a very low common denominator of agreement. Nevertheless, faith in the need for the concept of planning, if not in the procedures necessary for planning, continued on the federal level and found further expression in the Comprehensive Health Planning and Public Health Service Amendments of 1966 (Public Law 89–749), which went into effect on November 3, 1966.

This law, together with amendments to it in 1967, reveal a concerted effort on the part of the federal government to consolidate the large number of discrete programs operating side by side on state and local levels. More important was the apparent attempt to create a formal structure within which federal funds would be dispensed. The act enjoined the various agencies involved to establish communications and relations between various levels of government to encourage some "comprehensive planning." Staffs of planning agencies began to include economists, sociologists, demographers, and statisticians. The result was a tremendous increase in data and information, although not much else.

The slight impact of the areawide planning endeavors by 1967 was documented by Douglas R. Brown, who visited 30 hospital and health facility planning councils and interviewed 75 members of planning staffs. His main conclusion was that hospital planning at the local level was essentially a process enabling representatives of major business and industrial health care providers and planners to get together periodically. He wrote: "the process appeared to be incremental and designed to foster mutual adjustments among parties involved.[12]

Concurrent with the passage of the Comprehensive Health Planning legislation of 1966, which was intended to deal with the coordination and integration of facilities, mainly hospitals, was the passage of the Education, Research, Training, and Demonstrations Act (Public Law 89–239). This act was intended to coordinate and integrate the results of research in the university teaching and research establishments with clinical medicine. The idea was to facilitate the application of new techniques for treating heart disease, cancer, stroke, and related diseases. The prevailing delivery system was not to be modified, at least not directly, but its effectiveness was to be improved. The medical schools wanted money, and this was one way in which they could direct their efforts toward the community. The diseases mentioned are the chief killers and there was great public and political interest in attacking them frontally. After Johnson became president in his own right in 1965, his administration brought forth a spate of health legislation in the "war on poverty." This was a heady period for liberals and related social reformers.

Characteristically, Presidents work through commissions on various problems. This was done in the case of heart disease, cancer, and stroke, which led to the legislation described. Commissions, again characteristically, are composed of knowledgeable and dedicated people with special interests that do not necessarily coincide perfectly with the public interest, assuming the public interest can be defined precisely. This type of representation is understood and condoned, and it provides a legitimate forum for policy recommendations.

In the mid-sixties, more and more interest in the cost of the health services emerged. Still, cost was approached obliquely, through questions of supply and personnel, delivery methods, and, most sensitive, regulation.

President Johnson set up in 1966 a national advisory committee that was to deal with the question of supply of health personnel, but that actually ranged over all health services problems, particularly methods of delivery. The committee was composed, as usual, of the most eminent citizens and professionals the country could produce, and the task forces were staffed with well-qualified investigators, a category of personnel with which this country is well supplied. The report reflects the gung-ho style of the president and his search for quick solutions, which forced the committee to act in great haste. The result was a low level of theoretical and systems thinking, reflected in the report's naive suggestion that the health services be completely reorganized. Given the general sophistication of the staff and the members of the committee, it is hard to believe that they believed in what they had formulated. The report clearly indicates frustration. In neither the public nor the private sectors did the committee point to possible levers for reshaping the health system into the "rational" organization it sought. Although an overhaul of the system was suggested, the committee was fearful of giving control over construction of health facilities to areawide planning agencies, the very agencies the government was already funding, because "there is a long history of regulatory agencies becoming defenders of the status quo rather than promoters of innovation and change."[13] The committee was unwilling to give any agency leverage, while at the same time it was distressed with the prevailing and ineffective style of negotiation and bargaining between the parties at interest (ineffective, that is, in terms of cost control). Alternative models and their consequences were not evaluated; instead, the committee seemed to hope that a "rational" model could be an amalgam of all the advantages of the existing system with none of its disadvantages, a systems impossibility.[14]

A year later, the government made another attempt to consider the cost of health services. It limited the scope of its inquiry to hospitals because they were the largest and most rapidly growing cost component of health services. The inquiry could more logically have been directed toward physicians, who control hospital admissions and discharges and orders for services. This body was created by HEW Secretary John Gardner and was called the Secretary's Advisory Committee on Hospital Effectiveness. Apparently Gardner was not sanguine about being able to improve the health services immediately, as revealed in his instructions to the committee:

> There is not any agreement yet as to what more effective systems of health care ought to look like . . . certainly there isn't any agreement as to what

the organizing focus should be. But it is clear that there is going to be some kind of organizing focus. The system is going to be more interdependent than it is now, more interrelated, the various institutions are going to relate to one another in more orderly ways, and this suggests that there is going to be some order.[15]

The committee's aim was to create some order out of the presumed "nonsystem," which did not exhibit any clear bureaucratic structure. The reasons stimulating the investigation were the same as those that led to similar efforts in countries whose delivery systems were far more ordered than ours, such as Great Britain and Sweden: the sharply rising costs of hospital care.

The committee was assembled and chaired by the dean of the School of Business of Northwestern University, presumably to emphasize the managerial and economic aspects of the hospital industry. To avoid the global pretentions of previous reports, both private and public, the committee agreed "that its specific recommendations would be few in number, high in priority, and pregnant with potential consequences." The pregnancy metaphor suggested that something tangible had to result. Recognizing that their recommendations could be nothing more than a litany of desirable goals, the committee also decided that its calls for action must be stated specifically and that they should be capable of implementation in the foreseeable future. Finally, it was decreed that the recommendations must be "doable" rather than conceptual in nature (as if "doable" did not require a concept of what is practical) and that they must identify the persons and groups required to act.[16] This was raw pragmatism, but look at the recommendations.

The committee started with a premise and followed up with principles of implementation, which were to be applied through particular techniques of management:

> Given the extraordinary circumstances resulting from the nature of the health services [the need for community and professional "thrusts" rather than the profit motive], the Committee is convinced that the service must remain complex and pluralistic, and that its problems are not susceptible of solution either by the introduction of competitive forces or by monolithic centralized planning and controls. No such simplistic solution is sought or proposed in the recommendations here, and none is considered feasible.[17]

This premise puts the committee in a dilemma, given the Secretary's directive that there be some order:

> Instead, the Committee has considered that the key to solution of the problems of the health service as it exists, with the hospital already established as a central core of medical intelligence and activity, must lie in the

introduction of motivation and controls that can be expected to bring shape and a system to a service that has remained formless and disjunctive. The Committee believes an element of planning may be injected into the service in such a way as to compel improvements in effectiveness without directing the application of specific methods.[18]

This seems to suggest a variety of incentives rather than direct orders or regulations that would provide a framework in which details could be worked out. The gist of the recommendations is as follows:

1. All facilities should be in an areawide health service planning agency, and the facilities should each submit an institutional service plan to the planning agency annually. In turn, the planning agency should publish an areawide plan and guidelines for determining needs and programs.

2. The franchising and licensing powers of the state should be used for construction in connection with capital funds from the federal government, which are to be filtered through the local planning councils.

3. Physicians should be brought into the budget planning of the hospitals so that they acquire an understanding of finance. There should be more detailed internal budget reviews and cost accounting, as well as joint purchasing by groups of hospitals.

4. Health insurance agencies should formulate benefit packages that encourage the use of outpatient services rather than inpatient services.

The ideological underpinning of these recommendations is revealed in the following passage, a clear expression of the preferred American style:

> The Committee is convinced . . . that areawide planning should be done by voluntary nonprofit agencies whose governing boards are composed of leaders of decision-makers representing all elements of the community, including users as well as providers of health services. State authority should be called on only when the areawide planning agency isn't functioning [a nonfunctioning agency was not defined].[19]

The recommendations confirmed and sanctioned trends already established. They would lead to some degree of "structured pluralism," but the extent to which they would bring about a generally acceptable degree of order is hardly clear. There was faith in the very process, and this, presumably, is what the American political process is all about.

The committee's recommendations reflected the emergence of "corporate rationalizers," to use Alford's term.[20] Corporate rationalization is promoted by insurance agencies, hospitals, health planning agencies, medical schools, and public health agencies. They do battle with what Alford calls professional monopolists—that is, physicians in private or group practice and other health occupations holding or striving for professional status and who differ in their relations to each other and to the bureaucratic types of agencies mentioned. A third group striving to have some say in the operation of the health services is the various citizens' groups, the committee's "leaders of decision-makers representing all elements of the community."

In the American context, "order" is an acceptable and tenuous equilibrium between contending and cooperating interests. Also in 1967, and seemingly continuing the trend toward greater corporate rationalization, another national commission on health facilities was set up, with the usual array of distinguished experts and citizens; it was called the National Advisory Commission on Health Facilities. Its report went to the president and seemed less concerned with facilities, as such, than with their systematic organization into regional areas and comprehensive services.[21]

In July 1969, the Secretary of HEW set up the Task Force on Medicaid and Related Programs. This task force appeared to pick up the pieces after the fiasco of the Manpower Committee, in that it attempted to approach the financing, administration, and planning of health services as a total system. The task force was originally charged with examining the status of Medicaid, the health services program for the low-income segment of the population that was administered by the states and funded approximately one-half by the states and one-half by the federal government. Later in 1969, the charge to the task force was broadened to deal with the entire health services enterprise on the assumption that health care for the poor was an integral part of health care for the entire population. The traditionally residual nature of health care for the poor was to be erased, and the poor were to brought into the mainstream of health services.

Since its inauguration in 1966, Medicaid had expanded tremendously—beyond all predictions. It was now clear that Medicaid had perpetuated a patchwork of inadequate and underfinanced services among a great majority of the states. Expanding the review of care for the poor to a review of care for everybody was a logical sequence and was politically attractive.

This task force was made up of leading authorities in the health field, representing voluntary health insurance, government, all providers, and the social services. The chairman at that time was Walter J. McNerney, who headed the Blue Cross Association. McNerney had a thorough grasp of the health field, operationally, politically, and financially. In this task force's report, in contrast to previous ones, there emerged the basic structure of the health delivery system, involving concepts of competition, incentives, management, and performance indicators.[22]

For the first time in either public or private commission reports on the health services, the nature and structure of American social and political life was taken into account, as well as how a health service must relate itself to society in order to bring about reform. Although the task force claimed it "had no prescription for a new health care delivery system," it came very close to suggesting one; the ideal implicit in its report was group practice prepayment for the entire population. The task force's immediate objective was to suggest competition among a variety of delivery systems from which consumers could choose. A precedent had been established for federal employees in the Federal Employees' Health Benefits Program, which was inaugurated in 1961.[23]

Presumably, various methods of delivery would emerge from the explicit specifications as to range of services, accessibility, and so on to be established by the federal government, but prices should be competitive:

> . . . to provide all consumers with a greater range of choice among alternative forms of delivery and with the information to make the purchase decision a meaningful one. By thus subjecting the system to increased consumer-purchasing power, responsiveness can be increased without relying solely on centralized planning and direction.[24]

Although "there are no easy solutions," competition may well promise greater efficiency in the system:

> But competition within the health-care system also has obvious risks. The first risk is that choices made by consumers may be misguided by ignorance. The second risk is that competition among organizational modes may of itself tend to separate the parts and obscure the view of the system as a whole; one man's pluralism is another man's incoherence.[25]

In order to mitigate both risks, however, the report continues: "To safeguard the system against the hazards of provider self-interest, consumer ignorance, and pragmatism, it must be managed."[26] This managing was to be entrusted to HEW, the only agency charged with brooding over the entire "public interest," on the assumption that providers and consumers cannot manage for themselves. As far as looking after the "public interest" goes, the report stated a series of incompatible objectives, a common problem in recommendations to change the organization of health services delivery:

As it is envisioned and recommended here, the management function for the health-care system is to be innovative, but not prescriptive; bold, but not authoritarian. It is the intention that the federal leadership as far as possible shall guide, not direct; motivate, not demand; assist, not provide; and evaluate, not ordain. . . . Somewhere between the extremes of Adam Smith's "invisible hand" and a monolithic governmental health care system is an imposition of logical structure by Government on the health system.[27]

This philosophy stems directly from the concept of limited government and the balancing of the private and public sectors in some kind of interrelated whole. The ability of any central agency to be as judicious as this quotation implies is another question. The recommendation for the competitive model implies that it is not easy to specify consumer needs and wants and provider performance.

The Medicaid task force's report essentially sets up the pluralistic model of competition, negotiation, and bargaining while at the same time assuming that the agency acting in the public interest can specify what that is. The task force called this the "performance-contracting" approach and stated that it required expertise in contract administration and the ability to define objectives and indicators of performance.[28] In the very next sentence, however, the task force stated: "It is generally agreed that the state of the art in measuring the performance of healthcare services organization is still relatively primitive." The task force found at least a partial solution in the creation of Health Maintenance Organizations (HMOs), group practice prepayment plans and fee-for-service variants. HMOs are excellent examples of performance contracting in the health field. They sell a total package of health services at a contract price for a specified period. Providers police themselves. Given the primitive status of performance indicators, guidelines for performance could be quite general and limited: range of services, price of services, and access to services.

Although the report visualized greater efficiency resulting in net savings, nevertheless:

If the nation is serious about a commitment to a basic plan of health care for all citizens, a considerable amount of financing and a larger investment of manpower and facilities resources are required. By a simple extension of the $5 billion cost of providing service for 10 million people, for example, one can approximate the cost of providing the same service for 25 million. While this would not be all "new money" and while some economies may certainly be anticipated from the more effective methods of organizing and providing service that have been recommended here, the recommendations for better and more comprehensive service for all who are covered would have a countervailing effect.[29]

This pointed to the need for a reference point beyond the mainstream model of delivery. Basically, the report suggested the setting up of a structured pluralism, within which various delivery options would compete with each other under governmental guidelines. This model would require government regulations in order to assure competition.

NOTES

1. Herman Somers and Ann Somers, *Doctors, Patients, and Health Insurance, The Organization and Financing of Medical Care* (Washington, D.C.: Brookings Institution, 1961).
2. Marie Jahoda, *Current Concepts of Positive Mental Health* (New York: Basic Books, 1958).
3. Joint Commission on Mental Health and Illness, *Action for Mental Health* (New York: Science Edition, 1961).
4. Surgeon General's Consultant Group on Nursing, *Toward Quality Nursing— Needs and Goals*, U.S. Public Health Service Publication No. 992 (Washington, D.C.: Government Printing Office, 1963).
5. National Commission on Community Health Services, *Health Is a Community Affair* (Cambridge, Mass.: Harvard University Press, 1966).
6. Ralph W. Conant, "The Politics of Community Health" in National Commission on Community Health Services, *Report of the Community Action Studies Project*, (Washington, D.C.: Public Affairs Press, 1968), p. 104.
7. National Commission, *Health*, p. 221.
8. Much of my material on planning is drawn from J. Joel May, *Health Planning, Its Past and Potential*, Health Administration Perspectives No. A5 (Chicago: Center for Health Administration Studies, Graduate School of Business, University of Chicago, 1967).
9. Joint Committee of the American Hospital Association and U.S. Public Health Service, *Areawide Planning for Hospitals and Related Health Facilities* (Pub. No. 855) (Washington, D.C.: U.S. Public Health Service, 1961).
10. Ibid., p. 37.
11. Ibid., p. 9.
12. Douglas R. Brown, *The Areawide Planning Process*, Publication No. PB-197–267 (Springfield, Va.: National Technical Information Service, March 1971).
13. National Advisory Committee on Health Manpower, *Report* (Washington, D.C.: Government Printing Office, 1967), vol. 1, p. 69.
14. A detailed critique of this report appears in Odin W. Anderson, "Book Report" *Health Services Research* 3 (Spring 1968):65–70.
15. U.S. Department of Health, Education, and Welfare, Secretary's Advisory Committee on Hospital Effectiveness, *Report* (Washington D.C.: Government Printing Office, 1968), p. 1.
16. Ibid., p. 4.
17. Ibid., p. 10.
18. Ibid.

19. Ibid.
20. Robert R. Alford, *Health Care Politics: Ideological and Interest Group Barriers to Reform* (Chicago: University of Chicago Press, Phoenix, 1977), pp. 191–92. This book deals with attempts to reform the health services in New York City (a prototype of the national picture) and reveals the intensity of local health politics.
21. National Advisory Commission on Health Facilities, *Report to the President* (Washington, D.C.: Government Printing Office, 1969).
22. U.S. Department of Health, Education, and Welfare, *Report of the Task Force on Medicaid and Related Programs* (Washington, D.C.: Government Printing Office, 1970).
23. Odin W. Anderson and J. Joel May, *The Federal Employees' Health Benefits Program, 1961–1968: A Model for National Health Insurance?* Health Administration Perspectives No. A9 (Chicago: Center for Health Administration Studies, Graduate School of Business, University of Chicago, 1971).
24. U.S. Department of Health, Education, and Welfare, *Task Force*, p. 5.
25. Ibid., p. 3.
26. Ibid.
27. Ibid., p. 53.
28. Ibid., p. 60.
29. Ibid., p. 13.

15

Emerging Regulatory Methods

During the Eisenhower administration, political concern with the operation of voluntary health insurance and the organization of service began to appear in the form of legislation and litigation. The legal framework for delivering and buying services was taking shape. (Even a free enterprise system needs a legal framework in which to operate, a basic element of which is the enforcement of contract freely agreed to by buyer and seller.) Although the health services system in the United States in the 1960s was essentially nongovernmental, government operated at strategic points for special groups and problems, with increasingly legal implications.

The legal basis for the system is the laws that apply to all organized activities, such as those established for incorporation, which focus on public accountability. In the case of health professionals, state licensing laws designate who is qualified to engage in specified activities, in order to protect the public. (Another, less charitable school of thought points out that licensing laws, in contrast to registration laws, create a monopoly for those who qualify.) Within this framework, the health services system had operated with little official scrutiny from public agencies.

Third party payers left a host of legal and regulatory problems in their wake. For example, when nonprofit prepayment plans were developed in the 1930s, the laws applying to private insurance companies with respect to cash reserves, adequacy of premiums, form of incorporation, and so on were found lacking. Most states felt the need for enabling legislation to declare that the nonprofit plans provided a quasi-insurance that did not need the high reserves generally required. Thus the plans were to be exempt from taxes.[1] Such laws stemmed from the charitable and nonprofit traditions rather than the profit-oriented sector of the economy, and they became an example of social innovation in the public interest.

An attorney who served as legal counsel for the group practice plans in their formative years, Horace R. Hansen, observed:

> State legislation specifically authorizing prepaid medical care plans has only two basic purposes: to obtain release from the prohibition against corporate practice of medicine and to avoid application of the insurance laws of the state. As of the end of 1961, there are 18 states having enabling statutes suitable for either doctor or consumer sponsorship; there are 5 states having acts intended for use only by consumer-sponsored plans; and there are 17 states having acts restricted to use by doctor-sponsored plans. The balance of states and D.C. have no special statutes in the field. . . . [A]s one looks generally at all of the laws affecting group health plans throughout the United States . . . a trend toward a clearer legal climate for group health plans is discernible. Each year that passes clears away a little more of the legal obstacles. . . . [O]ur situation in the common law is good and getting better.[2]

Hansen's observations reveal the underlying legislative and legal support countervailing the attempts of organized medicine to monopolize not only diagnosis and therapy, but also methods of delivery.

Although certain types of health insurance have been fit into old legal modes, what is still unresolved is what constitutes the corporate practice of medicine.[3] There is consensus that, as professionals, physicians should be personally responsible and that no agency should engage them and "profit" from the services provided by them. Yet these traditional concepts are encountering new situations. Having more parties involved with big money diffuses accountability. With the development since World War II of more hospital and medical centers offering more new services and with the widening range of medical specialties, diverse organizational structures have arisen and various ways of engaging and paying physicians have resulted. These varying and often complex methods must hold up not only in courts of law, but also in the court of prevailing principles and ethics. Whenever a new technology emerges in medicine, questions that seemed to have been settled arise again in the new context.

By the 1960s, the United States had entered an era in which health services and their prices added up to an increase in expenditures. We began to look for "waste" and "inefficiency" and "duplication" in the system in order to reduce overall expenditures, or at least to slow their increase. We began to reconsider the nature of a professional service in terms of "proper" level of use, how quality is measured, and "proper" levels of expenditure. These issues were just beginning to be raised; attempts to quantify them remained far in the future.

The following developments illustrate what was taking place in the sixties.[4] The pharmaceutical industry came under heavy fire at the end of the 1950s from the Senate Subcommittee on Antitrust and Monopoly, headed by Senator Estes Kefauver (D-Tenn.). The industry had become very visible with effective and profitable development of antibiotics. The hearings were lively and evoked tremendous publicity. The issues in the 1960–61 hearings were the price of drugs and allegations of monopolistic practices. The fallout was an attempt to tighten laws on standards and adequacy of field trials before products were marketed. Quality as such was not in question; rather, Kefauver was trying to attack prices and profit margins.

Kefauver was not in favor of price control, nor did he intend to undermine the prevailing structure of the industry. He used the legislative privilege of investigation as a countervailing power against an industry that was becoming more and more important to the health services of the nation and that had experienced spectacular growth and development during the previous 20 years. In fact, the pharmaceutical industry was directly responsible for a great deal of the improvement in health indexes relating to communicable and infectious disease during those years.

The pharmaceutical industry is "clothed with the public interest," and Kefauver exploited this fact skillfully, keeping himself and his cause in the headlines. The publicity subsided eventually, but government had shown how it could affect prices indirectly by "jawboning"; the allegation of monopolistic pricing was not proven.

The Blue Cross plans' first serious encounter was with a state insurance commissioner in Michigan in November 1955. The Michigan Hospital Service filed a request with the state commission of insurance for a 23 percent rate increase. This request was startling and unprecedented in its magnitude. It sent shock waves through the hospital service enterprise and, as reported by a special study group, "the request triggered a series of quick responses from labor and government for investigation of hospital costs and prepayment."[5]

G. Mennen Williams, governor of Michigan, appointed a study group in February 1956 "to examine hospital and medical costs and coverages and make constructive recommendations." The Governor's Study Commission in Prepaid Hospital and Medical Care Plans made no startling disclosures regarding "waste," but it did find what could be regarded as normal slippage in a service as complicated as hospital care. This large-scale study increased our knowledge of the systems characteristics of the health services.

Expenditures for health services continued to rise in Michigan (and elsewhere), and a new insurance commissioner expressed alarm, feeling that there must be a basic solution. He believed that the burden of proof had to be "taken off the shoulders of the public. The hospitals and doctors have to accept a significant part of the problem and not just come back and ask for 20 percent more every two years."[6] The commissioner made the seemingly self-evident suggestion that the only way to recapture public trust and faith was to let the health plans be operated by public-controlled boards rather than boards dominated by providers.

Similar signs of unrest arose in Maryland, Pennsylvania, New Jersey, Massachusetts, and New York. In a sharply worded speech in September 1960, the insurance commissioner of Maryland, F. Douglas Sears, challenged the medical representatives to produce a "workable plan for curing hospital abuses within 60 days."[7] At the same time, acting in contradiction to his own mandate, Sears denied the Blue Cross of Maryland its request to include diagnostic procedures as a benefit. The plan's purpose was to encourage out-of-hospital rather than in-hospital diagnostic workups. In due course, the Maryland situation led to a study commission that, like the study group in Michigan, produced a range of pertinent data but hardly any startling evidence of rampant abuse.[8]

In Pennsylvania early in 1961, Francis R. Smith, commissioner of insurance, turned down a requested rate increase from Blue Shield of over 26 percent, reducing it to 21 percent. At the same time, he scolded Blue Shield, suggesting that the majority of the board of directors should represent the general public rather than practicing physicians. He asserted that "Blue Shield is not the doctor's plan; it is the public's plan."[9] He apparently assumed that a board dominated by citizens, in the manner of public utilities, would be more cost-conscious. Whether a public board would be more inclined or able to hold down costs than a board made up of doctors is problematical, but it would probably look better.

Other developments during this decade point to increasing public concern over the operation of voluntary health insurance because of increased use of services and rising prices. In November 1956, a joint legislative committee of the New York State Assembly headed by Republican senator George R. Metcalf reported that there were serious deficiencies in current health insurance. The particular deficiency at issue was the age limit imposed by many health insurance policies when a covered worker retired. Metcalf envisioned a bill prohibiting age limits on medical and hospital benefits and compelling insurance companies to allow individuals to continue their coverage when they left an insured group.[10] In 1963, legislation was passed enforcing these provisions.[11]

The Metcalf committee continued to exist and tied up with the School of Public Health and Administrative Medicine at Columbia University. The committee sponsored and financed the compilation of a great mass of data on health services and health insurance in New York State, expanding its initial charge to examine benefit and enrollment deficiencies. The committee considered the matter of noncancellable contracts—contracts that the insurance carrier could not cancel with an individual in a group unless the entire group contract was cancelled. This was designed to prevent discrimination against individuals who proved to be relatively frequent users of services.[12] The proposal, which had the backing of Governor Averill Harriman, would require that all group health insurance policies be convertible to individual policies at no increase in premium or decrease in benefits when the policyholder retired and that the policy be noncancellable. These requirements would result in increased rates for insured groups.

Evidence of widespread cancellation has never been impressive, but enough instances came to light to catch the attention of legislators. Naturally, this kind of legislation did not sit well with the insurance companies, for it meant government interference with the prerogatives of companies to experiment and protect themselves with various types of contracts.[13] This, of course, is the American way—to have private insurance companies take on the characteristics of government health insurance without the government's assuming the responsibility itself.

The skirmishes in New York over the regulation of health insurance contracts were minor compared to the stir caused by legislation to set up hospital planning regions by a state agency that would work through local voluntary hospital planning bodies. The local planning bodies were then granted the power to enfranchise new hospitals, whether financed from public or private funds. This action marked a new era in the voluntary hospital's prerogative to be autonomous in the community.[14] The franchise is a time-honored legal device applied when the body politic feels it is in the public interest to do so. In the New York instance, however, franchising power was delegated to private, voluntary bodies, illustrating further the marble cake of private and public sectors in the United States. The New York action was a precursor of the Health Resources Planning Act of 1974, which strengthened the role of the state and federal governments in determining need for facilities. In the United States, we start with a desire to solve problems and then move toward compulsion, trying to somehow balance the two.

In April 1963, New York State made further incursions into the heartland of medical practice with a law empowering the state health department to undertake "scientific medical audits" to determine the quality and availability of medical care. It was hoped that quality could be improved and costs lowered thereby. In this case, a government agency attempted (by means other than licensure) to measure the quality of a professional service beyond the educational and experience level of professional performance, a function heretofore left to professional associations and private professional bodies. These private bodies were not particularly adept at monitoring themselves: no matter who tries to do the monitoring, it is a complex task at best. The action in New York can be regarded as a precursor of utilization review in hospitals in the Medicare Act of 1965 and later in the Professional Standards Review Organization legislation of 1972. A general atmosphere of control over physicians' discretionary decision-making prerogatives was emerging as costs and imputed wastes were rising.

There were further interventions of public bodies in the operation of the health services. A case in point was the battle that raged between physicians practicing in the Health Insurance Plan of Greater New York and physicians in the local medical societies. Flare-ups continued in out-lying areas of Long Island and Staten Island regarding discrimination against HIP physicians in obtaining admitting privileges in local hospitals. Unlike previous instances in the history of HIP, however, the Staten Island and Long Island cases attracted the attention of public officials. The Metcalf committee held public hearings on the Staten Island case in July 1960.[15] As a result, the county commissioners adopted a regulation forbidding hospitals to refuse to appoint physicians to their medical staffs because of group practice, prepayment affiliations. This action probably set a precedent for medical societies in other areas. Henceforth, discrimination against group practice physicians would have to be more subtle.

Still another straw in the wind in the late fifties and early sixties was Governor Nelson Rockefeller's appointing a committee to look into the problem of monitoring hospital expenditures. Rockefeller chose as chairman Marion B. Folsom of Eastman Kodak, Secretary of HEW during the Eisenhower administration and a member of many committees and commissions in the health field. The committee's report, which became known as the Folsom report, had some controversial suggestions from a political moderate: obligatory hospital insurance for all employed persons; a state-controlled system for reporting hospital costs; seven-day-a-week use of hospital facilities such as laboratories and operating rooms to reduce unit costs; and the purchase of generic drugs by hospitals, which were regarded as cheaper than brand-name drugs.[16] Compulsion thus entered by the back door, through the employer and employee groups and admonitions to find methods for slowing the acceleration of costs.

NOTES

1. See the intensive treatment given the subject by Robert D. Eilers, *Regulations of Blue Cross and Blue Shield Plans* (Homewood, Ill.: Irwin, 1963).
2. Horace R. Hansen, "Laws Affecting Group Health Plans," in *Proceedings, Twelfth Annual Group Health Institute of the Group Health Association of America, May 14–16, 1962* (Washington, D.C.: Group Health Association, 1962), pp. 49–55.
3. Alanson W. Willcox, *Hospitals and the Corporate Practice of Medicine* Hospital Monograph Series, No. 1 (Chicago: American Hospital Association, 1957).
4. See U.S., Congress, Senate, Committee on the Judiciary, Antitrust and Monopoly-Administered Prices: *Hearings on S. Res. 238*, 86th Cong., 2d sess., 1960 and U.S., Congress, Senate, Committee on the Judiciary, Drug Industry Antitrust Act: *Hearings Pursuant to S. Res. 52 on S. 1552*, 87th Cong., 1st sess., 1961. Also see Richard Harris, *The Real Voice* (New York: Macmillan, 1964), pp. 139–245.
5. Walter J. McNerney *et al.*, *Hospital and Medical Economics: A Study of Population, Services, Costs, Methods of Payment, and Controls* (Chicago: Hospital Research and Educational Trust, 1962), vol. I, p. 5.
6. Ron Martin, "Blue Cross Shakeup Demanded," *Detroit Free Press*, 22 November 1962, p. 1.
7. "Maryland Doctors Are Told To Curb Alleged Hospital Abuses Immediately," *Washington Post and Times-Herald*, 22 September 1960, p. 28.
8. Maryland Commission to Study Hospital Costs, *Report* (Baltimore: State of Maryland, 1964).
9. "Pennsylvania Commissioner Tells Blue Shield To Loosen Ties with State Medical Society," *Modern Hospital* 96 (March 1961):77.
10. A. H. Raskin, "Gaps Criticized on Health Plans," *New York Times*, 27 November 1956, p. 33.
11. New York State Consolidated Law Service—1963, sects. 162, 253.
12. "Metcalf Committee Had 4–Point Program," *Eastern Underwriter* 58 (22 November 1957):33.
13. Douglas Dales, "Insurance Chiefs Hit Health Bills," *New York Times*, 31 January 1958, p. 80.
14. Norman S. Moore, in *Report of the First National Conference on Areawide Health Facilities Planning* November 28–29, 1964, Miami Beach, Fla., jointly sponsored by the State Hospital Review and Planning Council of New York and the American Medical Association: Department of Hospitals and Medical Facilities (Chicago: American Medical Association, 1965), pp. 57–62.
15. Morris Kaplan, "HIP Antagonists Charge Monopoly," *New York Times*, 12 July 1960, sect. M, p. 31.
16. "Crisis Facing Blue Cross Plans: Committee Headed by Marion Folsom Offers Recommendations for a Possible Solution," *Medical World News* 6 (25 June 1965):54–63.

16

The Nixon Administration Discovers Competition, Planning, and Other Complexities

It did not take long after Medicare and Medicaid were in operation for Congress and other decision-making bodies to realize that the open-ended, hardly-any-questions-asked funding mechanism was stoking the fires of rising expenditures for health services. From 1965 to 1970, for example, expenditures rose from $139 billion to $169 billion. The proportion of public sources of funding, mainly federal, rose from 25 to 37 percent of the total during that same period. The public sector—that is, payroll taxes and general revenues—absorbed the major impact of this increase, as did, in turn, Congress, the U.S. Treasury, and the body politic. A more comprehensible figure than these mind-boggling billions of dollars may be the increase in per capita expenditures: these rose from $198 in 1965 to $334 in 1970. If the average person did not feel this increase in payroll deductions or even in taxes, because they were so widely diffused, he or she would undoubtedly have felt it in increased out-of-pocket expenses. There was an increase of 75 percent between 1965 and 1970 in total expenditures and about 70 percent in per capita expenditures, the differential taking into account the increase in population during that period. Total expenditures increased faster than per capita expenditures.

The five years between 1965 and 1970 marked the transition from unquestioned payment to concern with the seemingly endless increase in expenditures for health services; these expenditures eventually threatened other goods and services that people wanted, both through the pubic and the private sectors.

The foregoing figures reveal the objective basis for the growing concern with expenditures. Lyndon Johnson's decision not to run for president in 1967 may have been a wiser one than he realized, for, beyond his troubles with the Vietnam War, he had helped to open the flood gates of public programs without controls. Johnson's Great Society and War on Poverty were the logical successors to Roosevelt's New Deal, Truman's Fair Deal, and Kennedy's social programs.

In 1968, Nixon inherited both the Great Society and the Vietnam War. Their combined drain on national resources fed the inflationary spiral. By the end of the sixties it was apparent that the Comprehensive Health Planning Act was not working: that is, it was not stabilizing the supply of hospital beds. Medicare and Medicaid expenditures were greatly in excess of expectations, although the programs were accomplishing their intended objectives: to increase access to services for the aged and the poor.

Government impotence in cost control was expressed through attacks on the providers, particularly the physicians and, more muted, the hospitals. A favorite method of attack was to publish annual gross payments to individual physicians from government programs in excess of, say, $100,000.[1] No attempts were made to determine if the payments went to one physician or were distributed among other physicians and support personnel in a clinic. The hope was apparently to control physicians' fees through exposure and shame. Other symptoms were large periodic requests from the Blue Cross and Blue Shield plans for premium increases as hospital and physician charges rose.

The uniquely American concept of usual, customary, reasonable fees was, to physicians locked into the Medicare Act, an invitation to raise charges; it probably influenced Medicaid fees as well. Conventional wisdom had it that Congress feared to impose a negotiated fee schedule because not enough physicians would treat the elderly. There were some grounds for this. An apparent clarification of the murky concepts of usual, customary, and reasonable, which in time became only usual and customary, was the AMA's definition:

> "Usual" is defined as the "usual fee" which is charged for a given service by an individual physician in his personal practice (i.e., his own usual fee). "Customary" is that range of usual fees charged by physicians of similar training and experience for the same service within a given specific limited geographic or socio-economic area. The definition of "reasonable" fee is a fee which meets the above two criteria, or, in the opinion of the

responsible local medical association's review committee, is justified in the special circumstances of the particular case in question.[2]

Possibly HEW's publication of highly reimbursed physicians' fees was a reaction to the difficulty of administering a program based on usual, customary, and reasonable fees.

On the hospital side, one request for a rate increase from a Blue Cross plan was 49.5 percent, in New York.[3] This was not an isolated instance; it reflected the nature of health services expenditures during that time and for some time into the future.

From the standpoint of persons who made public policy decisions, the health services were out of control. This was certainly the view of Walter Reuther, director of the United Auto Workers-Congress of Industrial Organizations, when he announced at the 1968 annual meeting of the American Public Health Association his intention of forming a Committee of 100 to formulate and press for a comprehensive national health insurance plan. His immediate officers were Texas heart surgeon Michael DeBakey, philanthropist Mary Lasker, and director of the National Urban League Whitney M. Young. Reuther hoped to build a coalition of organized labor, industry, civil rights organizations, consumers, farmers, educational groups, and health and related groups.[4]

On July 10, 1969, this sense of crisis was shared by Republican President Richard Nixon. While holding a press conference on health services, he commented:

> When this administration came into office in January, we initiated a major study of the nation's health care problems and programs. . . . The report that I have received from Secretary Finch and Dr. Egeberg indicates that the problem is much greater than I had realized. We face a massive crisis in this area unless action is taken both administratively and legislatively to meet the crisis within the next two or three years. We will have a breakdown in our medical care system which could have consequences affecting millions of people throughout this country. . . . [There is] a crippling inflation in medical costs causing vast increases in government health expenditures for little return, raising private health insurance premiums, and reducing the purchasing power of the health dollar of our citizens.[5]

According to Joseph L. Falkson, who was close to the federal scene, "rather than an orderly system of policy making, HEW in 1970 presented little more than an amorphic clustering of ad hoc work groups, poorly organized agencies, personalities, styles, and, as one observer noted, free lancers."[6] I take this to be less a criticism than a matter-of-fact description of the situation when a new administration takes over, one that is repeated every time there is a change in power.

When Nixon and his staff in HEW took over, the locus of health policy advice and formulation shifted from the health professionals who staffed the PHS and who automatically thought in terms of the public health model of programs, budgets, control, and regulation to the HEW offices of the assistant secretary for planning and evaluation and the undersecretary. These offices were staffed by nonmedical professionals such as Ph.D.'s, management specialists with M.B.A.'s, and lawyers. This new breed of professionals regarded the problems besetting the health services as essentially economic in nature; in their analyses, therefore, they might overlook the medical and health aspects of the problems. The health services, from their point of view, were already over-financed. There were no incentives for either the insurance agencies or the insured to contain costs.

By an unusual combination of circumstances, the concept of HMOs was introduced to the Nixon administration as an important step toward cost containment by Paul M. Ellwood, Jr., a physician from the American Rehabilitation Foundation, the research arm of the Sister Kenney Institute in Minneapolis. The foundation was finishing a comprehensive review of the health services and possible ways of reforming it. The timing was perfect, for the administration was casting about for an idea.

Cost containment by any means possible became the central concern of the Nixon administration. The major form of cost containment was to be some kind of local and national planning structure that would facilitate feedback among the local health service planning areas, the states, and the federal government regarding needs, supply of facilities, personnel, and priorities. This resulted in the National Health Planning and Resources Development Act, signed into law by President Gerald R. Ford early in 1975, to be described later.

The federal government encountered the hospital establishment head on in an attempt by HEW to revive an apparently ignored, if not forgotten, clause in the Hill-Burton Act requiring hospitals that were receiving funds under the act to contribute between 2 and 5 percent of their operating budget annually for indigent or nonpaying patients.[7] Also, Secretary of HEW Caspar Weinberger suggested that persons being admitted to hospitals should be screened to determine need for hospitalization. These actions represent the administration's grasping at anything that would dampen the rapidly rising expenditures.

Regarding the obligation of hospitals toward the indigent, Nixon's third Secretary of HEW, Elliot Richardson, announced a proposed regulation on April 18, 1972, setting forth guidelines for Hill-Burton-aided hospitals to determine a reasonable amount of service for those unable to pay. By June, the House of Delegates of the AHA was under full steam in opposition, holding a special meeting in Chicago. The house voted to challenge the proposed regulation relating to charity services. As is usually the case in the sensitive relations between the public and private sectors, someone claimed to have been misinterpreted, in this case HEW: "Until recently, it had been accepted that hospitals based on their own statements were providing free service and thus were in compliance."[8] Apparently, HEW was attempting to quantify this obligation. In any case, it hastily abandoned both the proposal that hospitals guarantee a certain amount of free care to the poor and the proposal that admissions be screened ahead of time.

The administrative massiveness of HEW in trying to manage problems was expressed eloquently by Richardson:

> As an administrative matter, the system [HEW] is at best inefficient. As a creative matter, it is stifling. As an intellectual matter, it is incomprehensible. And as a human matter, it is downright cruel.[9]

In the same interview, Richardson must have been referring to the interest groups that were attacking what they considered to be the callous stance of the Nixon administration:

> There is an unfortunate tendency on the part of many to view pragmatism and realism as somehow opposed to high promise and humanism. But we have reached a point at which high promise and humane concern can be responsibly expressed through operational performance which is pragmatic and realistic. To continue to pretend otherwise would be irresponsible.[10]

This was said at a time when the Nixon administration was coining the phrase, it is not enough simply to "throw money at the problem," as the Johnson administration had. Richardson eventually resigned as Secretary of HEW.

Nixon's Economic Stabilization Program (ESP), a short-term effort to control costs, lasted from August 1971 to April 1974. It began with a 90-day freeze on wages and prices in the entire economy, known as Phase I. Phase II was aimed at more specific controls for each major sector of the economy. HEW contended that the health care industry had sufficiently unique problems to be controlled separately from other sectors of the economy, but the administration did not buy that contention. As noted by Abernethy and Pearson, ESP caused problems because hospital reimbursement methods were in fact unique among government contracting methods for goods and services.[11] It was not clear whether the controls applied to charges or to cost-based payments from third party payers (usually whichever was lower). Regulations clarified this problem by defining cost-based payment as "prices." This clarification led to further problems, as usual when definitions become arbitrary.* The question was raised as to whether controls were to be applied to prices per unit of services per day or to admissions. I am less interested in going into the details of the regulations than in illustrating the results of them: it took nine months to refine definitions.

One problem with ESP became obvious immediately, according to Abernethy and Pearson:

> The ambiguity of the regulations, and the several attempts to clarify them, made it difficult for hospital administrators to comply with the directives. Furthermore, the program more than likely removed any incentives to comply since it was almost impossible to know if one was in compliance at any point in time.[12]

The Cost of Living Council formulated new regulations going into Phase IV in July 1973. These regulations, with innovative features, were never tried before controls ended abruptly on April 30, 1974. Two architects of ESP, Stuart Altman and Joseph Eichenholz, concluded that the experience showed that the federal government could not administer equitably a reimbursement system requiring the sensitivity needed for prospective reimbursement of hospitals. They felt it could be done more equitably on the state level.[13] Some states are very large, however, so the question remains, how local is local for hospital rate regulation purposes? In any case, because the states have the major responsibility for regulatory activities that do not cross their boundaries, rate regulations now exist in many of them.

Early in the Nixon administration there were three additional moves toward cost control: (1) legislation in 1972 mandating surveillance of physicians' decisions regarding length of their patients' stay in hospitals (PSROs); (2) the National Health Resources and Planning Act; and (3) an act to encourage the establishment and growth of HMOs. There was a conflict in Congress over whether costs should be controlled by regulations or by some kind of competition: PSROs represented regulations, and HMOs represented competition. The idea of competition as a means of controlling costs was rather new to Congress, and even though it had authorized the concept ten years earlier when it allowed federal employees to choose delivery options under the Fed-

---

*This is illustrated by an apparently true story I heard regarding freight regulations for air cargo. A shipper wanted to fly a rat to a certain destination, but regulations covered only birds. The regulation had to be stretched to include the rat: that is, for purposes of shipment, the rat became a bird.

eral Employment Health Benefit Program. It seems that the principle of choice had been adopted so as not to favor any particular health insurance agency for this new market of approximately 8 million federal employees and dependents nationwide.[14]

Congress was not sure which concept to endorse, so it in effect endorsed both; it passed the PSRO legislation in 1972 and the HMO legislation in 1973. According to Falkson, Paul M. Ellwood, Jr., the physician who had been promoting HMOs, tried to avoid the PSRO regulatory approach by proposing that Congress set up an agency to monitor outcomes of medical care. Neither approach had any general methodology that could be applied rapidly nationwide. The PSRO was a continuation of the utilization review mandate first applied in the Medicare Act in 1965, in which hospitals had to set up some sort of internal review committee to monitor admissions and length of stay.

The PSRO legislation, purported to be the brainchild of Jay Constantine, an aggressive, self-confident, dedicated, and bright Senate staff member, mandated that the country be divided into 200 or so areas, each staffed by a committee of physicians. Although this may seem to have given physicians unwarranted and monopolistic control over evaluation of their own actions, there appears to be no alternative to peer review in an activity where the key factor is professional judgment. Peer review was limited to Medicare and Medicaid patients, for whose care the government was responsible, both in terms of quality and cost. The PSRO concept was aimed at hospital use and has three components: (1) concurrent review of lengths of stay in order to prevent "overstay," the goal being to reduce hospital use; (2) evaluation of admitting practices and correction of them when necessary; and (3) comparative, or profile, analysis of the decisions made by individual physicians.

The PSRO concept was an extremely radical one from the standpoint of the medical profession. It went to the heart of the traditional discretionary privileges of physicians regarding diagnosis and treatment. It is ironic that the United States was the first country to review physician decision making, an intrusion into physicians' freedom usually attributed to countries with "socialized" medical systems.

It is of more than passing interest that politicians, aided by their staffs, are the ones who have promoted utilization review. Logically, the profession itself should have done so, but physicians have been notably reluctant to systematize peer review. In 1965, after the Medicare Act was passed, I queried Wilbur Mills, one of its chief architects, about the apparent contradictions in the act. The preamble read that there was to be no interference with the private practice of medicine, yet a few paragraphs later the act stated that the hospital admissions decisions of physicians would be monitored. I asked, "Is this not interfering with the private practice of medicine?" Mills leaned back in his chair and smiled: "Oh, no, this is to make the doctors talk to each other."

As far as HMOs were concerned, all programs or strategies that had been proposed or put into operation did little to reshape the structure or operation of the mainstream health services delivery system: fee-for-service payment to physicians, with no fee schedule to speak of; retrospective reimbursement based on costs to hospitals; and complete separation between providers and the insurance and government funding agencies. There were no incentives for efficiency or cost containment: in fact, the incentive structure encouraged use. The traditional method of control was regulation; the Medicare Act itself discouraged the government from changing the system.

According to Falkson, the HMO concept was foreign to the HEW establishment's way of doing things: "The idea of stimulating a competitive, private health care marketplace challenged HSMHA's [Health Services and Mental Health Administration] traditional role."[15] The Social Security Administration, led by the Bureau of Health Insurance staff, tended to think automatically in terms of detailed regulations for monitoring reimbursement to HMOs. After the Nixon administration took office, a critical meeting between Ellwood and high officials in HEW took place in Ellwood's hotel room in Washington, D.C., on February 5, 1970, according to Falkson. The under secretary of HEW, John G. Veneman, stated that the government's basic problem was how to deal with cost overruns in the Medicare and Medicaid programs. Ellwood remarked that federal tinkering with narrow aspects of the health services system or enacting more regulations would not solve the cost problem. In fact, federal interventions had so far made inflation worse. Further, "The full range of federal, economic, legal, and persuasive power had to be coordinated in an effort to restructure the health care delivery system." Finally, some means had to be found for the government to influence the future structure of the health services, not simply to rely on the voluntary characteristics of the existing comprehensive health planning and regional medical programs.

Remarkably, as soon as Ellwood had presented his analysis of the expansionary incentives built into the prevailing delivery system and had suggested replacing them with the HMO concept, Veneman accepted the idea. Veneman had had seven years' experience in the California legislature as chairman of the welfare committee and was therefore familiar with the Medicaid problems in that state. He then left the matter to his aides to work out.

Up to this time, Ellwood had visualized the HMO as essentially a group practice with salaried physicians who were prepaid by a known population. This type of organization was revolutionary from the viewpoint of mainstream medical and hospital care, even though group practice was becoming an increasingly common method of delivering physicians' services. Physicians, however, did not want to tie themselves organizationally to a known population that would pay them salaries. A variation of the HMO concept had appeared in Washington and in some provinces of Canada in the 1930s. These foundations, as they were called, disturbed the prevailing solo practice fee-for-service pattern relatively little. They did not receive any national publicity until they were established in California and Oregon after World War II, in order to compete with the pure HMOs such as Kaiser-Permanente. A foundation was created by a county medical association, which contracted with its members to deliver all physician services at agreed-on fees. The salient characteristic of these foundations, however, was their monitoring of physicians to reveal "excessive" office visits or laboratory procedures and diagnostic and treatment methods seemingly out of line with "normal" practice. Peer judgment was exercised by a committee of physicians in the foundation.

Lewis H. Butler, a top aide to the Secretary of HEW, was present at the meeting with Ellwood, and he responded to Ellwood's prototype of an HMO by asking if it were necessary for the government to support only one type of HMO in order to tie Medicare and Medicaid to prepayment. Butler was chary of government's telling people how to do something; he would rather have the government tell the people what it wanted to accomplish and let them choose the method. Butler said, as quoted by Falkson:

> Let the doctors—let everybody do it, figure out how to put it together. Let's specify what we want to do and we don't give a damn how they put it together. They can make a partnership, a corporation, they can make it one of 55 different organizational forms. Let's describe the thing by what we want it to do, not how it is formed.[16]

Ellwood accepted Butler's strategy "after only a moment's reflection." This simple variation on the group practice prepayment concept could have profound ramifications. Over 90 percent of private medical practitioners were already associated with Blue Shield plans, which had some sort of contracts with physicians. The same roughly 90 percent were being reimbursed by private insurance companies without a contract, simply by submitting their claims. Both sources of reimbursement operated within a range approximating "usual, customary, and reasonable" fee schedules.

What HEW wanted, as expressed by Butler, was any variety of organizational structure that would guarantee a fixed price for a specialized bundle of services for Medicare and Medicaid patients for a given period. The government wanted to avoid the open-ended, cost-plus funding that had been wreaking havoc with the payroll deduction and tax structures. Butler's concept was an eminently reasonable and conservative one that would effect changes in the status quo of the delivery system. The federal government was not interfering with the internal administration and structure of the delivery system, but was confining itself to the role of purchaser. As Falkson put it, the idea could be presented as a market reform strategy rather than yet another federal program requiring a large bureaucracy to administer.

> This would be exceedingly appealing to a Republican administration. It would be equally unappealing to a federal health bureaucracy committed to tinkering with small pieces of the delivery system and to the aggrandizement of its own role or to a Congressional system of watchdog Committees dedicated to tracking very precisely articulated programs involving the spending of the federal government.[17]

This purchasing concept required highly sophisticated politicians and civil servants, not to mention a sophisticated body politic and press.

The term "health maintenance organization" was coined by Ellwood. Although group practice prepayment had been around for 30 years, a new term was necessary to avoid raising the hackles of the medical establishment. The new term lent a positive note to prepayment, implying that this type of organization tried to maintain health through early diagnosis and prevention. It hit a responsive chord at that time, in part because acute care had become expensive. The premise was plausible: "HMOs have an incentive to keep you well in order to contain costs on a fixed budget."

The government's initial interest in the concept of HMOs was as a means of controlling the costs of Medicare and Medicaid. Since cost-plus reimbursement with private insurance plans had been a financial disaster, it might prove salutary to support alternatives that could compete with existing contracts with the private sector.

The rapidity with which the concept of HMOs surfaced in the new administration was remarkable. The top HEW policy-making staff began to run with the idea in order to put it into the president's message to the country in March 1970. The next group to convince was the HEW administrative staff, the people who had to put policy into effect and take the blame if it failed. The Social Security Administration staff were not enthusiastic. Aside from their being geared toward a regulatory and supervisory method of administering programs, they also feared according to Falkson, the ambitious nature of the HMO approach, which was designed to change the delivery system in a few years. They recommended an incremental approach. The staff feared the loss of direct accountability, which they saw as the bedrock of government administration, that would result from "delegating" responsibility of this magnitude to private operators. Further, the HMO concept seemed to weaken their control over an area they regarded as a responsibility to the public.

The House Ways and Means Committee, however, appeared amenable to the HMO concept and with little debate incorporated it into Medicare as Part C of the HMO Act.[18] Thus, with little fanfare the Nixon administration was authorized to make HMOs the cornerstone of its health policy. As stated in a press release:

> The Secretary announced that legislation would be proposed to authorize The Social Security Administration to enter into contracts [with HMO's] guaranteeing comprehensive health services for the elderly at a fixed annual rate. Our goal, the Secretary said, is that every elderly or poor person, covered by Medicare or Medicaid, be given the right to choose between receiving services under such a contract and receiving individual hospital and physician services in the traditional manner. We must promote diversity, choice, and health competition in American medicine if we are to escape from the grip of spiralling costs.[19]

Although the Nixon administration put itself squarely behind HMOs and competitive options, there was no guarantee that the ideas would have clear sailing in the Congress, not to mention the HEW bureaucracy. The administration turned the legislative development of the HMO concept over to a group of management specialists—that is, M.B.A.s recruited by HEW and oriented toward the private health care market.

As usual in a controversial measure that tries to break new ground in Congress, a horde of interest groups surfaced, as did differences among members of Congress—differences caused in large part by the interest groups. Three separate but related proposals were introduced in Congress in 1972, one by the administration, a second by Representative William R. Roy (D-Kan.) and Paul G. Rogers (D-Fla.), and a third by Senator Edward Kennedy (D-Mass.). The administrations' proposal was the most general of the three. The Roy-Rogers bill sought tighter definitions and controls than the administration bill, and Kennedy's bill exceeded both in its scope and specifications. The most basic difference among the three bills was what organizations could quality as HMOs.

The administration's bill permitted a wide spectrum of organizations to qualify for federal subsidy.

The Roy-Rogers bill would include the pure HMO type originally envisioned by Ellwood and the foundation type of HMO described earlier. (In the rapid evolution of terminology, the foundation type had become known as independent practice associations; these were grafted onto the existing structure of private practice.) Kennedy had an obsessive dislike of mainstream medical practice and did not want to encourage it in any way. His Health Security Act came close to mandating HMOs, although it allowed fee-for-service arrangements that would be phased out. Kennedy relented somewhat and allowed independent practice associations in rural areas, where it would be difficult to establish pure HMOs. He believed that the administration intended to mute agitation for national health insurance by touting HMOs; he grabbed the concept and made it the organizational centerpiece of his Health Security Act. The Nixon administration had no such strategy in mind. The Roy-Rogers bill was in between. Roy was a practicing physician (and lawyer) prominent in Kansas medical circles and politics who did not sit well with the AMA for fostering legislation to start HMOs. The AMA was curiously obtuse on this matter of encouraging competition.

Interestingly, given Americans' ambivalence regarding profit in the health services, all three bills allowed assistance to profit-making entities. Debate on this issue surrounded the very complex issue of formulas for controlling profits, or rate of retention. Kennedy did not want to encourage the formation of profit-making agencies, so he provided only loan guarantees for them. The administration's bill provided for contracts to plan and establish profit-making HMOs as well as loan guarantees to offset their initial losses. Roy and Rogers were unsympathetic to profit making, and their bill assisted only nonprofit and public organizations.

Also under consideration were quality control and assurance. The administration's bill recommended that arrangements be made to assure quality, undoubtedly assuming that higher quality would result from competition. The Roy-Rogers bill went further and specified that quality assurance procedures must examine medical practice processes and their outcomes. With predictable consistency, Kennedy's bill would establish a Commission on Quality Care Assurance, a federal regulatory agency. The Kennedy bill seemed to assume that quality assurance and control were a more or less ready-made process that lacked only full-scale application. The seemingly simple concept of the HMO was headed for an agonizing political pulling and hauling, the Democratic Congress not intending to let the Nixon administration dominate national health policy.

Obviously, the rising interest in HMOs resulted from intense concern about cost containment and cost-effectiveness in the health services. It is interesting to note, as Falkson does, that the strategy for change "was a product of the newer, rather than the older, established health interests." It emerged without benefit of guidance from the established health interest groups that had shaped the health policies of earlier periods. These policies, in fact, were being vigorously challenged by the advocates of HMOs: the energetic efforts of the American Rehabilitation Foundation (Ellwood's group) working closely with its professional counterparts at HEW; the Group Health Association of America; and the American Association of Foundations for Medical Care. Strategy development for HMOs in 1970 and 1971 was notable because of its insulation from most of the traditional health interest groups and for the ascendency of these newer groups. These groups can be classified as Alford's corporate rationalizers, a countervailing force to professional monopolists.

Consumers were not considered directly in the HMO debate in Congress, but they were heard from in another context—the National Health Planning and Resources Development Act then under deliberation by Congress.

As mentioned previously, the full legislative story can be found in Falkson's outstanding account. It is sufficient here to report that Nixon signed the HMO bill on December 29, 1973. This bill did not end up changing the private market structure of the health services: the seemingly simple HMO concept got mangled in the legislative process. The bill was encumbered with open enrollment; community rating, which hampered flexibility in setting rates for premiums; and an unrealistic range of benefits that made it difficult to compete effectively with other modes of delivery. As stated by Falkson:

> Feasibility of implementation, of course, was not foremost in the minds of the legislators responsible for the passage of P.L. 93-222. Liberals, moderates, and conservatives each had their own parochial motives as they pursued passage of the bill.[20]

The final legislation resulted in a sense of demonstration or experiment rather than reform, even though the concept of the HMO had proven viable for 30 years or more.[21] This was three full years after the Nixon administration had latched onto the HMO concept.

Like the jigsaw puzzle of the Medicare Act, the HMO Act was an administrative and health planning monstrosity. Yet it was a natural outcome of pluralistic politics when a consensus is lacking: in order to achieve consensus, there had to be such a low common denominator that the original objective was diluted altogether. The impact on mainstream health services delivery was minimized. The goals had been scaled down considerably, from the suggestion of the Nixon staff (resisted by HEW) to have between 5,000 and 10,000 HMOs in place in five years down to a proposed 250 HMOs in five years, with federal assistance of $375 million.[22] Two years later, a revised bill was passed and signed by President Ford, giving HMOs more flexibility to become competitive.

Lawrence D. Brown in his treatment of the politics of the HMO legislation is less critical of the political and legislative process than Falkson. Brown feels that the politicians and the government did not fail, that the American political process is too complex to deal adequately with as complicated an entity as an HMO. This is a reasonable observation, but it would seem to apply to most of the problems that enter the political arena.[23]

While the Nixon administration was trying to contain costs and rationalize the health services enterprise by the invisible hand of market controls, Congress was formulating and passing a wide-ranging health planning act—the National Health Planning and Resources Development Act, Public Law 93-641, signed into law in 1975 by President Ford. There was a great deal of dissatisfaction with the six-year-old Community Health Program, Public Law 89-749. The Regional Medical Program was not working either, and the Hospital Survey and Construction Act needed reformulation. The new act essentially replaced these three programs. It was hoped that the new act would enable interest groups to talk to each other and would serve as a source of information in thinking through their situations jointly and rationally. It was also hoped that this process would reduce duplication of services. Critics accused the Community Health Program of having wasted more than $100 million since it was enacted because local groups had floundered without direction.[24] As a matter of fact, a clear direction could not have been expected, given the permissive nature of the program.

A possible resemblance between the health planning act and the HMO market concept was the strengthening of consumer influence on the health services enterprise to assist in determining the relationship between need or demand, on the one hand, and supply, on the other. This would also affect to some degree the price of hospital services. In a sense, consumer sovereignty was the basis of both approaches, one depending on consumer choice in the marketplace and the other on consumer influence in the planning process. It seems reasonable to assume that Nixon would also have signed this bill, given the general congressional support for it.

The National Health Planning and Resources Development Act was exceedingly detailed in its specifications and certainly unprecedented in its scope and intent to influence the supply and distribution of facilities (and, indirectly, personnel).[25] The bill clearly reflected Americans' ambivalence toward planning of any kind, but Congress was forced into drastic measures in order to achieve some semblance of control over rising Medicare and Medicaid expenditures. It will be recalled that direct price controls had fizzled and the PSRO approach to rationalize physician decision making was as yet untested. Congress was trying to avoid issuing directives by placing the responsibility for major planning decisions on over 200 local planning groups which, in turn, would tell the state and federal governments what the people wanted. The federal government bypassed local political jurisdictions, or, at best, permitted a planning agency to be responsible to the local political jurisdiction. Planning activities were wholly financed by the federal government and were evaluated by it (HEW).

There were three tiers of planning—local, state, and federal (HEW). The major planning action was to take place in the 200 or so health service areas, which were more or less set up on the basis of health service market criteria as to range of facilities and population. These areas, therefore, did not necessarily coincide with political jurisdictions within the states.

Each Health Service Agency (HSA) had a board of governors with 10 to 30 members, at least 60 percent of whom were to be "consumers." The remainder could be providers and local political representatives. The consumers were to mirror the population of the planning area in regard to income levels, racial and ethnic composition, and even language. The providers could be physicians, hospital administrators, nurses, dentists, and pharmacists. Consumer representatives, for example, could not be physicians' wives or even educators who trained health services administrators. The HSAs were given negative planning powers for facilities expansion and development: in states that had certificate-of-need laws for hospital improvement and construction, HSAs could recommend, or not recommend, a plan to the state planning agency.

The act did not place an easy charge on the planning process when it practically mandated "equal access" to "quality" health care at "reasonable" costs. The implicit assumption was that much more value could be squeezed out of the medical dollar through reduced duplication of facilities, greater efficiency of operation through multiple organizations, deemphasis on institutional care, greater emphasis on out-of-hospital services, and better education of the public, which would reduce the pressure on services. This was all to be done without direction—by local consensus integrated into state and eventually national consensus.

In summary, between 1968 and 1976, the Nixon and Ford administrations played with the Economic Stabilization Program (1971 to 1974), an extremely unpopular endeavor of short duration; mandated utilization control through PSROs (1972); got the HMO concept started as a possible cost-control measure (1973); and adopted the National Health Planning and Resources Development Act (1974). Meanwhile, national expenditures for all health services rose from $54 billion to $139 billion; per capita expenditures from $264 to $638; and expenditures on health care as a percent of GNP rose from 6.5 percent to over 8.6 percent. Further, because Medicare and Medicaid had been in effect since 1966, federal, state, and local governments were accounting for 40 percent of all personal health expenditures. The health services price index climbed from 107 in 1968 to 179 in 1975, an increase of 60 percent in prices alone. Hospital prices virtually tripled.

During the Nixon administration, Congress authorized unlimited appropriations for kidney dialysis for all patients needing it. The bill was passed in the fall of 1972, and the program began July 1, 1973. This program was estimated to have cost $5 billion in five years and was a model for groups concerned with other diseases. At the same time, as part of the ethnic heterogeneity of American politics, Congress pushed for programs on diseases that appeared to afflict certain ethnic and racial groups. Kennedy supported research on Cooley's anemia, which affects mainly Greeks and Italians, a politically important segment of the population of Massachusetts. There was also some support for a program directed at sickle-cell anemia, a disease affecting mainly blacks.[26] Lacking a relatively comprehensive and universal national health insurance program, special interest groups focused on various diseases. It is possible that these groups would exert political pressures within a universal health insurance program as well, but the lack of a national program would seem more likely to generate such interests.

NOTES

1. Selected references include: "Medicare Incomes of Doctors Cited," *New York Times*, 17 May 1968, p. 16; Thomas Powers and Ronald Kotulak, "State Medical Costs Up 300 Percent in 4 Years," *Chicago Tribune*, 3 June 1969; Dennis Farney, "Medicare Rematch," *Wall Street Journal*, 27 February 1968, p.1; "Medicare Payments and the Tax Collector," *Congressional Record* 115 (17 June 1969):S6603.
2. "AMA defines 'Usual Fees'," *AMA News* 11 (16 December 1968):12.
3. Murray Illson, "Blue Cross Asks a 49.5 Percent Rise for Most in Plan," *New York Times*, 23 May 1969, p.31.
4. Stephen Cain, "Health Plan for All Asked by Reuther," *Detroit News*, 15 November 1968, p. 1.
5. Joseph L. Falkson, *HMO's and the Politics of Health System Reform* (Chicago: American Hospital Association, 1980), pp. 6–7. Quotation taken from Robert H. Finch, Secretary of HEW, and Roger O. Egeberg, M.D., assistant

secretary-designate for health and scientific affairs, *A Report on the Health of the Nation's Health Care Systems* (Washington, D.C.: Department of Health, Education, and Welfare, 1969).

6. Falkson, *HMO's* p. 51. Another book on HMOs has since appeared: Lawrence D. Brown, *Politics and Health Care Organization: HMO's as Federal Policy* (Washington, D.C.: Brookings Institution, 1983). Although Brown takes a broader view of the HMO movement (dealing with competition and regulation as well as politics), he essentially agrees with Falkson.

7. I am indebted for much of my information to David S. Abernethy and David A. Pearson, *Regulating Hospital Costs: The Development of Public Policy* (Ann Arbor, Mich.: AUPHA Press, 1979). Unless specifically attributed, interpretations are my own.

8. *Hospital Week* 8 (9 June 1972):1

9. Elliot L. Richardson, "The Image of Social Programs," *Washington Post and Times-Herald*, 21 January 1973, p. 3.

10. Ibid.

11. Abernethy and Pearson, *Regulating*.

12. Ibid., p. 57.

13. Ibid., p. 55.

14. See Odin W. Anderson and J. Joel May, *The Federal Employees' Health Benefits Program, 1961–1968: A Model for National Health Insurance*, Health Administration Perspectives No. A9 (Chicago: Center for Health Administration Studies, Graduate School of Business, University of Chicago, 1971).

15. Falkson, *HMO's*, p. 74.

16. Ibid., p. 31.

17. Ibid., p. 32.

18. Ibid., p. 42–43.

19. Ibid., p. 43.

20. Ibid., p. 134.

21. Ibid., p. 163.

22. Ibid., p. 55, and Jonathan Spivak, "Nixon Signs Bill To Foster Health Plans Emphasizing Preventive Care," *Wall Street Journal*, 31 December 1973, p. 2.

23. Brown, *Politics*, pp. 401–41.

24. Nancy Hicks, "U.S. May Tighten Health Planning," *New York Times*, 14 June 1973, sect. C, p. 11.

25. I suggest that persons who want greater detail read the entire law. A useful interpretation is Herbert H. Hyman's *Health Planning: A Systematic Approach* (Germantown, Md.: Aspen, 1975), pp. 417–35.

26. Jonathan Spivak, "Congress Pushes Fight on Ailments that Afflict Ethnic Groups, Some Doubt Wisdom of Such Acts," *Wall Street Journal*, 29 September 1972, p. 26.

17

The Carter Administration Encounters More of the Same

The Carter administration inherited problems in the health field that had been gathering momentum since the Johnson administration. They seemed to be beyond the capacity of any administration to solve, given the sources of funding and the persistent attitude among Americans that more is better, although no one can tell what is enough.

Federal agencies are remarkable and useful gatherers of statistical information. No other country in the world has the solid statistical base for considering public policy in the health field that the United States does. Reports published under federal auspices appear to be neutral, although they do reflect the pluralistic nature of the American system in their styles of presentation. A particularly useful exercise has been the annual publication of the *Forward Plan for Health*, begun in 1974 and intended to coincide with the fiscal year.

The 1974 *Forward Plan*, which was projected to fiscal years 1978–82, can be regarded as a bridge between the Nixon-Ford administrations and the Carter administration, which began in 1976. There was probably no direct connection between the 1976 *Forward Plan* and the new administration, for such reports need a lead time of more than a year. The report published in 1976[1] appears to consider the process of implementation itself in addition to global goals. This increased sophistication may simply reflect the new kind of staff, who thought systematically and politically, as well as technically. Three criteria for establishing priorities were proposed: projects had to be needed, doable, and affordable. The criterion of need involved mountains of data and utopian goals, but the criteria of doability and affordability forced policy think-

227

ing into more concrete political and economic terms. The report seems to stress the need for a conceptual framework:

> Activities directed toward the development of a more systematic framework for the analysis of the health domain are a very high priority and are designed to increase our power to forecast and to predict the consequences of alternative policies. . . . With respect to our health sector phenomena, we are a long way from being able to make such predictions with even a minimal degree of certainty.[2]

The *goal* in the *Forward Plan* was to improve the health of the American people. The *objectives* were scarcely more specific: to assure equal access to quality care at reasonable cost and to prevent illness, disease, and accidents. These led to (1) improving the apparatus and process of policy making in the health field, (2) containing the cost of care, (3) implementing an aggressive preventive strategy (against smoking, for example), (4) improving the quality of care, and (5) strengthening the essential resources.[3]

Medicare and Medicaid were in full swing, presumably accomplishing some of these goals and objectives and certainly providing more nearly equal access. Charles C. Edwards, under secretary of health for Nixon-Ford, stated cogently the problem of meeting the criteria of doability and affordability:

> Medicare is a financing plan, and it is likewise a health care program, even though some tend to think of it only in terms of payment for services. . . . But you can't pay for services that you can't define and develop standards for. Tremendous medical judgments must be made within Medicare and Medicaid.[4]

The Nixon-Ford administrations made a frontal assault on costs through general price regulation, later limited to hospitals and physicians, and failed. There was no political enthusiasm for it. President Carter picked hospitals alone as the target because of their obviously high cost relative to other components of the health services. The political history and conflicts created by Carter's Hospital Cost Containment Act have been amply described by Abernethy and Pearson, so I will simply summarize them and add some interpretations of my own.[5]

President Carter proposed the Hospital Cost Containment Act on April 25, 1977. He asserted that it would restrain increases in reimbursements that hospitals received from all sources: Medicare, Medicaid, Blue Cross, private insurance companies, and direct-pay patients. A limit on the pace of rising costs would be set by a formula reflecting general inflation, with considerations for the quality of care: that limit was set at 9 percent. The legislation would also put capital expenditures below where they had been in recent years, with local planning agencies assisting in determining appropriate levels. Obviously, this legislation would attempt to control both price and supply. Since the government was responsible for at least 50 percent of hospital expenditures, Carter's motivation was understandable. Further, since he was contemplating a form of national health insurance, he had to have a cost containment measure already in place. Carter wanted to cover all payers, not simply Medicare and Medicaid, for he feared, justifiably, that hospitals would pass the controlled costs of the poor and elderly on to other patients. Accordingly, he wanted all patients covered by cost controls.

Leadership for the cost containment measure was assumed by Carter's ebullient and abrasive Secretary of HEW, Joseph A. Califano, Jr. Califano was widely quoted as calling hospitals "obese." The Carter administration estimated that, in fiscal year 1978, the legislation would save $1.86 billion out of total hospital expenditures of $50 billion or so, for Medicare, Medicaid, and other patients. By 1980, the estimated reduction in expenditures would be $5.53 billion.[6]

Early in 1978, while attempting to get his hospital cost control bill through Congress, Carter said that he was opposed to mandatory economic controls in general: he supported a voluntary approach instead. Carter felt that hospital costs were feeding the inflationary spiral; at the same time it seemed unreasonable to expect hospitals to be controlled or to control themselves while the rest of the economy remained free. As a bow toward labor, Carter allowed hospitals to increase their labor costs without restriction, even though labor normally accounts for two-thirds of the cost of hospital operation. It was felt that, unlike other sectors of the economy, hospitals had no incentive for being efficient: they operated on cost or charges and retrospective reimbursement arrangements, with patients paying little or nothing at the time of service.

As usual, although there may have been agreement in Congress that hospital costs should be controlled, there was no agreement on how. Five other major proposals were introduced in the next few months. Carter's bill, H.R. 6575, was introduced by Paul G. Rogers (D-Fla.) and Dan Rostenkowski (D-Ill.). In the Senate, a bill, S.1391, was introduced by Edward Kennedy (D-Mass.), William D. Hathaway (D-Me.), and Wendell R. Anderson (D-Minn.). The four additional proposals accepted the original one in principle, but added incentives for good performance by hospitals, a program to identify and close down excess beds, however defined, and an exemption from the revenue cap for all small hospitals. The latter was a concession to rural constituencies, who were worried about the fate of their hospitals. Representatives Tim Lee Carter (R-Ken.) and Richard Schweiker (R-Pa.) went further, encouraging the establishment of state rate and budget review programs.

As the debate on hospital cost containment continued, it became increasingly clear that the problem was exceedingly complicated and that formulas could not be easily devised and applied. Hospitals differed in size, case-mix, and mission (whether teaching, research, or service). Some were operating with a surplus whereas others were running deficits, others were breaking even. Was one to be punished and the other rewarded when standards of efficiency were undeveloped? The conclusions of Abernethy and Pearson appear reasonable:

> The proposal rejected the cost-push theories by basing the revenue increase upon the GNP deflator and by making the wage pass-through optional. It clearly assumed that the extent of unneeded services and excess utilization was great enough to withstand reductions in the rate of increase in hospital revenue and in capital expenditure. Moreover, the proposal recognized the important role of the provider by assuming that the imposition of the revenue cap would force hospital administrators and medical staff into making the hard choices necessary to increase efficiency in the production of health care services.[7]

These appear to be reasonable expectations, but they do not take into account the nature of the health services enterprise as it exists in this country. There are no measures of input or output. The concept of a budget cap is economically and politically reasonable, since costs cannot go up indefinitely, but that such cost controls result in more efficient services is not easy to determine. All that can be determined with certainty is that costs will be less if budget caps are imposed.

Quoting Abernethy and Pearson further:

> Perhaps the most important point is that the administration's bill recognized that the inflationary spiral in hospital cost is unjustified in the face of a great deal of evidence suggesting that hospital care is not providing the benefits expected [improved health indices] as a result of the increased investment. Unfortunately, the legislation proposed to apply these concepts in a vague and nonspecific fashion to an important social commodity.

The authors assume that hospital cost accounting and performance indicators had become sophisticated enough to be useful. Apparently they also believed this when they wrote: " . . . the theoretical base for the bill is not widely known nor generally accepted by observers of the health care system."[8]

Providers' reaction to the Hospital Cost Containment Act of 1977 was immediate and hostile. Alexander McMahon, president of the AHA, described the bill as "inequitable in design, wrong in concept, and impossible to administer."[9] He was most nearly correct about the last. Michael Bromberg, director of the Federation of American Hospitals (FAH), the growing for-profit contingent of the American hospital system, was more foreboding:

> If Congress votes to place a ceiling on hospital revenues and on hospital-based technology, then Congress will be voting to establish itself as the moral judge of the dollar value of increased life spans, fewer fatal heart attacks, reduced infant mortality, significantly higher survival rates for cancer patients, and every livesaving device or technique.[10]

Congress has the constitutional right, if sustained by the people, to judge the appropriateness of hospital costs. As it turned out, however, Congress as a whole did not seem to believe in cost control either.

Despite the seemingly uncompromising assaults of McMahon and Bromberg, the AHA settled down to discussing with congressional committees the technical problems of hospital cost control. The AHA pointed out that it had supported health planning, certificate-of-need, and rate review programs, but it objected to the current bill because it was impractical to administer.

Before long, Congress was flooded with protests from other hospital organizations (the American Protestant Hospital Association, the American Catholic Hospital Association, the Council on Teaching Hospitals, the National Council of Private Psychiatric Hospitals, the National Council of Community Hospitals) and from prestigious individual hospitals. Their common appeal was that the proposed containment bill would lower the quality of care, a contention that is difficult to support or refute. The clear tendency is to give providers the benefit of the doubt.

A maverick among hospital organizations was the National Council of Community Hospitals, founded in 1974 to give nonprofit community hospitals a more vigorous voice in Washington. John Horty, a health care lawyer, formed the council with Everett Johnson and William Wallace, both hospital administrators. Their mission was to come up with constructive alternatives to those proposed by the AHA and the FAH.[11] Horty testified that the council recognized and endorsed the need for immediate cost control measures. At the same time, however, it believed that structural reform was so important it should not be subordinated to cost control programs, which could become a permanent control system.[12]

The council recommended that a 24-month freeze be placed on hospital employment and on labor costs and capital expenditures. More tellingly, the council proposed that the income of both hospital and physician be reduced if a PSRO review found an admission or continued stay unnecessary. In the meantime, there should be a national debate on the nature and components of a permanent control system. The council's proposal was introduced as H.R. 8295 on July 13, 1977. A detailed justification of it was written by Paul Feldstein, an economist in the health field. The National Council of Community Hospitals was a small organization and scarcely able to make a national splash, but it is interesting as a group within the voluntary hospital system proposing "its own system of controls or a means of reducing controls."[13]

Lobbyists for the AMA were relatively quiet until it was proposed that control be extended to the establishment of physicians' offices as well as hospital beds. The AMA was also concerned with federal control of local hospitals. There was no significant lobbying on the part of groups that carried a great deal of the costs of hospital care, that is, Blue Cross plans, private insurance companies, large employers, labor (through collective bargaining), and state and local governments. They were more likely to make statements on specific issues. Thus leadership for hospital cost control lay with HEW—that is, with Califano and the president. The administration had no visible constituency supporting hospital cost controls.

The deliberations and debates in Congress dragged on. Congress could not or would not come up with a hospital cost containment bill that could be passed. In November 1977, Dan Rostenkowski, a cosponsor of the administration's original bill, hinted at the possibility of breaking the logjam. He told the House that many pressing problems required their attention and that the hospital cost containment bill was not getting anywhere. He suggested that, between November 1977 and January 1978, when Congress would reconvene, the administration and the hospital industry reconsider the entire matter:

> And because Congress has not passed legislation on the subject this year, the hospitals in this country have been given a brief grace period. With the knowledge that we will not resume consideration of the issue until early next year, hospitals have the opportunity to demonstrate that they can effectively and significantly restrain cost increases on a voluntary basis. . . . If the industry is as confident as their representatives have indicated to me that they can solve the hospital cost problem on a voluntary basis, they should be in a position to develop and to begin to implement a responsible alternative before Congressional debate on this issue resumes in February.[14]

Rostenkowski's proposal might be regarded as a brilliant maneuver on his part: Congress was unenthusiastic about the bill, so he threw responsibility for containing costs back on the providers. The AHA, FAH, and AMA were not slow in responding. Within three weeks, these provider organizations had established a National Steering Committee on Voluntary Cost Containment, and on November 23, 1977,

AHA sent mailgrams to its members enjoining "an immediate reassessment by each institution of planned budget and charge adjustments . . . to see if anything further can be done in the short term to reduce these increases."[15] By the end of December 1977, the steering committee had met and agreed on the general nature of voluntary effort. More specifically, the hospitals committed themselves to a national goal of reducing by 2 percent the rate of increase in costs for both 1978 and 1979. This was a far cry from the administration's original goal of 9 percent, but it was probably a more realistic one. It is not surprising that the providers were able to act so quickly; spearheaded by the FAH, they had been contemplating a voluntary effort for some time.[16]

By the middle of January 1978, the Voluntary Effort, as it was called, had a logo and stationery. Letters were sent to all chairpersons of hospital boards, executive officers, and chiefs of medical staffs. Within two weeks of the program's being made public, 40 or so state hospital associations had formed voluntary cost containment committees. The AHA, FAH, and AMA showed that they were serious in implementing an alternative to mandatory cost controls.

The program proposed by Voluntary Effort had, at last, the virtue of being understandable. It proposed (1) a goal of 2 percent annual reduction in hospital cost increases for two years, (2) no increase in hospital beds in 1978, and (3) a reduced rate of capital expenditures, to 80 percent of the average capital investment for 1975 through 1977 (adjusted for price). This program would be carried out at the state level through voluntary cost containment committees. The National Steering Committee for Voluntary Effort suggested that state committees establish some criteria for screening and reviewing hospitals, for example, hospitals that were in the top 15 percent of growth in cost per admission, hospitals that had rates of increase of more than 10 percent in 1978, and hospitals that had a rate of increase in total budgeted income or expenditure that was less than 2 percent below the rate in the last fiscal year. Goals for capital expenditures were less explicit.

Rostenkowski, as might be expected, responded favorably to the Voluntary Effort. Nevertheless, he proposed to his subcommittee that legislation for cost control be formulated as a standby measure, in case the hospitals failed to slow increases by 2 percent in 1978 and 1979. As reasonable as Rostenkowski's proposal seemed to be, providers and labor opposed it. According to Abernethy and Pearson, providers opposed the proposal because it was more likely to pass than the original one and they believed that the very presence of standby controls would undermine the Voluntary Effort. Hospital representatives claimed that standby controls would act as an incentive for hospital administrators to increase their costs because they feared that mandatory controls might be imposed. Labor opposed the Rostenkowski proposal because it felt that hospital administrators would cut wages in order to meet the goals of the Voluntary Effort.

These frustrating and fantastic crosscurrents make it difficult to try to reduce hospital cost increases: no one wants to take risks, and no one wants to fail or to suffer relative loss. Rostenkowski appeared to be suggesting reasonable compromises for all parties concerned, certainly for the Carter administration. The original bill would die anyway, and the administration could save face and show the public that it cared about rising hospital costs. Yet the public did not seem to care. Even though the White House lobbied vigorously for Rostenkowski's standby bill, Rostenkowski was finally able to muster only 7 votes out of 13. After adding several amendments that watered down even this proposal, the subcommittee at last reported a bill to the Ways and Means Committee on February 28, 1978, by a vote of seven to six. Small hospitals were excluded from controls if they were the only local providers, and the wage pass-through was not made mandatory. The most significant difference between the original bill and the new one was the provision of federal controls.

The hospital cost containment bill was not enacted in 1978. The Carter administration tried again in 1979 and failed again. The reasons are both simple and complex. The simple one was that there was no visible support. Congress, therefore, proceeded cautiously, in response to the interest groups speaking for the hospitals.

A more complex reason, which is impossible to document but which seems plausible, has to do with the mission of the general hospital and the nature of personal health services. The general hospital is deeply rooted in the community. It is the symbol of succor and healing, a postponement of death and the last resort for the body. Money is not allowed to interfere with the hospital's sacred mission—to heal the body regardless of cost. Further, most members of Congress are over the age of 50 and are increasingly vulnerable to illness and death.

Abernethy and Pearson give reasons for the demise of the cost control act:

> A significant problem in passing this legislation is that it applies a relatively arbitrary control in a nonspecific fashion to the production of an important, highly regarded set of personal services. There is no way to defend, or attack, the use of 150 percent of the GNP deflator limit, or the administration's original declining limit, because the necessary evidence was not made available, if it exists. Of course, it may not be possible to arrive at a limit for hospital costs which is actually based upon an acceptable measure of need, and, therefore, it may be necessary to use an arbitrary figure and assess its impact after the fact. Regardless, in terms of the

present controversy, the lack of any acceptable measure of the proper level of resources which should be provided for hospital care made it easy for opponents to attack the proposals, and difficult for proponents to defend it.[17]

This is a rationalistic, secular argument—that, given the proper facts, differences of opinion and values could have been reconciled. No amount of facts can reconcile our feelings about alleviating pain and postponing death unless our entire attitude toward death becomes reconciled to increasingly scarce resources.

The Carter administration centered its efforts on hospital cost containment because hospitals were very visible, and because it seemed possible to get such a piece of legislation enacted. Carter had promised some kind of national health insurance program during his campaign, and now labor and the liberal members of Congress were asking him to deliver. Like the Nixon-Ford administrations, the Carter administration was not enthusiastic about national health insurance, certainly not the more comprehensive kind envisioned by Kennedy. In addition to the Hospital Cost Containment Act, Carter tried to reorganize the health services delivery system.

Carter revived interest in HMOs. He talked about comprehensive national health insurance as a long-range goal that could be met by phasing in various measures that had general appeal and that solved generally recognized problems. Catastrophic health insurance is an example. All in all, the administration, like Congress, was frightened at the possible cost of national health insurance in terms of the federal budget, the take-home pay of the labor force, and the profits of employers for reinvestment and dividends. Politicians like Kennedy, however, saw national health insurance as a means of controlling costs. The Kennedy-Corman proposal would set up a regionalized structure with budget caps controlled by a federal agency. It would be backed by appropriations from Congress, and it would eventually cause the delivery system to be reorganized into a prepaid group practice sort of arrangement, something similar to the HMO.

The Carter administration introduced a national health insurance bill in September 1979, late in Carter's term. The proposal took a more or less middle-of-the-road position, starting out with continued coverage of the poor, the elderly, and the disabled and providing catastrophic coverage for those unable to obtain such insurance in the private sector. The other part of the bill required employers to provide employees and their dependents with benefits meeting uniform federal standards, including catastrophic coverage and a high deductible, such as $2,500.

The range of proposals for national health insurance introduced

in Congress was approximately the same as during the previous administration, from a very comprehensive proposal to one for catastrophic
coverage only. There were, however, more sponsors and proposals than
before, because the possibility of some kind of legislation seemed imminent (as it had for the last 30 years) and no one wanted to be left out,
just in case. In 1976, there were 125 congressional sponsors of 21 national health insurance bills.

It would serve no useful purpose to go into the proposed bills in
great detail, since others have done so.[18] I will borrow, with some modi-
fication, the useful classification found in the book by Feder, Holahan,
and Marmor.[19] There are several ways of classifying proposals, depending on their purpose. If, for example, the purpose is administrative
control, who is vested with control? Another classification is scope of
benefits: Who is to receive what services? A third is fiscal: Who pays
what and how much?

For the purposes of this book, the different political perspectives
on national health insurance can best be understood when proposals are
classified by source of funding, population to be covered, and scope of
benefits. These three aspects are particularly important because they
indicate the extent to which government becomes directly involved with
both providers and recipients of services. They also reveal the extent to
which government becomes involved in the private sector as a buyer or
provider of services.

Proposals for national health insurance can be classified along a
spectrum of government involvement, as follows:

1. Narrow coverage of the population and limited federal role in
   financing
2. Wide coverage and limited federal role in financing
3. Wide coverage and large federal role in financing

Scope of benefits would seem, for the purpose at hand, to be subordi-
nate to coverage and federal financial involvement, although benefits
do, of course, affect total fiscal requirements. The three classifications
involve three different sets of cost estimates: (1) to individuals directly,
if they pay part; (2) to employers; and (3) to the local, state, and federal
governments.

In the first category, an explicitly defined segment of the population is the target. Expenditures for health services in the event of catastrophic illness in a family is an example. Several legislative proposals,
including the bill proposed by the Carter administration, were directed
toward that problem. Other target populations have been the elderly,

the poor, or the very young. Some bills combine both expenses and special segments of the population.

Proposals in the first category have in common (1) their focus on a particular problem or segment of the population and (2) their limits on the federal government's financial responsibility. They will have greater benefits for some segments of the population and will have relatively little effect on tax sources.

Proposals in the second category would provide wider benefits and population coverage than proposals in the first. The federal financial role would still be relatively limited. This limitation would be achieved by diffusing premiums among employers, employees, and government and by relying on private insurance companies as underwriters. Plans in this category could be either voluntary or mandatory.

The Medicredit plan sponsored by the AMA in the early 1970s is an example of a voluntary plan. Under it, the federal government would provide incentives for enrollment by offering individuals and employers a tax credit for insurance premiums instead of the existing tax deductions. Credits to individuals were to vary with income. Employers were given tax deductions if they offered their employees qualifying health insurance policies.

The mandatory approach is exemplified in a proposal made by the Nixon-Ford administrations, the Comprehensive Health Insurance Plan. It would tax wages for health insurance, but the tax would not be reflected in the federal budget. The tax would be shared between employees and employers. The scope of benefits would also be relatively broad. The poor and the elderly would be brought in, thus the entire population would be included in some way.

Plans in the second category are national in scope. Participation is voluntary or compulsory, although the financing of a mandatory proposal does not show up in the federal budget. They are universal in that all Americans are included one way or another. They constitute an aggregation of plans rather than a single, uniform plan for everyone.

The third classification is illustrated in its pure form by the Kennedy-Corman bill. It is the opposite of the AMA Medicredit plan. The federal government would monopolize the entire health services enterprise, offering universal coverage and comprehensive benefits; it would eventually use its power to reorganize the delivery system into prepaid group practices. There would be a single health insurance program for everyone, with no division into old or young, rich or poor, employed or unemployed. The plan would be financed jointly by payroll taxes and general revenues. It would be administered by the federal government through regional tiers of management. The Kennedy-Corman plan is very close to the National Health Service of the United Kingdom. The politics of health insurance in the United States, however, is almost beyond comprehension. The "rational" model of the British would be impossible.

Some insight into these complexities is provided by Lawrence Brown, who observes that post-Medicare politics takes place within three distinct subsystems: (1) the old subsidy program, (2) the financing programs, and (3) reorganization and regulation. These three subsystems involve six different committees and at least as many Congressional "health leaders," with little coordination among them:

> Once a bill finds its way into law, it bears the marks of executive uncertainty and obligation, extensive Congressional reworking to build a majority coalition, and considerable interest-group accommodation. Bureaucratic powers are often unclear or sharply constrained at crucial points, reflecting executive fears of bureaucratic subversion. Congressional fears of bureaucratic dictation, and interest-group fears of bureaucratic high-handedness.[20]

The Carter administration inherited an obligation to carry out the National Health Planning and Resources Development Act of 1975. Over 200 health service areas, and health services agencies to administer them, had to be put in place, and guidelines for them had to be written by the Secretary of HEW. These guidelines were to suggest criteria for the number of hospital and nursing home beds, the mix of these beds (maternity, pediatrics, and so on), and the amount of high technology equipment, such as CAT scanners.

Perhaps Secretary of HEW Califano had to wait until all the areas and agencies were in place and functioning before he issued guidelines, but he did not issue any until September 23, 1977. When he did so, they recommended:

1. There should be no more than four general hospital beds per 1,000 persons in the population (exclusive of federal hospitals).

2. Average annual occupancy should be at least 80 percent.

3. Maternity units in population clusters of more than 100,000 persons should each handle at least 2,000 deliveries a year and have an average annual occupancy of 75 percent.

4. There should be at least 20 beds in an inpatient pediatric unit, and units should have an average annual occupancy rate of 65 to 80 percent, depending on the total number of beds.

5. There should be four neonatal (first month of life) intensive care units for every 1,000 live births per year in a defined service area, with no fewer than 20 beds in each unit.

6. At least 200 open-heart procedures should be performed annually in any institution providing open-heart surgery; no new open-heart units should be started unless existing or previously approved units in the area are operating at a minimum of 350 cases per year.

7. At least 300 heart catheterization procedures should be performed annually in any adult cardiac catheterization unit, and at least 150 should be performed annually in any pediatric unit; there should be no new adult units unless there is enough demand to do more than 500 studies per year.

8. There should be one megavoltage radiation unit for every 150,000 persons, or one for every 7,500 treatments per year.

9. Each CAT scanner for head and body should perform at least 2,500 procedures per year; no new scanners should be approved unless existing scanners perform 4,000 patient procedures a year.

10. The health service agencies' plans should be consistent with established HEW standards and procedures governing kidney dialysis and organ transplantation

The guidelines were to become final early in 1978, after a 60-day period for comments from the field. HEW was careful to call them guidelines rather than directives, even though, if they were to be effective, they eventually had to be enforced as directives within the framework of the state certificate-of-need laws.

The National Council on Health Planning and Development, the committee appointed to advise HEW at the national level, asked HEW for staff to take a hard look at the guidelines. The council apparently did not want to depend entirely on reports from HEW staff. Undersecretary of HEW Hale Champion said there was no appropriation for such staff. When the council convened in October 1977, it deferred any endorsement of the guidelines until further reviews had been conducted.[21] An estimated 50,000 letters and protests followed the release of the guidelines. Califano sent a clarifying statement to every member of Congress. The statement said, in essence, that only state and local planning agencies had the authority to review major new capital expenditures; HEW did not. HEW was to offer numerical guideposts, as mandated by the Health Planning Act, to help states and local communities in their planning. Actually, HEW had been mandated to issue guidelines by mid-1976, but the Nixon-Ford administrations had not done so.

Califano emphasized further in his memorandum to Congress that the guidelines were tentative and had been put forth to obtain comments:

> ... we are pleased the comment has been spirited. We intend to listen and to learn from these comments. Not only have the comments helped us learn, they have also started in earnest a debate that must occur if we are to stem spiralling medical costs. We simply must develop appropriate standards to measure the real need for medical facilities and equipment in this country.[22]

According to an HEW summary of the 50,000 comments, they expressed three major concerns: (1) small rural hospitals might be forced to close; (2) standards for obstetrical units might be too strict; and (3) the guidelines would tend to take decision making out of local hands. I suspect the last was the most important concern; the matters of small rural hospitals and obstetrical units required mainly compromises in arithmetic.

A month or so later, on January 18, 1978, Secretary Califano published a revised set of proposed planning guides. He also published his findings about the 55,000 written statements that had come to HEW from the field: about 80 percent of them came from three states—Texas, Iowa, and Montana. These states have large, sparsely settled areas with small hospitals.

Califano reminded the country that HEW had not picked these proposed standards out of the blue. Each was based on a recommendation, guideline, or standard previously developed by one or more of the following groups: the Institute of Medicine of the National Academy of Sciences, the Office of Technology Assessment (a federal agency reporting to the White House), the American College of Obstetrics and Gynecology, the American Academy of Pediatrics, the American College of Radiology, the Committee on Perinatal Health, and the Inter Society Commission on Heart Disease. These latter associations are private professional organizations.

Although the guidelines had not come out of the blue, they nevertheless represented professional judgments, which err on the side of optimum conditions. Very few of the guidelines had scientifically established reference points. This is not to argue that guidelines are not necessary for planning and operation, but they can be spuriously specific. Years ago, as a result of the Hospital Survey and Construction Act (Hill-Burton), 4.5 general hospital beds per 1,000 persons in the population was accepted as a standard. The country was used to this supply of beds, and there were no long waits for hospital admissions. In any case, the revised standards allowed more local flexibility. One must remember that HEW was paying for Medicare and Medicaid, which consumed almost 10 percent of the federal budget and almost 40 percent of expenditures for all personal health services, and spending guidelines were very much in order.

NOTES

1. U.S. Department of Health, Education, and Welfare, Public Health Service, *Forward Plan for Health FY 1978–82* (Washington, D.C.: Government Printing Office, 1976).
2. Ibid., p. 114.
3. Ibid., p. 2.
4. Interviewed by Michael Lesparre, in "The Federal Role in Health" *Trustee* 26 (October 1973):18.
5. David S. Abernethy and David A. Pearson, *Regulating Hospital Costs: The Development of Public Policy* (Washington, D.C.: AUPHA Press, 1979), pp. 54–72.
6. Ibid., p. 74.
7. Ibid., p. 93.
8. Ibid., p. 93.
9. U.S. Congress, House, Committee on Ways and Means, Subcommittee on Health, and Committee on Interstate and Foreign Commerce, Subcommittee on Health and Environment, *President's Hospital Cost Containment Proposal: Joint Hearings on H.R. 6575*, 95th Cong., 1st sess., 1977, p. 657.
10. Ibid., p. 262.
11. *Modern Health Care* 9 (July 1979):52.
12. Abernethy and Pearson, *Regulating*, p. 103.
13. Ibid., p. 104.
14. Honorable Dan Rostenkowski, *Congressional Record* 123 (2 November 1977):H12086.
15. Abernethy and Pearson, *Regulating*, p. 149.
16. Abernethy and Pearson citing John K. Iglehart, "The All-Volunteer Cost Control Plan," *National Journal* 10 (11 February 1978):236.
17. Abernethy and Pearson, *Regulating*, p. 186.
18. See "Battle Lines Drawn on NHI," *Health Security News*, 14 May 1976; Laurence K. Altman, "Costs Are Found Similar in National Health Insurance Plans," *New York Times*, 7 May 1976, sect. C, p. 15.
19. See Judith Feder, John Holahan, and Theodore Marmor, eds., *National Health Insurance: Conflicting Goals and Policies* (Washington, D.C.: Urban Institute, 1980) pp. 686–705.
20. Lawrence D. Brown, "The Formulation of Federal Health Care Policy," Brookings Institution General Series Report No. 334 (Washington, D.C.: Brookings Institution 1978).
21. "Planning Council Vows Hard Look at Guidelines," *Health Resources News* 4 (November 1977):1.
22. *Medical Care Review* 35 (January 1978):12–14.

18

The Decade of the Eighties: The Reagan Administration and "Explosions"

At the end of the Carter administration in 1980 and the beginning of the more conservative Reagan administration, the expenditures for health and health-related services in the United States stood at an all-time high of $249 billion, or $1,075 per capita and 9.5 percent of the GNP. Reagan felt he had a conservative mandate to slow government expenditures and reduce taxes. The portion of the health services bill paid by federal and state governments was around 40 percent, with the federal government paying most of that through Medicare. The expenditures for both Medicare and Medicaid were rising very rapidly, as was the outlay of the private insurance sector.

In 1987 the total expenditures for all health services and goods, program administration, capital expenditures, and research stood at $496.6 billion. The prediction for 1990 is $647.3 billion. Personal health services alone stood at $438.9 billion in 1987, and the prediction for 1990 is $573.5 billion. A more understandable figure is that in 1987 total expenditures for personal health services per capita were $1,744, and the predicted expenditures for 1990 are $2,225 per capita, an increase of 22 percent in three years. We are in a continuing cost explosion, apparently for the indefinite future. Extrapolating to the year 2000, given no drastic changes in fiscal and volume controls, expenditures will be $5,075 per capita. The sources of payment in 1987 were as shown in Table 18.1, along with the predicted distribution for 1990.

The continuing cost explosion of the eighties coincided with other policy issue explosions. In addition to the overarching issue of cost, there were pressing issues of equity, regarding the portion of the popu-

TABLE 18.1   Sources of Payment for U.S. Health Services by Percentage, 1987 and 1990

1987 (Actual)		1990 (Predicted)	
Third parties		Third parties	
Government		Government	
Federal	24.9	Federal	27.0
Other	5.4	Other	5.2
	30.3		32.2
Private insurance	41.9	Private insurance	41.3
	72.2		73.5
Direct payment	27.8	Direct payment	26.5
Other sources	0.1	Other sources	0.1

Source: Figures from Office of the Actuary, Health Care Financing Administration, "National Health Expenditures," *Health Care Financing Review* 8 (Summer 1987):1–36.

lation without health insurance; bioethics, as in the transplantation and supply of organs and the saving of anencephalic fetuses as organ donors; abortion (when is the fetus a person?); seemingly boundless technology driving up medical costs; the possible erosion of the quality of medical care in the face of cost constraints; the cost of malpractice insurance; and the changing of lifestyles to incorporate healthful habits presumed to lessen demand for health services. The concept of prevention was touted more and more in such forms as early diagnosis, immunization, and the detection and management of high blood pressure.

Resolution of some of these issues would, of course, result in higher expenditures, as in the case of the uninsured. Resolution of other issues, such as lifestyle and prevention, might lower costs, but only in the long run, if at all. Many believed that there was a great deal of waste in the health services system which, if eliminated, would enable the country to have more care for less money. The overriding paradigm for cost control and management was competition. Policy makers turned to the business and competition model, the model that made the United States the productive, affluent, and high-consumption economy it is. The industrial management model was to be applied to the health services enterprise largely through the incentives of the profit motive rather than through regulation and medical professional judgment.

The application of the competitive model to what was already being described as the medical-industrial complex, however, aroused mixed emotions in both the health services establishment and the body politic. Leading off early in the decade was Arnold S. Relman, editor of the *New England Journal of Medicine*. In a blistering editorial, quoted frequently by those who supported his view, he wrote,

It seems to me that the key to the problems of overuse [hence high expenditures] is in the hands of the medical profession. With the consent of the patients, physicians act in their behalf, deciding which services are needed and which are not, in effect serving as their trustees. The best kind of regulation of the health-care marketplace should therefore come from the informed judgments of physicians working in the interests of their patients. In other words physicians should supply the discipline that is provided in commercial markets by the informed choices of prudent consumers, who shop for the goods and services that they want, at the prices that they are willing to pay.

But if physicians are to represent their patients' interests in the new medical marketplace, they should have no economic conflict of interest and therefore no pecuniary association with the medical-industrial complex.[1]

Relman repeated his view in 1989 in an interview in the *Reece Report:* "We don't have a clear vision of what we want our health care system to be. Do we want it to be a business, or do we want it to be a social service?"[2]

Americans are schizophrenic toward medical care as a business. In our economic and political philosophy, how do we interrelate the private profit, the private nonprofit, and the governmental sectors in the health services to form a functioning composite? How do we identify private and public responsibility and accountability in a service that is essentially clothed with the public interest and that therefore requires a great deal of government involvement?

The private profit and private nonprofit sectors are not capable of assuring services to all segments of society. In the final analysis, only government responsible to the electorate can assume this task. But what is the public interest? Long ago Walter Lippmann, tongue in cheek, defined it as follows: "The public interest may be presumed to be what men [and women] would choose if they saw clearly, thought rationally, acted disinterestedly and benevolently."[3] I would presume that the last attributes—disinterest and benevolence—are the most difficult ones to practice.

The foregoing composite of problems was synthesized by Jack D. McCue, in his 1989 volume.[4]

COST CONTAINMENT METHODS

As stated, the model applied to cost containment was competition. But to exercise the consumer sovereignty fundamental to classical economic competition, consumers of health care would have to have free choice and perfect information. Thus, employers, the main source of funding for private health insurance, would offer employees a choice of several health insurance plans; employees would choose among them; and employers would pay a percentage of the premium with employees paying the balance.

This was the theory, although like all theories it was not applied in its pure form. The major theorists were Paul Ellwood of InterStudy and Alain C. Enthoven of Stanford University. A more embracing regulation-and-competition theorist was Clark C. Havighurst of Duke University. The competitive option concept did not surface in the early eighties—it was embodied in the HMO Act of Congress in 1973—but the full import of the concept did not become apparent until the eighties. Numerous macro and micro evaluations of the operation of the concept were undertaken in the eighties, and most of them seemed to be inconclusive.[5]

A rather extensive literature appeared in the eighties on the increase in costs that occurred despite attempts at introducing competition. A general feeling pervaded this literature that perhaps the federal and state governments were not deregulating the health insurance industry enough so that the classical theory of competition could be tried in an at-least-approximately-pure form. It seemed that regulatory measures were held in reserve in case the competition concept did not contain costs. For example, Minnesota, to facilitate fair competition, mandated a standard range of health insurance benefits to include alcoholism and chemical dependency care and psychiatric services in physicians' offices. What was not mandated was the standardization of employee groups by age; employers with younger, healthier employees could still benefit from lower premiums.

Enthoven, incidentally, recommended that the premiums for employee groups be standardized by age to avoid that competitive advantage for employers (and certain employees). In this connection, I have felt that Enthoven, Ellwood, and Havighurst devised a competition and regulation theory as complex as a Swiss watch, a theory well beyond the political sophistication of our interest-group political process. A watch built by politicians would not keep time—the necessary compromises would be intolerable in a functioning timepiece.

Many states have kept their certificate-of-need laws (for control of hospital beds and hospital rates) on the books and not applied them rigorously. Minnesota went so far as to abolish its certificate-of-need law, considering it no longer necessary given the proliferation of HMOs in that state. The whole stance of the federal government through its annual budget for Medicare, however, is in effect regulatory given that the health services cannot in all practicality have an open-ended reimbursement system as they had before the seventies.

The classical economic concept of competition is an illusion in the health services because, in the main, the public does not regard health care as a commodity like any other. This basic confusion over the nature of health care leads to policy schizophrenia in a heavily market-oriented culture.

The budget policies to repress the federal deficit are massive examples of macro financial regulation on the part of the federal government during and after the Reagan administration. They had a direct effect on all of Medicare and at least half of Medicaid, and these two entitlement programs in turn have an indirect effect on the rest of the health services economy. The Omnibus Reconciliation Act of 1981, the Reagan administration's first budget, established a prospective payment system for hospital services rendered to Medicare patients, replacing the traditional retrospective payment system. Medicare patients, on average, account for some 40 percent of a hospital's annual income.

Next the Tax Equity and Fiscal Responsibility Act of 1982 established the method for controlling hospital costs through the diagnosis-related group (DRG) system in the Social Security Amendments of 1983. Very briefly (because the DRG reimbursement system is now so well known that an elaborate description is not necessary), Medicare pays the hospital a flat, per case amount for the care of patients with diagnoses that have been shown to be quite similar in terms of hospital costs. With 475 or so DRGs in effect, there are thus 475 separate budget caps in American hospitals as opposed to a single global budget for a year as prevails, for example, in the Canadian health insurance system.

The Omnibus Deficit Reduction Act of 1984 froze Medicare reimbursements for physician fees and reduced DRG rates for hospitals. The Act affected mainly Medicaid, which experienced massive reductions in federal spending—3 percent in fiscal year 1982, 4 percent in 1983, and 4.5 percent in 1984. Free choice of provider, enshrined in the Medicaid Act of 1965, was waived for Medicaid patients although it was retained for Medicare patients. States were given the discretion to limit Medicaid patients to a choice of HMOs, curtailing their option to seek care from providers in the mainstream, fee-for-service system.

At the end of 1985, Reagan signed the Gramm-Rudman-Hollings bill requiring that the federal deficit be eliminated through the conventional legislative process of debate and compromise or, failing that, through automatic, across-the-board budget cuts over a five-year period. Exempt from automatic cuts were Medicaid; Aid to Families with Dependent Children; the Women, Infants, and Children program; food stamps; and child nutrition programs. Congress was, in effect, opting out of its responsibility to the people if its members could not agree.

There was obviously a passionate desire to cut costs, which crossed political party lines—the distinction between parties being that the Republicans were by and large more passionate than the Democrats.

Despite these massive attempts to "take the federal government off the backs of the people," the federal presence continued strong, indicating the historically inherent drive for government to take an active interest in the health and welfare of the public. Barry G. Rabe observed in 1987,

> The endurance of a significant government role in health care into the late 1980s is remarkable given the factors which seemed so likely to herald a new era of reduced central government involvement in health and countless other areas of domestic policy.
>
> This resiliency of the federal government in health care extends to all aspects of its relations with the nation's health care system, state and local governments, and health-related social and economic activity. This pattern encompasses federally funded and regulated categorical and block grant programs in health care as well as direct federal regulation of health care delivery and public health functions, such as environmental protection. It suggests an enduring role for the central government in health policy albeit one that increasingly emphasizes cost containment rather than service expansion or equalization.[6]

Even though the role of the federal government in health care remained substantial, however, cost shifting and consolidation in the second half of the eighties were real. For example, health programs were compressed into four new block grants so that the states received significantly less federal funding. Previous programs on high blood pressure, risk reduction and health education, venereal disease, immunization, fluoridation, rat control, lead poisoning, and family planning were consolidated into a preventive health services block grant.[7]

In 1983 the National Health Planning and Resources Development Act of 1974 was abolished by lack of appropriations. The federally mandated PSROs, which had monitored use of hospital services in Medicare, were also abolished, although legislation still mandated that agencies contract utilization surveillance out to private peer review organizations (PROs) so that regular monitoring of hospital care would continue. The DRG control mechanism mentioned above was a profound incursion into the professional decision-making prerogatives of physicians.

Later in the decade came the results of the study of physician reimbursement funded by the Health Care Financing Administration (HCFA) and conducted by William C. Hsiao and colleagues at the Harvard School of Public Health. The results were released in 1988 and created a sensation in the health services establishment, particularly among physicians.[8]

The reimbursement study attempted to measure three resource inputs to what physicians do: (1) the time they spend before, during, and after the provision of a particular service and how that time is spent; (2) average practice costs by specialty; and (3) the cost of physicians' training. The researchers concentrated on 23 services in 18 specialties. The results took the form of a resource-based relative value scale (RBRVS) and indicated more pay would be in order for cognitive physicians (those who talk more with their patients) and less pay would be in order for procedural physicians (those who talk less, presumably surgeons and radiologists).

The RBRVS is not supposed to be in place until 1991, before which time there will be much haggling between parties of interest and undoubtedly some softening modifications. Some physicians complain that the RBRVS uses purely resource-cost criteria and ignores the quality of the physician-patient relationship. The industrial model mentioned earlier, however, embraces the concept of costing out a service, minimizing if not ignoring the human relations component.

THE COMMISSION METHOD

American society is so large and has so many interest groups that a large variety of commissions and committees are in constant operation, in overlapping and rapid succession, and each trying to reach a policy consensus of one kind or another on issues ranging from bioethics to universal health insurance.

Bioethics is a profound and difficult area of study, having a long history and deep roots in human values. About 20 years ago, bioethical issues began surfacing in general discussion and debate. The Hastings Center, founded in 1969 as the Institute of Society, Ethics, and the Life Sciences, is the major private vehicle for furthering this debate. Over the years, the Center has become increasingly visible and effective in bringing to public attention and discussion the ethical issues raised by advances in medicine, the natural sciences, and the behavioral and social sciences. These advances, to name a few, include organ transplants, human experimentation, prenatal diagnosis of genetic diseases, life-extending technologies, and recombinant DNA research.

A clear spinoff of the activities of the Hastings Center was the appointment of the President's Commission for the Study of Ethical Problems in Medicine and Biomedical and Behavioral Research, chaired by Morris B. Abrams. This commission was created during the Carter administration in 1978 but did not report until the early eighties, during the Reagan administration. The reports totaled 16 volumes, and each of the reports drew from the advice of experts on the spectrum of issues listed above.

The purpose of the commission was to establish a rational philosophical framework in which to think about and formulate public policy on these thorny problems, but not to make explicit recommendations. The intention behind this mandate was to promote rational policy discussions on a clearer ethical base than usually obtained. Daniel Wikler, a bioethicist at the University of Wisconsin–Madison, was a "house philosopher" for the division of the commission that considered the ethical implications of differences in the availability of health services. I heard him say in a lecture that policy makers seem incapable of formulating public policy within a conscious and explicit ethical framework because they are not fully aware of the roots of their own ethical behavior. This made for great difficulty in formulating a policy on access to health services—which would seem to be one of the simpler issues in public policy (compared to, for instance, the issue of when a fetus is a person).

Alexander Capron reflected on this vagueness in 1983, shortly after all the reports had been submitted to the president. He wrote,

> If Shaw's suggestion that Englishmen think themselves moral when they are actually only uncomfortable applied to the life services today, we should all be feeling very moral. Rather than confirming our morality, however, the uncomfortable dilemmas we've had to confront of late have seemed merely to multiply our uncertainties. From a few thin volumes on "medical ethics" twenty years ago, the literature on the newly styled subject of "bioethics" has grown at a spectacular rate. Does such an explosion of application justify or contradict the need for a federal Commission? Having just spent more than three years as executive director of the President's Commission . . . , I am still unsure of the answer—or, rather, unsure that any general answer is possible.[9]

Capron's observation is borne out by the ethical problem of the continuation of life support systems in obviously irreversible cases, or of life support measures' being rationed by ambiguous criteria. It is not my purpose to dwell at length on this issue but to offer extreme examples as illustrations of its inherent complexity.

A most dramatic and poignant incident took place in 1989 at Rush–Presbyterian–St. Luke's Medical Center in Chicago, involving Rudy Linares whose 15-month-old son had been kept alive for 8 months via a life support system. The child was comatose and reportedly had no chance of recovery. Linares walked into his son's room at the hospital, held the staff at bay with a gun, and disconnected the life support system. Understandably, the hospital had kept the boy alive because of fear of legal action. The Rush officials tried to get the Linares family to talk with "an array of physicians, nurses, chaplains, social workers, psychiatrists and lay people."[10] But the family—Linares's wife and two other children—refused, as well they might given this "array." The father had little insurance, and he was not poor, so he struggled with the double burden of a completely incompetent son and huge debts. The father was charged with first-degree murder, but the charge was dropped when a grand jury found inadequate cause to support it. Linares was put on probation for a year when he pleaded guilty to a misdemeanor charge of carrying an unlicensed gun. The case, naturally, hit the news media, and a legal precedent was presumably established that has many ambiguous ramifications. Value norms and public policies are often set in this way when no clear-cut resolution seems possible.

In the state of Oregon in 1987 a policy stemming from scarce resources, or at least an unwillingness to raise taxes for Medicaid, aroused national ethical attention.[11] The state legislature bit the bullet of rationing scarce resources for the poor (the population with whom rationing usually starts) and decided to eliminate Medicaid payments for organ transplants in favor of funding basic health services for thousands of pregnant women and young children. One of the first dramatic results of this policy, which was set by a body representing the people, was the death of seven-year-old Coby Howard who was waiting for funds for a bone-marrow transplant.

John Kitzhaber, a physician and also president of the Oregon state senate, reaffirmed his support of the legislation and killed an emergency proposal to refund the transplant program, a proposal offered presumably to prevent similar cases in the future. He is quoted as saying, "I don't oppose transplants; what I oppose is refunding that program out of context, without making a judgment about whether other people might be squeezed out of the program as a consequence."[12] What Kitzhaber wanted was a control, since the state had no policy at all on how limited health care resources were to be applied. The significance of the Oregon action was that the state was not going to engage in ad hoc policy making based on the merit of individual cases, a fact that may begin to assure Capron that a general answer is possible.

As a close to discussion of this intractable issue—which is far from resolved nationally—I offer the observation by Ron Kovener, vice president of the Health Care Financial Management Association, that the federal government has no priority guidelines for services to Medicare beneficiaries: "Clearly the federal government doesn't want to pay for all the service Medicare beneficiaries may want to use. But formulating overt rationing policies would be politically risky. Instead, the government shifts the decision to hospitals by underpaying them."[13] Obviously the Medicare population has much more political clout than the Medicaid population. (As an aside it should be observed that countries with national health insurance have no rationing policy, as such, either; they depend on the physicians, particularly the hospital-based specialists, to do the rationing within the budgets they are appropriated to work with.)

Two privately financed and sponsored commissions deliberated on the health services issues of the nation during the eighties. The National Leadership Commission on Health Care, inaugurated in 1987, studied for 30 months and reported in 1989. The Health Policy Agenda for the American People, sponsored by the American Medical Association, started rather quietly in 1982 and began to report in 1988.

The leadership commission's 35 members were well-known leaders in health care, business, law, economics, and public affairs, and they were assisted by 20 advisors. The commission was a private and self-designated multipartisan effort and included former policy makers from both national and state levels as well as former presidents Gerald Ford, Jimmy Carter, and Richard Nixon. The commission's recommendations covered the waterfront: (1) a universal access (UNAC) plan, entitling all citizens to a basic level of health services; (2) a national quality improvement initiative for health services practices; (3) cost control, through economic leverage in the purchase of care and through economic incentives including cost sharing; and (4) reform of medical professional liability to control costs and discourage the practice of defensive medicine.[14] Most of the members of the commission endorsed the recommendations. Several, however, dissented, and the dissenters were mainly from business and industry, medicine, and insurance—hardly unimportant interest groups.

The national health insurance plan was the most controversial recommendation, the others being easier initiatives on which to achieve consensus both in concept and in implementation. The concept of universal access—not to mention its funding and implementation—will be intensely debated, from basic services to sources of funding to type of agency. It is clear, however, that a "made in America" approach to health insurance for everybody, aided and abetted by government in one way or another, is emerging beyond Orwell's "non-think" stage.

The second private policy body, the Health Policy Agenda for the American People, was an elaborately conceived and mounted agency. (It did not use the term "commission.") That the AMA took leadership in sponsoring this forward-looking effort is significant given the AMA's usual image of reluctant leadership. The Health Policy Agenda was an impressive coalition of 172 public- and private-sector organizations committed to improving health care services. The rancor associated with the national health insurance legislation proposed before President Dwight D. Eisenhower took office in 1952, and with the miniature version of national health insurance for the elderly that began in 1965, had apparently subsided as providers, payers, and the public began to realize that they have problems in common that require consensus solutions.

Like the leadership commission, the Health Policy Agenda wished to set forth a broad framework (although boundaries were not entirely clear) in which policy makers and the public could consider policy with respect to equity, funding and benefit levels, and universal coverage. The reader will recall that the President's Commission for the Study of Ethical Problems in Medicine and Biomedical and Behavioral Research, described earlier, also attempted a sort of superstructure in which to address the equity issues: this is a highly philosophical but profoundly necessary task.

The Health Policy Agenda reports included two significant policy recommendations, one of them dealing with the important concept of basic benefits and the other dealing with health services for the poor, that is, a reformation of Medicaid.

The recommendation regarding basic benefits in health insurance was surprisingly elaborate. It seemed to include almost every type of service, and it greatly emphasized preventive services and early detection of disease, maternal and child health, immunizations, and medical examination. There was a relatively generous inclusion of mental illness in private offices and other out-of-hospital settings. Virtually all emergency services (not clearly defined) were included, as were home settings for hospice services for the terminally ill, short-term home care, up to 90 days of care in skilled nursing facilities, and up to 90 visits of home nursing care. These services would be subject to deductibles and coinsurance, and there would be maxima for out-of-pocket expenses.[15] What the Health Policy Agenda skirted was what might be called long-term care in long-term facilities—it appears that this type of care was to be shifted to Medicaid.

The report on Medicaid "Including the Poor" became a thorough description and examination of the current status of Medicaid federal-state program sharing, with its state-to-state inconsistencies in poverty levels served and benefit ranges. The recommendations had substance certainly as to a national concept of equity. They included an uncoupling of the Medicaid program from cash assistance programs, eliminating the categorical eligibility definitions, using 100 percent of the federal poverty level as the minimum standard for uniform eligibility, and developing federal incentives to close coverage gaps for individuals and families with incomes between 100 percent and 200 percent of the poverty level.

The report said also that there should be a "medically needy" program for those above the national poverty level. Medicaid should be restructured so as to be governed by national standards and goals, with each state providing a standard, federally mandated benefit package that is quite basically comprehensive and includes institutional care for the elderly and long-term care services. And, very importantly, the federal government should bear a greater burden of the funding, supporting the program through general revenue. The federal formula governing reimbursement to the states should be revised to correct for tax burden inequalities.[16] Interestingly, though, the Health Policy Agenda sidestepped the issue of universal coverage, except possibly implicitly through its heavy emphasis on private-sector funding by employers for their uncovered employees.

The commissions were established and in session when attitudes and actions were changing significantly with regard to the presence of the 37 million or so persons among us who are uninsured for one reason or another: they are self-employed, employed in small firms that offer no insurance, or ineligible for Medicaid. Morally if not legally, the providers of health care have had to serve the uninsured who presented themselves at hospitals, resulting in a great deal of cost shifting to privately insured patients and recourse to reserve funds.

In other words, the private sector, largely through the employers and employees, was in effect subsidizing a public responsibility through higher premiums and fees. The pressure on hospitals and physicians to provide free care represented a moral blackmail of the private sector. This situation is an interesting example of the persistence of the private, noblesse oblige charity that goes back to the beginning of the Industrial Revolution. In the United States, at least, the funding of public responsibility through general revenue or special taxes has not proved congenial with the politics of taxation; funding has not been able to keep pace with the increasing costs of modern, high-technology medical care.

The Reagan administration was cutting back on the federal and federal-state programs—in the case of Medicare by capping the costs of hospital stays and increasing deductibles and coinsurance, and in the case of Medicaid by reducing funding to the states—thus forcing the states to tighten income-eligibility standards and curtail benefits in order to save money. The results were documented by a nationwide survey sponsored by the Robert Wood Johnson Foundation in 1986. To quote the general conclusions of the report, "The most disturbing findings of the

. . . Survey involve the deterioration in access to medical care among the nation's poor, minority, and uninsured citizens compared with 1982."[17] Since funding has not improved since then, one may reasonably assume that access conditions have deteriorated further. The reduction in funding was a clear administration policy with, it seems, the intent of changing the definition of the poor to "the really poor."

The Medicare constituency had more political clout than the poor as seen in the 1965 legislation establishing universal entitlement for the elderly, supported by a stable financial base of earmarked payroll taxes. The act was in effect catastrophe health insurance for acute care rather than long-term care. Long-term care became the responsibility of Medicaid, which used a means-test criterion for elderly persons who could not afford nursing home care.

By early 1988 bipartisan action emerged to extend the benefits of the Medicare Act of 1965 to include additional catastrophic costs, although it left the substance of the problem of long-term care for the elderly to Medicaid and the means test. Under this legislation, the elderly would still have had to "spend down" to the income and assets criteria of the various states. The number of covered hospital days was, however, increased, as was the number of nursing home days, filling out here and there. The most important additional coverage was the pharmaceutical benefit, which the original act had excluded altogether.[18] The Medicare Catastrophic Coverage Act was passed on July 1, 1988[19] and, due to public outcry and intense lobbying over both its limitations and its funding—a tax on the population served—repealed on November 22, 1989. The flood of protests from the elderly to the members of Congress was so traumatic that politicians are being reported as predicting that the repeal of the Act will delay indefinitely any legislation covering chronic care.

The pressure to contain the federal budget deficit in the late 1980s was tremendous. The constant drive to expand health services through legislation necessitated finding sources of funds for the catastrophic health insurance legislation that would not draw from general revenue and the personal income tax. (This is not to say that payroll taxes could be open-ended either without an employer tax revolt.) The new costs were not to be added to either the employer-employee payroll or the general revenue, but spread over the 29 million or so persons in the Medicare population, according to income.

Economic statisticians had discovered that, since 1965, a segment of the U.S. population 65 years of age and over had become so affluent as to more or less parallel the population under age 65. The welfare state had created a population of elderly persons with higher incomes than they had ever had in history! In 1965, roughly two-thirds of the elderly were classified as poor. By the 1980s, one-third or less could be so classified.

The elderly were set apart to finance their "catastrophic" health care plan out of their own pockets. Estimates were made that the low-income elderly would pay nothing in added taxes. Ten percent or so of the upper-income elderly would be paying the maximum, or $800 per person per year. This arrangement promised to have future repercussions to general revenue and to distribute the cost over everybody. In short, the method devised to pay for the increased benefits was pragmatically ingenious, but, as far as the elderly were concerned, politically explosive. One of the important long-view byproducts of the Medicare Catastrophic Coverage Act of 1988 was the establishment of the Bipartisan Commission on Comprehensive Health Care. This commission was based in Congress, and thus had direct connections with political power sources. It was established by since-deceased Representative Claude Pepper (D-Fla.), for decades a champion of the elderly, and its mandate was to examine the nation's health care system, specifically long-term care and access to health care for all Americans.

Senator John D. Rockefeller IV (D-W.Va.) chaired the commission, which released its report on March 2, 1990.[20] The report and the reaction to it were widely described in the press; I draw here from an article by Merit C. Kimball.[21] Kimball described vividly the political response to the report.

> It was billed as the main event, one that could break the logjam on what to do about the battered U.S. health care system and launch the nation toward a broad-based solution.
>
> Instead, the eagerly awaited effort by a blue-ribbon congressional committee, the Pepper Commission, turned out earlier this month to be just another report by a virtually deadlocked group of politicians.[22]

The commission approved proposals to assure all Americans access to health care and to provide long-term care, "but failed to come to grips with the key question of funding."[23] The overall cost was $66 billion, but the commission offered no specific recommendations as to how this money would be raised. The report simply listed all the conventional sources, from general revenue to deductibles charged to patients at the point of service.

Kimball reported that President Bush "enjoined" Republican members of the commission (by last-minute phone calls) not to accept any package calling for new taxes. They complied, along with two Democrats, Representative Fortney "Pete" Stark (Calif.) and Senator Max Baucus (Mont.).[24] So much for the ability of this country to agree on a national health policy as long as new taxes are not to be considered.

At the outset of the nineties, ferment outside of Congress over the issue of the uninsured has the potential for a political ground swell from the grassroots. Another ground swell is the increasing restiveness among employers who are shouldering a major portion of the costs for their employees. Employers are complaining about the difficulties in maintaining their necessary profit margins in a competitive economy.

Employers are not getting much sympathy yet, but the drive toward universal coverage of some type is gathering support. Past opponents of universality are supporting those who are supporters. James Todd, president of the AMA supports the policy that employers should be taxed for the uninsured. Former Representative Paul Rogers (D-Fla.), co-chair of the National Leadership Commission described earlier, fears that the middle classes may lose their insurance.[25] There seems to be increasing support, then, for the warhorse liberals such as Senator Edward R. Kennedy (D-Mass.) and Representative Henry A. Waxman (D-Calif.).

In 1989 the *Wall Street Journal* reported that Bethlehem Steel and the Steelworkers Union jointly would recommend a national health policy. AT&T considers backing a similar Communications Workers bid for a national health plan. Lee Iacocca of Chrysler says that it may be time for the United States, the only major remaining nation without national health insurance, to enact such insurance. The Ford Motor Company, seeing its health costs top $1 billion, calls for some "public sector cooperation."[26]

At current writing it is difficult to describe adequately the trend among states toward covering the uninsured, but the trend is there. Many states are making surveys of who the uninsured are and for what reasons they are uninsured. The conventional and probably accurate enough figure for policy thinking is that 37 million people—around 12 percent of the U.S. population—are uninsured, with the percentage varying some by state.

The first problem to attack is that of the employed uninsured, which automatically means small firms of 100 or fewer employees, possibly leaving out very small firms such as under 15 employees. The next group is the segment of the population that is uninsured and either unemployed or self-employed. Demographic statisticians have been at work in various states trying to tease out these uncovered segments of the population, toward the end of matching them with any available sources of mandated health services coverage and thus lessening the states' need to draw on general revenue to fund their health care. This process is a remarkable example of salami slicing, trying in the usual incremental fashion to get enough slices of coverage out of current insurance arrangements to obviate the need for national health insurance. Massachusetts in 1987 was the first state to mandate employer-financed health insurance for the employed and unemployed uninsured (the latter through pooling a separate fund). (When Governor Michael Dukakis was a presidential candidate, he tried to make much political hay of his expansion of insurance coverage in Massachusetts.)

THE QUALITY OF CARE ISSUE

Another area of concern since the middle to late 1980s is the possible effect of cost containment on the quality of patient care. Are hospitals and physicians cutting quality corners to reduce costs? Given the inherent difficulty of defining quality of care in operational terms, there is a great deal of speculation as to what is actually happening. Providers are likely to believe that the quality of care in hospitals and in physicians' offices is eroding in Medicare and in HMO-type practice under "managed" care, whereas funding agencies such as the Health Care Financing Administration press ever more on cost reduction and claim that quality is being maintained.[27] Employers wonder if they are getting adequate quality for the increased premiums they pay, and so it goes. There are plenty of anecdotes about "premature" discharge from hospitals for Medicare and Medicaid patients and about the loading of nursing homes with sicker patients than before.

A survey in Minnesota, an HMO-saturated and group practice-intensive state, of physicians' perceptions of the effect of managed care on quality reveals at least their impressions. It would seem that physicians are a logical source and important reference point for such views. Of a representative sample of physicians polled, 57 percent said that third party payers had limited treatment that the physicians would otherwise have recommended. On the face of it this percentage seems high, but what does it mean? As a patient I find it disturbing. Another aspect of the quality question is the physician's ability to function as an advocate for the patient. Among Minnesota physicians, the survey revealed, 62 percent believed that prepaid plans have reduced their ability to act as advocates for their patients.[28]

In seeming desperation, HCFA in the late 1980s caused a media explosion by reporting mortality rates for a very substantial number of hospitals, from standard community hospitals to high-technology teaching hospitals. Not surprisingly, the rates revealed that there were wide and unexplained differences among hospitals.

This fascination with numbers as such, flowing from the industrial model, would seem to have premature application to the many variables that go into hospital service decision making. I suppose, however, one must start somewhere with a shotgun technique, given that neither the medical profession nor the medical schools have taken the initiative to develop quality of care indicators. HCFA did open up the subject by following the precept that how to get the attention of the mule is to hit it over the head with a two-by-four. Both DRGs and the published mortality rates stimulated as nothing else interest in quality control methodology.

In time a competent team of health services researchers made an intensive review of hospital mortality rates as indicators of quality of care, putting the matter into a larger and more adequate perspective.[29] They concluded that hospital discharge abstract data are insufficient information from which to determine the extent to which differences in severity of illness or quality of care account for variability in mortality rates. Thus data on hospital death rates cannot now be used to draw inferences about the quality of care. The researchers suggest, however, that the magnitude of variability in death rates and the clustering of facilities with low death rates argue for further study of hospital death rates. These data may prove most useful as a screening mechanism to identify patterns of potentially poor quality of care.

The authors of the study ask, practically, "Until more definitive data become available what are potential patients to do when they read in their local newspapers that one or more of their hospitals have greater-than-expected death rates for one or more specific conditions? We urge such concerned persons to seek specific answers from their physicians."[30] The assumption is that patients are generally associated with a physician, not with a hospital directly. Such is the state of the art for lay judgment of quality.

HCFA's shotgun method may have been salutary in that apparently sensible moves are being made in the country in the direction of systematic, empirically grounded quality control methodology, but they will take time. In this connection a very thoughtful and balanced review of quality control standards and methods appeared in *GHAA News* by June H. White, managing editor of *Health Affairs*.[31] She reports that the Harvard Community Health Plan (HCHP) is working out specific practice guidelines. HCHP has 30 algorithms in the pipelines, which it is putting into computers, and supporters of the practice guidelines are impressive: HCFA, Congress, the Physician Payment Review Commission (PPRC), and the AMA.

The algorithm-computer approach is not without its sophisticated critics, however. White reports that Philip Caper, who heads the

Codman Research Group, said that this approach is the wrong way to solve the problem of controlling costs. Caper explained that "standards will be either narrow and specific and will gain little support, or they will be broad and vague and will have wide support, but little effect."[32] There are good reasons for using guidelines, but not for cost control. Further, White quotes Alan Rosenberg, a physician at Michael Reese Hospital, as saying that "for many of the most controversial areas [of medicine] there are just not good standards,"[33] by which I take it he means there is too much disagreement among professionals.

White herself takes the long view:

> As more research is conducted and more public and private resources committed to the issue, medical practice patterns and development guidelines will move even closer into the spotlight of health policy debate. Whether practice guidelines will be the magic pill to cure the inefficiency, wide practice variations, fluctuating quality, and rising costs across the U.S. health system or for individual providers remains to be seen.[34]

In any case there is, in both houses of Congress, a rising tide of interest in legislation promoting medical practice outcomes research.[35] The Senate bill at the time of this writing is the Patient Outcomes Research Act of 1989 (S. 702), and the House bill is the Medical Care Quality Research and Improvement Act of 1989 (H.R. 1692). Both bills have the same objectives, and both have clear bipartisan support. The areas of research specified in these bills are patient survival, clinical outcomes, complications, morbidity, the effect of medical treatment on symptoms, and, significantly, the effect of medical treatment on the quality of life. This last introduces the concept of "is the procedure worth it?"

Carolyne K. Davis and Frederick B. Abbey, in a 1989 article, warned and implored the providers of care not to underestimate the importance of what the authors called this "wave" of interest toward health services quality control.[36] Davis and Abbey said that the government hopes state-of-the-art data bases will enable it to expose individual cases of poor care, make profiles of the performance of providers to identify "aberrant behavior," establish boundaries to investigate variations in overall practice patterns in a community, and establish national practice guidelines. They went on to observe that there is nothing new about the desire to measure quality in health care. What is new is the intensity of the interest and effort in doing so, combined with the capability to apply computer technology to the process—faith in computers is unbounded.

With some passion Davis and Abbey admonished the providers:

> Practical use of quality indicators of the sort described here requires intense institutional and individual self-examination by management and

practitioners. Even this process, however, holds the promise of something worthwhile: the creation of better collegial relationships among medical, nursing and administrative staff, enabling the hospital to serve its community more effectively.[37]

Since cost is the driving force, despite Caper's earlier-cited caution, it seems that there must eventually be formulated some relationship between these numbers and quality of care translated into costs: from the best possible care, to good care, to adequate care, with dollar signs for each level.

At the risk of opening up a whole new area of discussion without space for adequate qualifications, I must point out that what all the foregoing selections of writers and articles on the subject of quality appear to overlook or, by implication, take for granted is that basically the provision of medical care rests on a trust in the providers that they will try to perform at their optimum day after day. No matter how much monitoring there is and what quantity of data computers spew out, trust is a central ingredient of service. What monitoring and computers can do is to expose the quite bad practice patterns and leave the great majority of practitioners alone. (It is by the way, entirely conceivable that the "bad apples" are already known via proper surveillance within institutions and insurance agencies, without all the hardware and data that seem to be wanted almost as ends in themselves.)

Finally, to round out discussion of the quality of care issue, one must consider the related and intransigent problem of medical malpractice litigation. Fortunately, a good review of this thorny problem was published in 1989, by Frank A. Sloan and Randall R. Bovbjerg.[38] The authors observed that the mid-1980s malpractice crisis was the second in 10 years. They cited an AMA study that estimated the total costs of the professional liability system for 1985 at $15.4 billion. That amounted to 17 percent of the $82 billion paid to physicians during that year. The breakdown by categories was as follows:

— $3.7 billion for malpractice premiums paid by physicians
— $0.1 billion for physician time spent in court and other related activities
— $11.7 billion in defensive medicine (i.e., services provided to decrease the margin of error within which physicians may be sued).

The malpractice insurance premiums paid by physicians constituted 4.5 percent of their gross incomes, and these estimates apparently did not include institutional liability insurance bought by hospitals exclusive of physicians.

Sloan and Bovbjerg speculated as to the reasons for the malpractice crisis. They saw no evidence of any across-the-board decline in quality; they believe it is more likely, in fact, that a general improvement in outcomes has occurred. They believe that sudden jumps in the frequency of litigation result from changing social and legal attitudes about lawsuits and from shifts in medical outcomes (e.g., newborns who earlier would have died now survive and need expensive, lifelong care).[39] (There may also be the "deep pocket" phenomenon of large, rich insurance companies and enormous medical centers dealing in billions of dollars.) The authors also raised the issue of trust when they observed that physicians are distressed by what they regard as the new climate of litigiousness eroding the therapeutic trust between physician and patient.

It may be noted parenthetically that all my citations—and many more could be included—regarding bioethics and the quality of care came from 1988 and later publications, a fact that must be symptomatic of underlying ferment.

One more commission, this one having to do with the labor shortage in nursing, should be mentioned to symbolize the range of problems being faced simultaneously in this country. The secretary of Health and Human Services created in 1988 a Commission on Nursing, in response to the difficulties hospitals reported in filling nurse positions, even though in 1988 there were more staffed nurse positions than ever.[40] The commission's report estimated that 137,000 hospital nurse positions were unfilled in 1988 because of a shortage of nurses.

The nursing market, like the market for all professional health personnel, is volatile. As recently as 1983 the Institute of Medicine completed a study of nursing personnel and reported to Congress that the supply of and demand for nurses should be in "reasonable balance" by the end of the decade and that the nursing shortage of the 1960s and 1970s had largely disappeared.[41] I include this finding here as an illustration of the continuing difficulties of projections and estimates. According to the AHA in its 1988 Human Resources Survey, shortages of a range of allied health personnel appear to be chronic. The hardest allied health personnel to recruit are physical therapists, pharmacists, radiology technicians, medical technicians, and respiratory therapists.[42] On top of the felt nursing shortage, these recruiting difficulties would indicate that the health services delivery system is staggering along.

Concurrent with the problem of shortages, there is the perverse opposite problem in the supply of physicians. Early in the decade, based on massive studies on the contemporary and future supply of physicians and their practice patterns, the Graduate Medical Education National Advisory Committee (GMENAC) headed by Alvin R. Tarlov predicted that by 1990 there would be in the United States, 536,000 physicians—70,000 more than "needed."[43] (The most recent actual number is 588,000.) This prediction received a great deal of publicity and distressed current and future physicians.

The practical outcome of this "surplus" is still not clear. Many factors enter into the concept of surplus. Medical practice is changing. Possibly the most important factor is the reduction in the hours physicians work; they are shifting from the traditional fee-for-service style of practice to part-time and full-time salaried positions. The steady increase in the number of women in the medical profession is expected to decrease hours of practice from the traditional 60 hours a week to 40 hours or so. Offsetting these trends, of course, are the omnipresent increase in the number of the elderly persons and in the incidence of chronic diseases—notably AIDS—that require a great deal of time from physicians as well as from allied health professionals.

THE PREVENTION ISSUE

Overarching all the foregoing issues and problems has been the steady promotion of prevention by the Department of Health and Human Services, beginning with the Carter administration. By the latter part of the 1980s, DHHS had issued an avalanche of publications on the subject, the most salient of them *Disease Prevention/Health Promotion: The Facts*, which appeared in 1988. It was put together by public health and epidemiological experts in and out of government, and it dealt straightforwardly and factually with the entire range of behavioral and environmental elements affecting the health of the public—those caused by lifestyles and those caused by factors beyond individuals' control.[44] Certainly, the American people suffer no lack of information by which to guide personal behavior and policy regarding the promotion of general public health.

This concludes the presentation of simultaneous policy explosions. In Chapter 19 I will continue with the current status of cost control, HMOs and their variants, and competition.

NOTES

1. Arnold S. Relman, "The New Medical-Industrial Complex Policy," *New England Journal of Medicine* 303 (October 23, 1980):968.

2. Richard Reece, ed., *Reece Report* 3 (March 1989):1.
3. Walter Lipmann, *The Public Interest* 1 (Fall 1965):5.
4. Jack D. McCue, ed., *The Medical Cost-Containment Crisis: Fears, Opinions, and Facts.* (Ann Arbor, Mich.: Health Administration Press, 1989), pp. 3–14.
5. Stuart H. Altman, Susan Goldberger, and Stephen C. Crane, "The Need for a National Focus on Health Care Productivity," *Health Affairs* 9 (Spring 1990):107–13. Stephen H. Long and W. Pete Welch, "Are We Containing Costs or Pushing on a Balloon?" *Health Affairs* 7 (Fall 1988):111–17. Victor R. Fuchs, "The Competition Revolution in Health Care," *Health Affairs* 7 (Summer 1988):5–24.
6. Barry G. Rabe, "The Defederalization of American Health Care," *Medical Care Review* 44 (Spring 1987):37–38.
7. Ibid., p. 41.
8. See Douglas M. Fizel, "Physician Payment Reform," *GHAA News* 30 (May–June 1989):17–21.
9. Alexander Morgan Capron, "Looking Back at the President's Commission," *Hastings Center Report* 13 (October 1983):7.
10. Frank Cerne, "Life-Support Withdrawal Creates Ethical, Legal Dilemmas," *AHA News* 25 (May 15, 1989):8.
11. Courtney Price, "Innovators and Entrepreneurs: 1989," *Hospitals* 63 (May 20, 1989):40.
12. Ibid.
13. Howard Larkin, "Finances Will Force Rationing Decisions in 1989," *Hospitals* 63 (January 5, 1989):22.
14. National Leadership Commission on Health Care, *For the Health of a Nation: A Shared Responsibility* (Ann Arbor, Mich.: Health Administration Press, 1989), pp. 25–71. See also J. Bruce Johnston and Uwe E. Reinhardt, "Addressing the Health of a Nation: Two Views," *Health Affairs* 8 (Summer 1989):5.
15. American Medical Association, Health Policy Agenda for the American People, *Framework for the Future* (Chicago: The Association, 1988).
16. American Medical Association, Health Policy Agenda for the American People, *The Final Report of the Ad Hoc Committee on Medicaid Including the Poor* (Chicago: The Association, 1989).
17. Robert Wood Johnson Foundation, *Access to Health Care in the United States: Results of a 1986 Survey*, Special Report No. 2 (Princeton, N.J.: The Foundation, 1987). The survey was conducted by Louis Harris and Associates with analysis by the staff of the Center for Health Administration Studies, University of Chicago, Ronald M. Andersen, director.
18. See details in J. Bruce Johnston and Uwe E. Reinhardt, "Addressing the Health of a Nation: Two Views," *Health Affairs* 8 (Summer 1989):5.
19. Jeffery Finn, "Financing Difficulties Threaten to Undermine New Catastrophic Law," *AHA News* 24 (December 12, 1988):1.
20. U.S. Bipartisan Commission on Comprehensive Health Care, *Recommendations to Congress*. At the time of this writing, the report is still in typewritten

form; I obtained a duplicated copy from my Representative in the House, Robert W. Kastenmeier (D-Wisc.).

21. Merit C. Kimball, "Panel Divisiveness Negates Pepper Plan," *Healthweek* 4 (March 12, 1990):1, 55.
22. Ibid., p. 1.
23. Ibid., p. 1.
24. Ibid., p. 55.
25. Merit C. Kimball, "Universal Health Care Insurance Winning Solid Support," *Healthweek* 3 (May 1, 1989):9. This news article cites all individuals mentioned.
26. "National Health Plans Intrigue More Employers as Costs Soar," *Wall Street Journal* (May 16, 1989):A1. See also Milt Freudenheim, "Calling for a Bigger U.S. Health Role," *New York Times* (May 30, 1989):29.
27. Carol M. McCarthy, executive director of the American Hospital Association, is quoted as observing that "inadequate payment undermines high quality care," in "Arnett Emphasizes Policy Process and Members' Roles in It," *AHA News* 25 (January 9, 1989):4.
28. Stephen Dombrosh, "Competitive Medicine: A Survey of Minnesota Physicians," *Minnesota Medicine*, Special Issue 71 (January 1988):23.
29. Mark R. Chassin, Rolla Edward Park, Kathleen N. Lohr, Joan Keesey, and Robert H. Brook, "Differences among Hospitals in Medicare Patient Mortality," *Health Services Research* 24 (April 1989):1–31.
30. Ibid., p. 29.
31. June H. White, "Setting Standards for the Future of Medical Practice," *GHAA News* 30 (May–June 1989):9.
32. Ibid., p. 9.
33. Ibid., p. 9.
34. Ibid., p. 9.
35. *Health Services Research (HSR) Update*, May 1989.
36. Carolyne K. Davis and Frederick B. Abbey, "Keeping Score Alters the Game," *Health Management Quarterly* 11 (Second Quarter 1989):6–9.
37. Ibid., p. 9.
38. Frank A. Sloan and Randall R. Bovbjerg, "Medical Malpractice: Crises, Response and Effects," *Health Insurance Association of America Research Bulletin* R889 (May 1989):1–52.
39. Ibid., p. 9.
40. "137,000 Nurses' Jobs Vacant, HHS Nurse-Commission Report Finds," *AHA News* 24 (December 19, 1988):2.
41. *Medical Care Review* 40 (Spring 1983):15.
42. "AHA Tracks Shortage in Health Care Personnel," *AHA News* 25 (January 2, 1989):1.
43. Department of Health and Human Services, Graduate Medical Education National Advisory Committee, *Summary Report*, DHSS Publication No. (HRA) 81–651 (Washington, D.C.: Department of Health and Human Services, 1980).

44. U.S. Public Health Service, Office of Disease Prevention and Health Promotion, *Disease Prevention/Health Promotion: The Facts* (Palo Alto, Calif.: Bull Publishing Company, 1988).

19

The Reshaping of the American Health Services Delivery System

The decade of the 1980s began to reveal the potential shape of the American health services delivery system, a shape that began forming in the late 1960s and early 1970s. Spurred on by rapidly and constantly increasing costs, the various administrations tried several approaches simultaneously. The Nixon administration latched onto Ellwood's concept of competitive options and HMOs through employers. This policy found official expression in the HMO Act of 1973. From the passage of that legislation to about a year before the time of this writing (1990) national health insurance on the continental European or Canadian model was not regarded seriously as a cost containment option. Then, seemingly all of a sudden, during 1989 and since, interest began to be expressed toward the Canadian model at least on the part of liberal interest groups. Canada had been able to hold expenditures for its health insurance to 8 percent to 9 percent of GNP over the past years. In the meantime, in this country, employer sovereignty had replaced consumer sovereignty, and expenditures continued to rise. The result was a homogenization of the original pure HMO model, as will be described.

Ellwood's think tank, InterStudy, published in 1988 an overview of the current and future status of the HMO competitive option concept. Written by Judith A. Hale and Mary M. Hunter, the report was a refreshingly candid appraisal—disappointed with the pace of development of HMOs and their variants but quite optimistic that in the long run and in broad terms "managed care" would prevail.[1] In this chapter I will draw heavily on Hale and Hunter's review, and I will add to it my own observations and interpretations.

In the early days of HMOs, before they came to be seen as the vehicle for restructuring the American health services delivery system, there was mainly one generic type of HMO, the staff model: salaried physicians serving a known population and receiving premiums from one source or another, with no deductibles or coinsurance to speak of and quite comprehensive benefits covering the entire spectrum of professionally recognized services and goods, owning their own hospitals or contracting with hospitals in the service area, and with subscribers limited to the physicians in the HMO except possibly for some very unusual specialist services not available through the HMO. This model had a pristine quality, deviations from which were regarded as transgressions from the true way. The purest of the purest HMOs believed in consumer ownership and control and that the physicians were, in effect, the servants of the consumers.

An early evolution from the consumer-ownership-and-control model, paralleling and competing with the staff model, was the group model. The group model built on existing, physician-owned, private group practices. Physicians in the group were paid variously by salary, by fee-for-service, or by some combination of the two, as determined by internal policy. The group model's established clientele paid for services in a variety of ways, such as employed groups with insurance and direct-pay patients with fees. The group model added to these traditional sources of payment by establishing its own HMO and enrolling members from employed groups, with whose employers contracts could be made.

During the 1970s and into the 1980s occurred what the InterStudy authors describe as the "mongrelization" of the HMO. Big buyers of health services dominated the marketplace, competing for the best buys for their employees. Gone was the early milieu of special and relatively small groups of civil service employees and schoolteachers or a particular labor union, which seemed to desire small-scale, "homey" HMO operations. Such HMOs, moreover, grew more slowly than expected by their owners. So a new marketing and enrollment method was devised—dual choice—an arrangement by which an employer offered employees a choice of two plans. The Health Insurance Plan of Greater New York and the Kaiser-Permanente plans on the West Coast introduced dual choice to employers and employees in order to expand their markets faster. Previously, all of the employees of a given employer were expected to enroll—100 percent or not at all.

As the notion of competitive options gained popularity in the 1970s, pure HMOs found that their market—employers and employees—did not necessarily want pure HMOs. Buyers and consumers wanted price competition not only on a comprehensive range of services but on a narrower range of specific services in which they were particularly interested. They also wanted choice of physicians. The pure HMO concept supported comprehensive health services but stressed prevention, not insurance against particular contingencies, and choice of physicians was limited.

The cost control techniques of the pure HMO were impressive when total costs were compared with those resulting from the traditional, open-ended, fee-for-service insurance arrangement; HMO patients' use of hospitals was notably lower. Searching for cost containment methods, traditional insurers found they could use HMO cost control techniques without adopting the pure HMO structure. They began to require prospective utilization review, second surgical opinions, and for certain procedures, outpatient surgery. Hospital inpatient days decreased considerably, and outpatient surgery decreased. The effect of second opinions on surgery appears to be inconclusive, but the requirement is still popular as evidence that something is being done to reduce "unnecessary surgery."

While these cost control techniques—really volume control techniques—were unthinkable before the inflationary period of the 1970s, after the cost escalation the mainstream systems found that harnessing HMO-type professional decision making was not only possible but necessary to survival. Large, self-insured employers also realized they could incorporate cost and volume controls into their health benefit plans.

The medical profession, to counter the potential dominance of the pure HMO model, began to organize independent practice associations (IPAs). IPAs entailed the least changes in the fee-for-service, free-choice-of-physician (and hospital), mainstream type of practice. People did not have to change physicians, and start-up required relatively little capital because the physicians already owned or rented their own offices. The profession did not have to adopt the pure HMO structure. Naturally, a much higher degree of surveillance of physician practice patterns became necessary; IPAs had to control their "high" prescribers, particularly for hospital admission. But in fact it was plausible to assume that employers and employees might be willing to pay a higher price for the greater openness of the mainstream system.

For some time to come there will be severe market realities for HMOs: (1) growth capital will be limited, (2) employers' support will lack enthusiasm, (3) consumers will prefer to choose their own physicians, and (4) physicians will continue to resist any influence of capitation in their professional decision making. There will also be the marketing problem of community rating versus experience rating. Employers do not wish to be blanketed into an overall area premium rate, because they know that there are variations in rates of use between firms because selection factors such as the age and sex composition of employee groups create differential demand patterns—and hence differential costs. Employers want to be prudent buyers and not community collectivists, so to speak. Equity is regarded as a public responsibility not a private one.

A natural result of employer-consumer sovereignty in health insurance has been the desire for options not only in premium rates but in benefit ranges and openness of choice of physicians, both generalists and specialists. As the market has responded to buyers' preferences, there has been a blurring of distinction among HMOs and between HMOs and mainstream health providers. According to the InterStudy authors, four new kinds of managed care plans (the more generic term managed care having almost replaced the term HMO) have emerged. The first is the open-ended HMO, which offers the standard staff or group model plus special contracts at a higher price for free choice of physicians, particularly specialists outside the group. Open-ended HMOs are at risk. The second new kind of managed care plan is the preferred provider organization (PPO); the PPO is a contract between the insurer and a physician group. The group will provide specified services at a particular price to the employees selecting the group. In this model the insurance company is at risk. The third new type of managed care plan is the exclusive provider organization (EPO), which acts as the sole provider for an insurance agency. Presumably a fee schedule can be negotiated with the group, but it would seem likely that the financial arrangement would be capitation. (There is so much variety of payment now that it is difficult to generalize.) Finally, there is the multiple option plan, sometimes called a network, in which the insurer markets a range of options.

Hale and Hunter comment that over the past decade the emphasis in HMOs has shifted from managing *care* to managing *cost* (their emphasis). Indeed, what is behind the drive for managed care other than cost? It seems that the InterStudy group still regards HMOs as a health service rather than means of spreading risk for the consumer at an "affordable" cost. Quality standards and their control are not yet a burning issue, but they will undoubtedly become so.

In a survey of employers—well informed people in the field—Hale and Hunter asked for opinions on the future of managed care. There was a clear consensus that traditional, unrestricted indemnity insurance is dying and will represent at most a very small portion of the market. This would seem to be a safe prediction given the continuing cost push. At most the relatively open indemnity model may become a remnant, providing a luxury level service for the segment of the population that is affluent and wants total choice. Open-ended HMOs may also get some of this market.

Another prediction is that, in the short run (five years?), managed care plans with choice options will predominate. Some regard IPAs and PPOs as "stepping stones for both providers and consumers, as they accustom themselves to managed care and to defined provider panels."[2]

Reasonable as these predictions appear, the survey revealed a fair amount of dissent as well, indicating the unclear dynamics of a complicated and volatile enterprise. Respondents believed employers and government will continue to exert considerable influence, but they were not sure what the nature of that influence would be. They believed the 1973 federal HMO Act would have influence, but again they were not sure what kind. (At the present writing the HMO Act appears to be a more and more attenuated guideline.) Respondents felt that differences among HMOs were vague, that HMOs would survive in some form, and that both PPOs and HMOs must adapt to the market—although there was disagreement concerning who was best positioned to do so.[3] What seems apparent in all the foregoing is confusion.

The confusion is compounded in the meantime by the big employers' establishing self-insurance plans free from the usual regulatory measures. The self-insurance concept is one by which an employer acts as the sole insurer at risk for its employees; the employer usually contracts with a management firm to administer claims. The employers are introducing higher deductibles and coinsurance, which are not being unduly resisted by employees. Although information on this development is quite sparse, the trend seems clear. A 1986 study by Patricia McDonnell and others for *Health Care Financing Review* indicated that the trend started in the late 1970s and that by the middle of the 1980s the clear majority of large establishments used some form of self-insurance. The trend was also growing among smaller firms. In 1985, 62 percent of large companies were self-funded, up from 54 percent in 1984. Even though only 8 percent of all employment-related health plans were self-insured, more than 50 percent of all employees with health insurance participated in self-insured plans.[4]

Hale and Hunter, the InterStudy authors, reached some important conclusions and predictions given their objectives. They concluded that, "despite this massive restructuring of the health care industry, in certain important respects the 'competitive strategy' advocated by InterStudy and others has not fulfilled its original goals of cost containment, enhanced quality, and improved access to care."[5] One might ask, and not cynically, what else is new? It seems in the nature of social movements with high aspirations not to attain goals that are as vague as containment of cost, enhancement of quality, and improvement of access.

The authors continued, "The HMO structure facilitates managed care and cost containment but to date most HMOs have not taken full advantage of that potential: while HMOs are structured to encourage prevention and early detection, few embody a true preventive approach."[6] It might be observed, however, that HMOs have been so busy trying simply to compete and to increase their market share that they have not been able to work toward the ideal of prevention. Prevention requires a great deal of consumer interest and cooperation, factors over which medical plans by themselves have little direct control.

Hale and Hunter predicted that those HMOs that succeed in the next decade will have top quality management; they will be diversified (that is, to use economic jargon, they will offer a variety of product lines); and they will be large enough to realize economies of scale. Many HMOs will themselves become a product line of a large health management company. They will increasingly be identified by the broad names characteristic of big industry (GM, Kellogg, AT&T) such as Kaiser, Prudential, and Mayo rather than by the current generic acronyms of HMO or PPO.[7] These large corporations, however, will divide themselves into two categories that will retain the historical distinctiveness of their origins: staff- and group-model managed care plans on the one hand, and PPO- and IPA-like plans on the other.

Bold as these predictions are, the authors concluded that "a yet-to-be-determined *balance* of forces will shape the continuing evolution of health care over the next decade" (emphasis theirs).[8] What the authors seemed to imply is that the forces toward large, bureaucratic structures and those toward more open, fluid, and grassroots-oriented structures will be the two major types of delivery system struggling for market shares.

As for the relative status of the various types of HMO, in 1987 they were rank-ordered in terms of number as follows:

Staff-model	64
Group-model	74
Network	107
IPA	417
Total	662[9]

The number of (although not the enrollment in) staff- and group-model HMOs has been quite static since 1980. The network model was a new one for the 1980s. The IPA model had spectacular growth, from 97 in 1980 to 417 in 1987, and in 1987 had the largest share of the 29.3-million-person overall HMO membership. (This article did not show the distribution of membership by type of HMO.)

The 1980s were a period of take-off in HMO enrollment, with a two-million-member increase in 1988. The peak year for rate of growth was 1985, with a 26 percent increase in membership. Thereafter the growth rate decreased to 23 percent in 1986, 13.6 percent in 1987, and 8.7 percent in 1988.[10] Employers, as indicated earlier, are shifting to other types of managed care that offer wider choice of physicians and hospitals. It looks like the "balance" mentioned above is trying to work itself out.

Hospitals, of course, are feeling the effect of managed care in lower occupancy rates because physicians have altered their style of practice regarding hospitals to lower admission rates and shorter lengths of stay. The intent of the DRG method of hospital reimbursement is to put low-occupancy hospitals and small hospitals, rural and urban, out of business as being too small to be efficient.

Occupancy rates are low. The American Hospital Association reported early in 1989 that since 1980 445 community hospitals had closed. Seventy-nine hospitals closed in 1987, and 81 closed in 1988. Of the 81 that closed in 1988, 38 were urban community hospitals and 43 were rural community hospitals. The AHA attributed all of the closures to inadequate Medicaid and Medicare payments, that is, reimbursements lower than what the hospitals regarded as their costs of providing care.[11]

The rejoinder to the AHA was that the closure of hospitals stemmed from underuse and, furthermore, did not greatly diminish access to inpatient or emergency care. So stated a report from Inspector General Richard Kusserow to Secretary of DHHS Louis Sullivan. The statistics given were that the average occupancy rate for the rural hospitals that closed was 21.4 percent, compared with the national average of 36.9 percent in rural facilities. The patient census in the urban hospitals that closed hovered around 29.6 percent, compared with a national average of 61 percent for urban hospitals. And while the closures reduced the bed supply by 4,233 beds or about 0.5 percent, the report goes on to say that 13 new hospitals opened in 1987 and 8 hospitals reopened in 1988, offsetting the decline in beds.[12]

The trouble with government closure of hospitals through the reimbursement method is that many of the hospitals with low occupancy rates are in underserved areas, both urban and rural. The government seems to be at least partially successful in closing hospitals that are unable to sustain themselves in a competitive market, but the market is not intended to provide hospital care in underserved areas. If these areas are to be served, there must be a subsidy from public or philanthropic sources.

Perhaps the government, through HCFA, is trying to test the political feasibility of reducing the number of "inefficient" hospitals by the reimbursement method. Congress is now finding resistance to this method; protests are coming from rural areas. In true American grass-roots fashion, a rural interest group formed during the 1980s. One response took shape within Congress itself in the form of the Rural Health Care Coalition, started informally by Representatives Thomas J. Tauke (R-Ia.) and Micke Synar (D-Okla.) as early as 1984. This became the 100-member House Rural Health Care Coalition in 1987, with Tauke and Synar as co-chairmen. (It may be noted that both of these congressmen are from rural states.) Later in 1987, DHHS decided to establish an Office of Rural Health Policy and a National Advisory Committee on Rural Health.[13]

According to Timothy Size, executive director of the Rural Wisconsin Hospital Cooperative, the rural constituency has become very active politically in order to obtain what its members view as equitable reimbursement for Medicare patients, relative to urban hospitals. Rural hospitals feel the lower reimbursement to rural hospitals—on the presumption of lower capital and operating costs in rural areas—is jeopardizing the legitimate survival of many rural hospitals. Complicated formulas are being worked out as to the cost of labor, capital, and supplies in rural areas compared with urban areas.[14]

One of many examples of interest in the Congress early in 1989 was the action of the Senate Finance Committee. The committee rallied around a bill to increase Medicare payments to rural hospitals.[15] Actions toward this end are attempted both by legislation and, within the Health Care Financing Administration, by budget manipulations too complex to detail here. What I wish to present here is the apparent intensity of the activities of the rural constituency.

It is clear that hospitals operate in a hostile environment, with big buyers in particular—industry and government—contributing to that hostility. The traditional community hospitals feel themselves to be under siege, but they do not lack for loyal customers. Would-be patients are not boycotting the hospitals or the physicians as consumers may with the producers of automobiles, televisions, refrigerators, and other commodities important to the American standard of living. The health services system is the only gateway to the modern secular heaven of restoring health and daily functional ability (hearing, seeing, eating, walking, talking, interacting intelligently, and eliminating), abating pain, and prolonging life.

We once regarded general hospitals as community resources, like churches and schools. Hospitals were symbols of relief from suffering, and everyone had access to them at some level of dignity or other. Now the major objective of hospitals seems to be survival as an end in itself.

We have thrown them into a competitive marketplace, and we expect them to compete, survive, and do good.

A tangible expression of hostility toward hospitals are the growing attacks on their historical tax-exempt position, a position accorded them because they are "clothed with the public interest." In 1980 a scholarly article, not a polemic, raised questions as to the justification for hospitals' tax-exempt nonprofit status.[16] This drive toward modifying if not eliminating the hospitals' tax-exempt status stems in part from the fact that, to generate revenue, hospitals have made excursions into income from business unrelated to health care. At the same time that hospitals are placed in an environment in which survival—rather than the contribution to the general welfare of the community—is the ultimate test, they are asked to be magnanimous enough to fold up and die if they are not in some vague way serving the community beyond the bottom-line motive. The hospitals are not given an overall plan or grid by which to relate to other hospitals as a more or less total system. Hospitals are closed according to their profitability, not their location or their community's need.

Cynthia Ann Eisenberg and Ron Maroko made theoretical estimates in 1989 that a typical 300-bed hospital would lose more than 50 percent of its net income if taxed.[17] They observed, correctly, that the basic issue is competition with taxable commercial enterprises. Small business in particular has attacked hospitals' tax exemption, citing "unfair" advantages enjoyed by the tax-exempt entities. All levels of government are involved in addressing the issue of community benefit: does a hospital provide sufficient benefit in the form of indigent care, community health counseling, or whatever to warrant an exemption?[18] And then hospitals are asked to compete in rate negotiations with HMOs and the government with a vague bottom line of community benefit.

One of the apparent side effects of the presence of 37 million or so uninsured people and an indefinite number of underinsured people with high deductibles and coinsurance is the report that self-pay or partially self-pay patients are among the fastest growing sources of hospital revenue.[19] In fact, credit-reporting agencies have responded to this shift by jumping into the health care market.

I note in closing this discussion of the hospital situation that Stephen M. Shortell notes tremendous structural changes in American hospitals. Shortell describes what was once an industry composed of thousands of individual, freestanding, and largely not-for-profit hospitals as now "a crazy-quilt of health care systems, alliances, networks, federations, consortia and joint ventures."[20] Shortell uses the term "partnering" to refer to these arrangements, because their central characteristic is a desire to share one or more activities with one or more institutions. He reports that as of 1989 40 percent of the nation's community hospitals belonged to health care systems, which he defined as two or more hospitals with a common form of ownership. He predicts that 60 percent of community hospitals will be "partnering" by 1995. He regards this phenomenon as "fundamentally a response to a highly uncertain, highly complex, and increasingly hostile environment."[21] Hospital chief executive officers say that the challenge they face is survival.

NOTES

1. Judith A. Hale and Mary M. Hunter, *From HMO Movement to Managed Care Industry: The Future of HMO's in a Volatile Healthcare Market* (Excelsior, Minn.: InterStudy, 1988).
2. Ibid., p. 41.
3. Ibid., p. 44.
4. Patricia McDonnell, Abbie Guttenberg, Leonard Greenberg, and Ross H. Arnett, III, "Self-Insured Plans," *Health Care Financing Review* 8 (Winter 1986): 1.
5. Judith A. Hale and Mary M. Hunter, *From HMO Movement to Managed Care Industry: The Future of HMO's in a Volatile Healthcare Market* (Excelsior, Minn.: InterStudy, 1988) p. 47.
6. Ibid.
7. Ibid., p. 50.
8. Ibid., p. 51.
9. Lynn R. Gruber, Maureen Shjadle, and Cynthia L. Polich, "From Movement to Industry," *Health Affairs* 7 (Summer 1988):202.
10. Data for 1985 through 1987 drawn from Judith A. Hale and Mary M. Hunter, *From HMO Movement to Managed Care Industry: The Future of HMO's in a Volatile Healthcare Market* (Excelsior, Minn.: InterStudy, 1988), p. 47. Data for 1988 drawn from Marion Laboratories, Inc., *Marion Managed Care Digest: HMO Edition* (Kansas City, Mo.: Marion Laboratories, Inc., 1989).
11. Dona DeSanctis, "Struggling Rurals Gain Attention from National Policy-Makers," *AHA News* 25 (April 3, 1989):6.
12. Merit C. Kimball, "Little Effect on Access to Care after '87 Hospital Closures," *Healthweek* 3 (May 15, 1989):43.
13. Carol McCarthy, "AHA Closure Data Sound, But Not Cornerstone of Advocacy," *AHA News* 25 (April 3, 1989):4.
14. Telephone conversation with Timothy Size, executive director of the Rural Wisconsin Hospital Cooperative, on May 17, 1990. The organization is a coalition of rural hospitals in southwestern Wisconsin, based in Sauk City, Wisconsin.

15. Tinker Ready, "Senators Champion Medicare Bill to Aid Rural Hospitals," *Healthweek* 3 (May 15, 1989):9.
16. Robert C. Clark, "Does the Nonprofit Form Fit the Hospital Industry?" *Harvard Law Review* 93 (May 1980):1,416–89.
17. Cynthia Ann Eisenberg and Ron Maroko, "Protecting Tax-Exemption," *Health Management Quarterly* 11 (Second Quarter 1989):10.
18. Ibid., p. 11.
19. Paul Eubanks, "Finance: Patient Credit Checks Help Hospitals Minimize Bad Debt," *Hospitals* 63 (June 5, 1989):22.
20. Stephen M. Shortell, "Worried CEO's: The Real Reason Behind Health Systems Growth," *AHA News* 25 (June 30, 1989):4.
21. Ibid., p. 3.

PART V

Health Services Research

20

Toward an Understanding of the Health Services Enterprise

INTRODUCTION

Research in the health services has generally stemmed not from curiosity, but from a need to have facts on which to base organization, administration, and legislation. The search for facts has been frankly for public policy purposes, to provide a factual basis for a given policy. There has been little interest until recently in attempting to understand the structure and nature of the health services as an end in itself and to let policy flow from this understanding.

Necessary as it may be to understand the nature of the enterprise, it is hardly satisfying to policy makers who have an immediate problem. Recognition and acceptance of the intractability of a problem is not congenial to the American temperament. Policy makers turn to social scientists ostensibly to be guided in their policy formulations, but they get little guidance unless the social scientists are ideologically committed to solutions that agree with the policy makers' own viewpoints. Aaron points to the difficulties of social research relating to policy:

> Social scientists, in emulation of physical scientists and mathematicians, seek simplicity and "elegance," though the question whether the problems of social science *can* be solved elegantly remains unanswered. In order to permit simplicity and elegance, problems are separated into components that can be managed and understood. Such abstractions produce theory apparently detached from reality, [which] often provokes the lay-

man's scorn. Of greater importance, the impulse to isolate individual influences, to make complex social and economic [phenomena] statistically and mathematically manageable through abstraction makes it almost impossible to identify policies that may be necessary, but not sufficient to achieve some objective.

Possibly of greater significance, however, is that these characteristics of the people and institutions that produce research and experimentation, of the problems they address, and of the data and scientific procedures they use guarantee that over the long haul R and D [research and development] will be an intellectually conservative force in the debates about policy. The political liberalism or radicalism of many of those who produce R and D in education and labor markets makes this conclusion paradoxical, but the experience of the last decade [1967–1977] supports it. A problem that is both politically and intellectually interesting for a number of years must be difficult and must deal with matters about which people deeply and diversely care. It will typically involve a number of objectives that are hard to define or measure and that people will value differently. The interactions among various aspects of the problem are likely to be so numerous and complex as to overload existing capacities of the social sciences.[1]

Aaron suggests that there is a spontaneous resolution of this dilemma: "One can be fairly confident, however, that at any given time there will coexist several theories consistent with any given set of facts that are more or less congenial to persons with differing political or philosophical predispositions."[2]

By and large, reformers of the health services have been avid users of whatever disparate facts were available, such as infant mortality rates, hospital admission rates, physician visits per person, per diem costs of hospitals, and so on, with no attempt to correlate them. Systems thinking was not part of their strategy. They seemed to assume that people and health services organizations were almost infinitely malleable, provided that the appropriate facts were made available to them. Reasonable solutions would flow from reasonable people, who would see the implications of the facts as self-evident. If the infant mortality rate is high, correct it by maternal and child health programs. If low-income families have less access to health services than high-income families, redistribute the resources. Self-evident facts suggest self-evident solutions.

I imply, of course, that people are naive about the possibilities for social reform and social change. I believe this naivete is rooted in the tremendous production and distribution capacities of the liberal-democratic societies since the Industrial Revolution. This surge of goods and services—and, after 1900, of personal health services—appeared to come from nowhere. There seemed to be no limit to the cornucopia. It did not stem from planning; indeed, if some authority had tried to plan, it would have been a dismal failure. It stemmed from a belief in applied technology.

Not until recently have researchers in the health services become more interested in systems thinking—in relating variables to other variables, in probing the characteristics that are peculiar to the health services enterprise. The stimulus for this interest is the increasingly accepted view that resources are scarce and must be allocated on the basis of priorities, whether through pure market mechanisms, pure public mechanisms, or a mixture of both. It is therefore increasingly necessary to learn more about the nature and functioning of the health services enterprise itself. Sociologists have been the most prominent in this endeavor, for their discipline compels them to think in terms of social systems. They have not thought in terms of resources, as do economists. Sociological research in the health services has therefore been deficient: in studying the behavior of persons in the health services system, sociologists have acted as though resources were unlimited, which until recently they seemed to be.

Wide-open societies, such as those in the liberal-democratic countries, and especially in the United States, had so much leeway for success that there was scarcely any need for a political strategy for reform. The strategy was mainly one of exhortation to moral action. The clamor of a great many interest groups for a share of what seems to be a decreasing pie appears to be sharpening the conceptual and analytical tools of reform strategists. Even the process of implementing legislation has become an area of study. I therefore ask: On the basis of what we know about the nature and operation of the health services, to what extent is it manageable?

In the synthesis of health services research I present in this chapter and the next one, I have, I believe, mentioned every problem and issue that has been researched conceptually or empirically. I also believe that I have read, or at least riffled through, all the conceptual and empirical literature under the rubrics of history of medicine, medical sociology, the economics of health, the politics of health, equity, statistical studies in use, expenditures, facilities, personnel, and insurance coverage written since such literature first began to appear, in the early twentieth century. I have also read all the public health literature, which began to appear in the latter nineteenth century. Obviously, it is neither necessary nor practical to cite all of them. I have attempted to be fairly representative in my selection in order to validate my synthesis. Obviously, then, to some readers I will have left out references that should have been included or I will have chosen inferior examples. This is inevitable, but, to show how extensive the literature is, I refer the reader to three source books[3] and to the many bibliographies in professional journals.

To what extent is it possible to plan and direct the health services toward desired objectives? The American health services have not, so far, been planned or managed. The rush to do so has come about because they are consuming an inordinately large proportion of the social surplus.

RESEARCH BEFORE THE EARLY FIFTIES

Research has moved from straightforward inventories of the incidence of mortality and disease and the stock of facilities and personnel probings in complex systems and interactions. Building up a data base to comprehend the anatomy of an enterprise takes a long time; research into its physiology has to come later. Interest in the function and operation of the health services did not appear in the research until the 1940s or later. The compilation of data on personnel, particularly on physicians by the AMA, and emerging professional types was in good order by 1900. Systematic data on facilities began to appear toward the latter part of the nineteenth century. Most of this research was carried out by the AMA for accreditation of internships and residencies. Systematic national data on expenditures, although collected by the Department of Commerce since 1929, were not published until 1944.[4] They form an incomparable, detailed resource on expenditures for health services by component of service. After the appearance in 1946 of the monthly *Social Security Bulletin*, the Office of Research and Statistics of the Social Security Administration began to publish annually data on expenditures for health services; it also published, first sporadically and eventually annually, data on voluntary health insurance. These were extremely useful services.

The Committee on the Costs of Medical Care did systematic research into public need and demand for health services. The committee studied the incidence of morbidity, use of services, and expenditures on services by individuals and families at a time when health insurance was nonexistent and government support was minimal. See chapter 8 for a full description.

Epidemiology and Public Health

Research on delivery systems was preceded by research into the epidemiology of the common scourges, from the latter nineteenth century onward. After many of them were found to be caused by microorganisms, research on the incidence of mortality and morbidity began. This, in turn, led to the development of modern health departments. The general public's belief in the efficacy of personal health services, and their expenditures on them, led to research on the relationship between mortality and morbidity and the use of personal health services. Research on communicable diseases became somewhat subsidiary to research on personal health services. It seems that the optimistic belief of early public health workers that we could rid ourselves of diseases in general was carried over into the personal health services as medicine became more effective through surgery and specific therapies such as insulin for diabetes.

The following is a summary of epidemiological research before the 1930s.[5] Systematic formulation of the relationship between disease and social and economic conditions, as well as recommendations for some kind of social action to ameliorate conditions, was undertaken in Germany in the latter part of the 19th century. The relationship between disease and environmental conditions was further elaborated by cellular pathologist Rudolph Virchow in Germany, sanitarian Edwin Chadwick in Great Britian, and Lemuel Shattuck, a bookseller and publisher but a self-taught epidemiologist, in the United States. These men propounded a concept that was revolutionary at the time: many deaths are preventable.[6] The prevailing theory for the cause of many deaths—vapors rising from refuse heaps, garbage, and gutters—was wrong, but the remedy—clean up the physical environment—was right. After the discovery of bacteria by Pasteur, the correct solution was joined to the correct theory.

An early attempt in the United States to reveal the relationships between social factors and mortality rates was made by Charles V. Chapin with data for 1865 from Providence, Rhode Island.[7] Chapin found that, among almost all age groups, members of households paying an income tax had a much lower death rate than members of households not paying one. (This is not necessarily to conclude that paying taxes is good for one's health!) Joseph Goldberger and G. A. Wheeler uncovered the combination of circumstances that was causing pellagra in the rural south: low income and diets deficient in fresh meat and milk, relatively expensive commodities.[8] The specific factor was later found to be the absence of vitamin B.

As early as 1920, Edgar Sydenstricker and Wilford King collaborated on an article in which they attempted to devise a method of classifying family incomes in relation to disease prevalence. These authors recognized that, whereas communicable diseases can be traced quite easily to specific causes, other diseases result from multiple causes.

Today, however, the accepted concept is that there are reciprocal relationships between host, environment, and agent in all diseases.

Sydenstricker's primary interest was in producing a body of data that could be used to show where the health services, both public and personal, should be applied to reduce death, disability, and loss of income in the population. Sydenstricker's research and thinking centered on the interrelations of disease and the physical and social environments, the social environment being defined exclusively as economic.[9] Sydenstricker implies that variations in disease patterns and use of personal health services by the population were caused by variations in income. Twenty years later, sociologists and social anthropologists began to investigate cultural and social-psychological factors as well.

While Sydenstricker and others were probing the relation of disease to environment, the U.S. Children's Bureau was looking into a relatively specific area of population and disease, infant mortality. The Bureau was alarmed at the high infant mortality among low-income groups. It therefore sponsored studies of infant mortality in eight cities between 1916 and 1924 in an attempt to relate the death rates to family income and other socioeconomic factors.[10]

During the twenties and thirties, many studies showed the relations between income and mortality and morbidity. In 1927, Selwyn D. Collins provided a useful summary of data and studies on this relationship.[11] As an expression of the gathering interest in the possible cost-effectiveness of reducing mortality and morbidity in a population, Louis Dublin and Alfred Lotka published a book with the descriptive title *The Money Value of A Man*. Two chapters were particularly pertinent, "Disease and the Depreciation of the Money Value of a Man" and "Application to Public Health."[12] The first chapter tried to measure the economic liability to society of a sick man, and the other dealt with the economic gain to society if certain public health measures were carried out. The results of these measures were expected to be longer working life, reduced morbidity, and, therefore, increased productivity.

At the same time that these empirical studies were being done, other scholars were concerned with a broad conceptual framework for thinking and research. Complementing Sydenstricker's empirical work was the theoretical work of Henry E. Sigerist, a noted medical historian and philosopher. During the thirties and forties, when Sigerist was director of the Institute of the History of Medicine at The Johns Hopkins University, he wrote numerous articles and eventually a book developing the concept that health and disease are rooted in social conditions and that medicine is basically an applied social science, concepts that had been propounded by Frank and Virchow in Germany years before.

Sigerist helped to establish a salubrious climate for thinking about disease and population.[13]

One of the first sociologists to pay attention to disease, health services, and society was Bernard J. Stern of Columbia University. He wrote many papers and books showing the relations between specific diseases, such as heart disease, and social factors.[14]

These studies of social and economic factors drew largely on existing data published by public and private agencies. In only a few instances were studies based on data gathered specifically for that study. I point this out to show that research can begin simply and still have an impact, as long as an appropriate conceptual framework has been adopted to classify data.[15]

Relating Need and Demand

As interest and research in the relations of socioeconomic factors to mortality and morbidity grew, there followed an interest in the relations of expenditures for and use of health services to mortality and morbidity. It was reasonable to assume that an important way of reducing mortality and morbidity was by promoting personal health services.

Early in the twenties, a series of studies on morbidity and use of health services was conducted in Hagerstown, Maryland, by staff from the U.S. Public Health Service in Washington, D.C. Using data from these studies, Sydenstricker published in 1927 an article showing, for the first time, I believe, the extent to which a population received physician and hospital services, by diagnosis. He found that 46 percent of all illnesses reported by household respondents were seen to by a physician. This varied considerably, from 11 percent for headache to 100 percent for cancer.[16]

The Hagerstown studies undoubtedly led directly to the studies conducted by the CCMC between 1928 and 1931. These were the first nationwide studies of morbidity and health services use and expenditures, and they provided a synthesis of all related studies made up to that time and a point of departure for all subsequent studies.

The most important study was report No. 26.[17] It concluded that the incidence of illness was borne unevenly by families, regardless of income, and therefore expenditures for personal health services also fell unevenly. The obvious way to even out unpredictable expenditures was to establish some form of health insurance. The CCMC studies cost over a million dollars, which was contributed by six philanthropic foundations. They also required a large technical staff, virtually exhausting the pool of qualified personnel in the country.

Shortly thereafter, in 1935 and 1936, the PHS conducted the extensive nationwide morbidity and disability survey of over 1 million households known as the National Health Survey. Until the fifties, the data from the CCMC studies and the National Health Survey provided the rationale for the development of health insurance, whether privately or publicly sponsored.

Further research into illness and use of services and attitudes toward them was carried out by rural sociologists in the forties. The Agricultural Extension Service of the United States Department of Agriculture stimulated a large number of local studies through its extension departments in land-grant universities. These studies were staffed mainly by sociologists with an interest in rural life. Farmers were a powerful constituency in American politics, and they felt—as they still do—that their interests must be served as fully as those of city dwellers. Studies were showing that physicians in rural areas were getting older and fewer.

Interest in rural health was also stimulated by the Social Science Research Council, which in 1941 invited a number of rural sociologists to do some planning on social research in health. In 1943, this group met in Birmingham, Alabama, to discuss preliminary reports. A book followed.[18] Recommendations ran the gamut of social research, from use of services to attitudes of the public toward health and health services. No particular social priorities were set, but there was an underlying feeling that somehow the researchers should find out how low-income rural people could obtain more adequate health services than they were getting. Economic variables, although important, were regarded as only one among many.

Sociologists conducted many studies in rural areas of Missouri, New York, Michigan, Minnesota, Oklahoma, and Mississippi. These studies can be regarded as extensions of the CCMC studies and the National Health Survey to local areas. A noteworthy synthesis of data on rural health can be found in *Rural Health and Medical Care*,[19] which for many years was the chief reference on rural health. The authors were PHS medical officers lent to the Farm Security Agency.

A study in rural Michigan deserves special mention because it was the forerunner of methods to measure need for health services in a population. The research team devised a list of symptoms that, according to physicians' opinions, should be brought to the attention of a physician. The perception of symptoms on the part of the general public in this rural area was compared with results of a physical examination given by a medical team. The congruence was encouraging enough to warrant using respondents from the general public to measure need in an area.[20]

After the passage of the Social Security Act, there was quickening interest in some form of government insurance. The primary data used to portray the problems of the consumer were those from the CCMC studies and the National Health Survey. The polemics regarding the relative merits of government and private sponsorship could not be settled by facts.

Beginning Programmatic Considerations

Many position papers, at various levels of sophistication, were drawn up on the issues of medical education, medical services provided by government, medical research, voluntary health insurance, nursing and nursing education, medicine in industry, and preventive medicine. The New York Academy of Medicine sponsored a group with the portentous title of Committee on Medicine and the Changing Order. A series of books was commissioned to deal with the aforementioned topics. One of them described and evaluated for the first time the status of voluntary health insurance. Blue Cross and Blue Shield plans were then beyond their infancy and some kind of stock taking was warranted.[21] The verdict was that their growth was astonishing but they had a long way to go; the authors were cautiously sanguine about the plans' becoming the major health insurance vehicle for the country.

At the same time, a profusion of other books on the general problems of health services organization and financing was being published. Most of them were in the nature of considered opinions. Louis Reed, an economist on the staff of the CCMC and later in the PHS, wrote a book in which he advocated government-sponsored health insurance.[22] A few years later, he made as thorough a study of the impact of Blue Cross and Blue Shield plans as was possible with the existing data. To his own surprise, he became quite sympathetic to the Blue plans.[23] Herbert D. Simpson, a professor of finance at Northwestern University, wrote a monograph on government-sponsored health insurance; his appraisal was largely negative.[24] During the same period, Franz Goldmann, then on the faculty of the School of Public Health at Yale University (later at Harvard University), wrote two rather evenhanded books scrutinizing voluntary health insurance and public welfare medical care.[25] The Brookings Institution sponsored a critical review of the social insurance and government health insurance concepts.[26] I. S. Falk wrote a book on health insurance abroad, the only one attempting to draw on foreign experience.[27]

While these "global" writings were going on, other studies related to the health services enterprise were beginning to appear. Two of them that are of particular interest were premature. The health field was not ready to apply their findings or methods, and consequently they appeared to have been lost. Years later, the problems these studies anticipated are much with us.

One of these studies was conducted by Nathan Sinai and Marguerite F. Hall, of the School of Public Health, University of Michigan, on the medical care plan in Windsor, Ontario. In the 1930s, the Province of Ontario delegated to the Essex County Medical Society responsibility for providing health services on a capitation basis to the population on welfare, a sizable group during the Depression. The medical society wished to use the fee-for-service method of paying participating physicians, but it was fearful of the rising use and costs assumed to be inherent in the method. Sinai and Hall, together with a local physician, Roy E. Holmes, devised a statistical technique for monitoring the volume of services recommended by individual physicians and establishing a distribution of low to high prescribers. Physicians above certain levels would be brought to the attention of the medical review board. [28] This statistical technique was used in modified form in the Windsor plan until the introduction in 1968 of government health insurance for physicians' services.

The other study, conducted in Albany, New York, at the request of a legislative commission, was directed to the use of hospital care, anticipating concern with hospital utilization many years later. John Bourke, director of the state hospital planning and construction agency, was associated with this project. The study, based on hospital and welfare records of almost 3000 patients discharged from the wards of more or less representative hospitals in New York State, was an early attempt to study patterns of hospital use. [29]

In the 1940s, health services research in universities was gaining a foothold and grudging respectability. Michigan State University has been mentioned. At the University of Michigan School of Public Health, the Bureau of Public Health Economics, later the Medical Care Organization Department, was formed. The first publication was an analysis of emerging legislation to exempt Blue Cross and Blue Shield plans from the state laws governing private insurance companies. This legislation regarding nonprofit and provider sponsored plans was an expression of a public policy quite peculiar to American conditions. [30] A study of the comprehensive health services program for recipients of old-age assistance (OAA) in Washington anticipated the later frantic interest in health services for the aged. [31] There was also a study of the operation of the Emergency Maternity and Infant Care Program for the wives and children of servicemen during World War II. This program had all the elements of a national health program and the administrative problems inherent in any prepayment program regardless of sponsorship. Methods of paying hospitals and physicians were examined.[32]

The small group at the University of Michigan embarked on studies of administrative problems, picking up where some of the CCMC studies had left off.[33] Those who generalized from the CCMC reports had tremendous faith in the validity of group practice and prepayment. Sinai's group at Michigan was more pragmatic. It was willing to study the prevailing structure of practice and not wait for a basic transformation of the delivery system. (This may now be happening, but not in the pure form hoped for by early proponents of group practice.)

The laying out of the dimensions of the health services delivery system continued through special commissions and the prescient pioneer work of J. W. Mountin and associates in the PHS. These studies dealt with the distribution of hospital facilities and fed directly into the Hospital Survey and Construction Act of 1946. The most notable one was the report on a model for regionalization of hospitals.[34] World War II was being fought while these studies were going on, which reveals the faith of Americans in postwar domestic developments—it was a very heady and optimistic period.

The commissions were privately financed, private endeavors. One was the Commission on Hospital Care, funded by the Commonwealth Fund, the W. K. Kellogg Foundation, and the National Foundation for Infantile Paralysis. The commission was made up of persons from the entire range of major interest groups in the United States. The study director was Arthur Bachmeyer, superintendent of the hospitals and clinics of the University of Chicago. The commission was concerned with the total American hospital system, no less, and the maintenance of and planning for it. The commission was set up because legislation to provide grants-in-aid for hospital construction and improvement in the United States, presumably building on Mountin's work, was pending in Congress. Before the Hospital Survey and Construction Act (Hill-Burton) was passed in 1946, the state of Michigan was used as a model for other states in hospital planning. No new data were collected, but a formula to measure need for hospitals was devised by C. Horace Hamilton, a rural sociologist at North Carolina State University. Called the bed-death ratio, it was the first systematic attempt at establishing bed-population ratios. The method was apparently never applied.[35]

Data gathering and research on broad systems aspects of the health services culminated in the five volume report of President Truman's Commission on the Health Needs of the Nation.[36] These five volumes contain a compilation and synthesis of all studies and reports on the health services of the United States up to that time.

After World War II, several universities besides the University of Michigan established teaching and research units in health services administration that went beyond the traditional public health pattern. Among these were North Carolina, Yale, Harvard, the University of California at Berkeley, and Johns Hopkins. Because of the bitterness and rancor associated with the polemics on compulsory versus voluntary health insurance, research of this kind was inhibited and the researchers themselves were suspect. After Eisenhower's election, however, the imminent enactment of government-sponsored health insurance subsided and a much less controversial atmosphere for research and policy discussion emerged. Social research was then a possibility.

RESEARCH FROM THE EARLY
FIFTIES TO THE SIXTIES

The Eisenhower administration preferred to go slowly and to stabilize trends in social legislation that had taken place since the enactment of the Social Security Act in 1935. Voluntary health insurance in the early fifties covered almost 60 percent of the population and paid one-half of the general hospital bill, with employers paying an increasingly large proportion of the premium as a result of collective bargaining. Voluntary health insurance was permitted to fulfill its potential without hindrance from Congress. The compilations of data that had characterized the period before 1952 were no longer as relevant. The research now needed was (1) research to evaluate the benefit structure of voluntary health insurance in terms of helping the public to pay for services, and (2) research into the operational and organizational problems of the enterprise, which had gone through a phenomenally free wheeling period of expansion with little concern for costs, volume of use, or quality. The primary objective of the health services enterprise was simply "more." Although other ways of organizing physicians' services had emerged, their objectives appeared to be high quality at a reasonable price, not necessarily a low price. They were also operating in a flush economic period and did not have to pay close attention to costs.

Social research rose to this challenge; it helped considerably, of course, that there was research money around. A new generation of social researchers emerged to build on the work of Sinai, Reed, Roemer, Rorem, Falk, Goldmann, and Brewster. New social science disciplines had become involved, and new, more appropriate methodologies were employed. Sociologists, social anthropologists, and social psychologists joined the ranks of health service researchers. Economists and political scientists arrived on the scene later, the economists when they discovered that health services had become the third largest industry in the country, and the political scientists when they discovered that health services involved interest groups and political power. Expenditures for health services were channeled mostly through nonprofit production and distribution structures, a segment of the economy that is confusing to economists (and to others) and that does not lend itself to standard economic analysis.

In 1951, a commission was established to investigate the costs of general hospital care and voluntary health insurance, an example of the emerging concern with costs. Regarded as a natural sequel to the Commission on Hospital Care, which issued a report in 1947, the Commission on the Financing of Hospital Care was a private agency financed by private funds.* It was made up of 34 persons from the usual interest groups, and its objective was "to study the costs of providing adequate hospital services and to determine the best systems of payment for such services." Research was obviously moving into methods of financing the day-to-day operations of hospitals because of their steadily rising per diem rates (from $10 in 1946 to $17 in 1950 in voluntary hospitals). The previous commission had been primarily concerned with supply and distribution of hospitals. The 1951 commission was limiting itself to "voluntary" methods of financing hospital care. In due course, three volumes of new data and information were amassed on the financial problems of the American general hospital system, providing more insight into its operation.[37] As voluntary health insurance was paying for a larger share of the costs to employed persons, the commission explored how the hospital could help unemployed and low-income persons.

As the base of research in the health services broadened in the 1950s, two broad categories of problems emerged: (1) those dealing with general population's expenditures for and use of health services, including an evaluation of the effectiveness of contemporary health insurance benefits, and (2) those relating to the operations of the insurance agencies and the health services. At the same time, the nationwide morbidity studies of 1935–1936 were resumed on a permanent basis in 1956 by an act of Congress. Since then, a steady stream of excellent studies of morbidity and physical handicaps has been produced; the studies have been expanded to include use of and expenditures for health services as well. In due time, the National Center for Health Statistics was cre-

---

*The range of sources is of interest: Blue Cross Commission (AHA), Health Information Foundation, John Hancock Mutual Life Insurance Company, W. K. Kellogg Foundation, Michigan Medical Service (Blue Shield), Milbank Memorial Fund, National Foundation for Infantile Paralysis, and the Rockefeller Foundation.

ated. Further evidence of interest in general data gathering under government sponsorship was the creation in the early 1960s of a subcommittee on health economics by the U.S. Committee for Vital and Health Statistics. It published in 1964 an excellent report summing up the nature and sources of data on health economics in this country.[38] In 1968, the National Center for Health Services Research was created to fund work done both in federal agencies and in academic settings. The emphasis was and continues to be on research that has fairly immediate application.[39]

Chronic illness was viewed as warranting special attention, in contrast to the almost exclusive concern with services for the acutely ill. Accordingly, the Commission on Chronic Illness was established to investigate this problem. It was in operation from 1949 to 1956 and was sponsored by the AMA, the AHA, the American Public Health Association, and the American Public Welfare Association. Financing came from various private sources, ranging from insurance companies to voluntary health agencies for special diseases, and the PHS. The membership exhibited a great range of skills and interests. The technical staff was assembled under the direction of Morton L. Levin (1950–1951) and Dean W. Roberts (1952–1956). Four massive volumes were published, two of which set forth landmark standards for prevention and management of chronic illness and two of which dealt with the results of extensive field studies in Hunterdon County, New Jersey, and Baltimore, Maryland. These field studies reached a new high in sophistication of research methodology. Successful attempts were made to measure morbidity and unmet need. In this respect, the fourth volume, by Ray E. Trussell, a physician-administrator, and Jack Elinson, a medical sociologist and social survey expert, is of special interest:[40] the authors attempted to measure the extent to which chronic illness was preventable. They concluded that not much of it was preventable at that time.

By 1952, voluntary health insurance had come to be regarded as the chief vehicle for financing personal health services, particularly hospital care. It was being used increasingly often to pay for physicians' services such as surgery and obstetrics. Still, no systematic evaluation had been made of the impact of voluntary health insurance on families with relatively high expenditures, and no nationwide household surveys had been conducted to update the data on use and expenditure patterns in the general population since the days of the CCMC in 1928–1931. Only relatively crude evaluations were possible using the national aggregates from the Department of Commerce and the Social Security Administration. Beginning in 1948, the latter agency published annual summaries of total national expenditures, by component of service, in the private sector of the health services economy. Also, and very important in the political battle between compulsory and voluntary health insurance, estimates were made of what proportion of the total expenditures for personal health services went for voluntary health insurance. In December 1953, the Social Security Administration reported that, after 15 or more years, voluntary health insurance was paying only 15.3 percent of total private expenditures for all types of services.[41] To show that social research findings sometimes matter, this figure was attacked by AMA secretary and general manager George Lull as a "perversion of statistical information," in that voluntary health insurance was not intended to cover 100 percent of expenditures.[42] What this figure, as used, revealed was a lack of sophistication in the interpretation and evaluation of health insurance benefits. The figure was confirmed in a nationwide survey of households conducted by the Health Information Foundation, New York City, and the National Opinion Research Center, University of Chicago; a detailed treatment of its significance was also given.[43]

The Health Information Foundation was chartered in 1950 exclusively for research in the health services, primarily in the financing and delivery of services. It was privately funded, chiefly by pharmaceutical companies. In 1962, the agency and its staff were invited to move to the University of Chicago to become part of the Graduate School of Business and to take over its graduate program in hospital administration and establish a unit on health services research. Other such programs were being set up at the University of Michigan, Columbia University, the University of Minnesota, the Johns Hopkins University, the University of North Carolina, the Health Insurance Plan of Greater New York, and the Kaiser plans on the West Coast. Research was conducted at other sites as well, but the ones mentioned above established formal programs.

The Health Information Foundation's research strategy was to accept the prevailing health services and health insurance structure as a given, examine its problems, and find and examine innovations and deviations from the mainstream. When the foundation embarked on its large-scale field studies in 1953, the terms "comprehensive medical care," "subsidy," and to some extent "service benefits," "experience rating," and "means test," were dirty words separating the nonprofit prepayment plans from the private insurance companies and separating both from proponents of government health insurance. Research in the health services would be controversial if it dealt with the generic problems that these terms suggest.

The foundation's first project enabled health insurance agencies to evaluate their benefit structures in relation to the expenditure patterns of American households. Existing health insurance benefits were adequate for some services but inadequate for others, even given loose criteria.[44] Evaluations of the benefits offered by a private insurance company in Boston and by Blue Cross-Blue Shield health insurance plans in Birmingham and Boston were made.[45]

The foundation conducted or sponsored several studies to examine various types of medical prepayment plans that offered physicians' services either in a fee-for-service arrangement or in a group practice structure. The nationwide survey had indicated the need for some broadening of health insurance beyond hospital-based services. The intent was to evaluate the possibility of insuring home and office calls in the prevailing structure of medical practice as well as in the group practice type and to show the results of various alternatives.[46]

In the meantime, because of the rapid expansion of voluntary health insurance, the Health Information Foundation and the National Opinion Research Center mounted in 1958 a second nationwide survey of family use of services and the impact of voluntary health insurance on use.[47] Results showed that, although aggregate expenditures had increased by 42 percent, one-half of this increase could be attributed to increased use and the other half to increased price. Further, the proportions of total expenditures covered by insurance had increased to 19 percent (from 15), and families with high expenditures had a larger proportion of their costs covered. It appeared that one aim of voluntary health insurance—covering high risks—was working. A survey in 1963 revealed more or less the same trends.[48]

Since voluntary health insurance appeared to be working reasonably well for the employed segment of the population, the problem of the aged began to surface. The aged were usually out of the labor market and their expenditures were relatively high. Accordingly, the Health Information Foundation sponsored a nationwide survey of the aged conducted by Ethel Shanas, a sociologist engaged by the National Opinion Research Center. The issue of government-sponsored health insurance reemerged in debates about health services for the aged. A great deal of census and income data were available on this group, plus data from old-age assistance programs, public medical care programs, mental hospitals, and general hospitals. That serious social and medical problems existed among the aged was not doubted, but systematic, nationwide data on their social situation, their illnesses, and their use of and expenditures for health services were lacking. Shanas' survey revealed, as expected, that persons age 65 and over had lower incomes than younger people, were likely to have more illnesses, and were higher users of services; they consequently had high expenditures. Her study revealed the hard core of the problem, showing that, by an illness index, 14 percent of the elderly (including persons in institutions) were unable to care for themselves: they were bedridden, chair-ridden, in institutions, or housebound.[49]

The extensive fact finding and research done on the aged culminated in the White House Conference on Aging held in Washington, D.C., January 9–12, 1961. A budget was appropriated to be used by states for studies on the entire range of social, economic, and health problems of the aged and for state conferences. State after state carried out surveys, the findings of which were fed into state conferences and ultimately into the White House conference. If facts alone could have determined an appropriate policy, one for the aged would have been forthcoming. Majority and minority recommendations split along the familiar lines of financing, through the Old Age and Survivors' Disability Insurance section of the Social Security Act to the Public Assistance section described in more detail in chapter 13. The intent of the conference was to create a consensus.[50] In due course the Medicare bill was passed, but not without a great deal of political wheeling and dealing.

Two university-based research centers emerged in the late 1950s in direct response to politicians' and policy makers' requests for data and information to guide public policy and legislation. One was in the School of Public Health and Administrative Medicine, Columbia University (under Ray E. Trussell), and the other was in the Bureau of Hospital Administration, School of Business Administration, University of Michigan (under Walter J. McNerney). These two centers and the Health Information Foundation did the most research directly related to policy. Trussell's studies were funded by the state legislature through a legislative committee; McNerney's studies, though requested by the state government, were funded by the W. K. Kellogg Foundation. Each of these research agencies reflected the direction and general style of the persons who set research policy.

A brief description of Trussell's research situation, main sources of funds, and research policy is in order as an example of the "politics" of social research. The New York State departments of insurance and public health engaged Trussell as a university-based consultant by commissioning the School of Public Health and Administrative Medicine at Columbia University to conduct a series of studies on use, costs, and quality of personal health services in the state. Trussell quickly assembled a staff of sociologists, statisticians, physicians, and health service administrators. They studied the massive records of hospitals, prepayment plans, and related agencies. Voluminous reports were published, along with recommendations based on the staff's findings.[51] Trussell himself fused the roles of fact gatherer and policy proposer, a feat seldom accomplished by researchers in the social sciences. Trussell's reports made good newspaper copy. This was particularly true of the study on quality of care received by Teamsters' Union families in New York City. An examination of the hospital and medical records of board-certified internists performing surgery in New York hospitals revealed a high proportion of what the evaluators judged as unnecessary procedures, particularly hysterectomies.[52]

The Michigan project, published in two large volumes, embodied a series of studies on the entire health services system of the state, in various degrees of depth.[53] It was the first attempt to view the health services of a state as a total system, with a statewide household survey serving as a framework. Since the studies were precipitated by Blue Cross' applying for a rate increase, possibly the most important single study among them was the one attempting to establish criteria for the "effectiveness of hospital use." This was the first systematic attempt to apply medical criteria to hospital use. Medical specialists in practice and in medical school formulated the criteria for 18 diagnoses comprising 46 percent of all hospital admissions in a year. Applying these criteria to a representative sample of hospital discharges showed that less than 3 percent of them were inappropriate.[54]

Concurrently, research reports on quality of services, regulations governing Blue Cross and Blue Shield Plans, and differences in use of hospitals in various organizational concepts were being published. The group practice plans were showing lower and purportedly more efficient use of hospital services than plans using the fee-for-service method of paying physicians. The report that probably received the most initial attention in this regard was prepared by I. S. Falk. In it, he compared hospital utilization rates in various delivery systems in several parts of the country, showing relatively low use of hospitals in prepaid group practices.[55]

During this period from the early fifties to the early sixties, beginnings were made in the exceedingly difficult problem of measuring the quality of medical care. Studies of rural general practitioners in North Carolina by Peterson and associates and evaluations of premature births in the Health Insurance Plan of Greater New York by the plan's research staff deserve mention.[56]

One gratifying development, in view of the generally chronic neglect of this area, was the creation of the Joint Commission on Mental Illness and Health in 1955, financed by grants from the National Institute of Mental Health and a number of private sources. The director was Jack R. Ewalt. The commission was a nongovernmental organization representing a variety of national agencies concerned with mental health. It sponsored an impressive series of books, from the conceptual to the empirical.[57]

NOTES

1. Henry J. Aaron, *Politics and Professors: The Great Society in Perspective* (Washington, D.C.: Brookings Institution, 1978), p. 156.
2. Ibid., p. 158.
3. Theodore Litman, *Sociology of Medical and Health Care: The First Fifty Years, Research Bibliography* (San Francisco: Boyd and Fraser, 1976); Harold E. Freeman, Sol Levine, and Leo G. Reeder, eds., *Handbook of Medical Sociology*, 3rd ed. (Englewood Cliffs, N.J.: Prentice-Hall, 1979); David Mechanic, ed., *Handbook of Health, Health Care, and the Health Professions* (New York: Free Press, 1983).
4. William H. Shaw, "Consumption Expenditures, 1929–43," *Survey of Current Business* 24 (June 1944):6–22.
5. See some elaboration in Gerald Gordon, Odin W. Anderson, Henry P. Brehm, and Sue Marquis, *Disease, the Individual, and Society, Social-Psychological Aspects of Disease: A Summary and Analysis of a Decade of Research* (New Haven, Conn.: College and University Press, 1968), pp. 10–21.
6. George Rosen, *A History of Public Health* (New York: MD Publications, 1958), pp. 135, 254.
7. Charles V. Chapin, "Deaths Among Taxpayers and Non-Taxpayers, Income Tax, Providence 1865," *American Journal of Public Health* 14 (August 1924):647–51.
8. Joseph Goldberger and G. A. Wheeler, "A Study of the Relation of Family Income and Other Economic Factors to Pellagra Incidence in Seven Cotton-Mill Villages of South Carolina in 1916," *Public Health Reports* 35 (November 1920):2673–714.
9. Edgar Sydenstricker, *Health and Environment* (New York: McGraw-Hill, 1933).
10. Robert M. Woodbury, *Causal Factors in Infant Mortality: A Statistical Study Based on Investigation in Eight Cities*, Publication No. 142 (Washington, D.C.: Government Printing Office, 1925).
11. Selwyn D. Collins, *Economic Status and Health: A Review and Study of the Relevant Morbidity and Mortality Data*, Public Health Bulletin No. 165 (Washington, D.C.: U.S. Public Health Service, 1927).
12. Louis I. Dublin and Alfred J. Lotka with Mortimer Spiegelman, *The Money Value of A Man*, rev. ed. (New York: Ronald Press, 1936).
13. Henry E. Sigerist, *A History of Medicine: Primitive and Archaic Medicine* (New York: Oxford University Press, 1951).
14. Bernhard J. Stern, *Historical Sociology: The Selected Papers of Bernhard J. Stern* (New York: Citadel Press, 1959).
15. Examples can be found in Gordon *et al.*, *Disease*, p. 15.
16. Edgar Sydenstricker, "The Extent of Medical and Hospital Service in a Typical Small City, Hagerstown Morbidity Studies No. 3," *Public Health Reports* 42 (14 January 1927):121–31.
17. I. S. Falk, Margaret C. Klem, and Nathan Sinai, *The Incidence of Illness and the Receipt and Costs of Medical Care Among Representative Family Groups*. CCMC Publication No. 26 (Chicago: University of Chicago Press, 1933).

18. Otis D. Duncan, *Social Research on Health* (New York: Social Science Research Council, 1946).
19. Frederick D. Mott and Milton I. Roemer, *Rural Health and Medical Care* (New York: McGraw-Hill, 1948).
20. C. R. Hoffer *et al.*, "Health Needs and Health Care in Michigan," Michigan State College Agricultural Experiment Station, Section of Sociology and Anthropology, Special Bulletin No. 365, 1950, East Lansing, Michigan; Charles R. Hoffer and Edgar A. Schuler, "A Measurement of Health Needs and Health Care," *American Sociological Review* 13 (December 1948):719–24. Milton Roemer had done some earlier, preliminary work on the method which contributed directly to the larger studies of the Michigan State University sociologists.
21. Nathan Sinai, Odin W. Anderson, and Melvin L. Dollar, *Health Insurance in the United States* (New York: Commonwealth Fund, 1946).
22. Louis S. Reed, *Health Insurance: The Next Step in Social Security* (New York: Harper, 1937).
23. ———, *Blue Cross and Medical Service Plans* (Washington, D.C.: Federal Security Agency, 1947).
24. Herbert D. Simpson, *Compulsory Health Insurance in the United States: An Analysis and Appraisal of the Present Movement* (Evanston, Ill.: Northwestern University Press, 1943).
25. Franz Goldmann, *Voluntary Medical Care Insurance in the United States* (New York: Columbia University Press, 1948) and *Public Medical Care: Principles and Problems* (New York: Columbia University Press, 1945).
26. George W. Bachman and Meriam Lewis, *The Issue of Compulsory Health Insurance* (Washington, D.C.: Brookings Institution, 1948).
27. I. S. Falk, *Security Against Sickness: A Study of Health Insurance* (Garden City, N.Y.: Doubleday, Doran, 1936).
28. Nathan Sinai, Marguerite Hall, and Roy E. Holmes, *Medical Relief Administration: Final Report of the Experience in Essex County Ontario* (Windsor, Ontario: Essex County Medical Economic Research, 1939).
29. *Report of the Temporary Legislative Commission to Formulate Long-Range State Health Programs*, New York State Legislative Document No. 91 (Albany: State of New York, 1940).
30. Odin W. Anderson, *State Enabling Legislation for Non-Profit Hospital and Medical Plans, 1944*, Research Series No. 1 (Ann Arbor: University of Michigan School of Public Health, 1944).
31. ———, *Administration of Medical Care, Problems and Issues: Based on an Analysis of the Medical-Dental Care Program for the Recipients of Old-Age Assistance in the State of Washington, 1941–45*, Research Series No. 2 (Ann Arbor: University of Michigan School of Public Health, 1947).
32. Nathan Sinai and Odin W. Anderson, *EMIC: A Study of Administrative Experience*, Research Series No. 3 (Ann Arbor: University of Michigan School of Public Health, 1948).

33. See C. Rufus Rorem, *Private Group Clinics*, CCMC Report No. 8 (Chicago: University of Chicago Press, 1931); I. S. Falk, *Organized Medical Service at Fort Benning, Georgia*, CCMC Report No. 21 (Chicago: University of Chicago Press, 1932); Michael M. Davis and C. Rufus Rorem, *The Crisis in Hospital Finance* (Chicago: University of Chicago Press, 1932).
34. J. W. Mountin, E. H. Pennell, and V. M. Hoge, *Health Service Areas—Requirements for General Hospitals and Health Centers*, Public Health Bulletin, No. 292 (Washington, D.C.: Government Printing Office, 1945).
35. Commission on Hospital Care, *Hospital Resources and Needs: A Report of the Michigan Hospital Survey* (Battle Creek: Kellogg Foundation, 1946).
36. The President's Commission on the Health Needs of the Nation, *Building America's Health*, Five volumes (Washington, D.C.: Government Printing Office, 1952).
37. Commission on Financing Hospital Care, *Financing Hospital Care in the United States;* Vol. 1, *Factors Affecting the Costs of Hospital Care;* Vol. 2, *Prepayment and the Community;* Vol. 3, *Financing Hospital Care for Non-Wage and Low-Income Groups* (New York: Blakiston, 1954–55).
38. United States Committee on Vital and Health Statistics, *United States Statistics on Medical Economics: Present Status and Recommendations for Additional Data* (Washington, D.C.: Government Printing Office, 1964).
39. Details can be found in Paul J. Sanazaro, "Federal Health Services R&D Under the Auspices of the National Center for Health Services Research and Development," in E. Evelyn Flook and Paul J. Sanazaro, eds., *Health Services Research and R&D in Perspective* (Ann Arbor, Mich.: Health Administration Press, 1973), pp. 150–83.
40. Commission on Chronic Illness, *Chronic Illness in the United States:* Vol. 3, *Chronic Illness in a Rural Area, The Hunterdon Study* (Cambridge, Mass.: Harvard University Press, 1954).
41. "Voluntary Insurance Against Sickness: 1948–51 Estimates," *Social Security Bulletin* 15 (December 1953):3–6.
42. *New York Times*, 4 January, 1953, p. 512.
43. Odin W. Anderson and Jacob J. Feldman, *Family Medical Care Costs and Voluntary Health Insurance: A Nationwide Survey* (New York: McGraw-Hill, 1956), p. 24.
44. Ibid.
45. Odin W. Anderson et al., (staff of the National Opinion Research Center), *Voluntary Health Insurance in Two Cities: A Survey of Suburban Households* (Cambridge, Mass.: Harvard University Press, 1957).
46. Benjamin J. Darsky, Nathan Sinai, and Solomon J. Axelrod, *Comprehensive Medical Services Under Voluntary Health Insurance: A Study of Windsor Medical Services* (Cambridge, Mass.: Harvard University Press, 1958); George A. Shipman, Robert J. Lampman, and S. Frank Miyamoto, *Medical Service Corporations in the State of Washington* (Cambridge, Mass.: Harvard University Press, 1962); Odin W. Anderson and Paul B. Sheatsley, *Comprehensive Medi-*

cal Insurance—A Study of Costs, Use and Attitudes Under Two Plans, Research Series No. 9 (New York: Health Information Foundation, 1954).

47. Odin W. Anderson, Patricia Collette, and Jacob J. Feldman, *Changes in Family Medical Care Expenditures and Voluntary Health Insurance: A Five-Year Resurvey* (Cambridge, Mass.: Harvard University Press, 1963).

48. Ronald Andersen and Odin W. Anderson, *A Decade of Health Services: Social Survey Trends in Use and Expenditures* (Chicago: University of Chicago Press, 1967).

49. Ethel Shanas, *The Health of Older People: A Social Survey* (Cambridge, Mass.: Harvard University Press, 1962).

50. U.S. Department of Health, Education, and Welfare, *The Nation and Its Older People: Report of the White House Conference on Aging* (Washington, D.C.: Government Printing Office, 1961).

51. Columbia University School of Public Health and Administrative Medicine, *Prepayment for Hospital Care in New York State: A Report on Eight Blue Cross Plans Serving New York Residents* (New York: Columbia University Press, 1961) and *Prepayment for Medical and Dental Care in New York State: A Report on the Seven Blue Shield Plans and Health Insurance Plan of Greater New York, Group Health Insurance, Inc., and Group Dental Insurance, Inc., Serving New York Residents* (New York: Columbia University Press, 1962).

52. Ray E. Trussell, J. Ehrlich, and Mildred A. Morehead, *The Quantity, Quality, and Costs of Medical Care Secured by a Sample of Teamster Families in the New York Area* (New York: Columbia University Press, 1962).

53. Walter J. McNerney *et al., Hospital and Medical Economics: A Study of Population, Services, Costs, Methods of Payments and Controls,* 2 vols. (Chicago: Hospital Research and Educational Trust, 1962).

54. Ibid. and Thomas Fitzpatrick, Donald C. Riedel, and Beverly C. Payne, "Character and Effectiveness of Hospital Use," *Hospital and Medical Economics* 1 (1962):361–588.

55. In George St. J. Perrot and Nancy E. Maher, "The Federal Employees' Health Benefits Program: Third Term Coverage and Hospital Utilization," *Group Health and Welfare News,* Special Supplement (February-March 1965).

56. Osler L. Peterson, *et al.,* 'An Analytical Study of North Carolina General Practice, 1953–54," *Journal of Medical Education* 31, Part 2 (December 1956):1–165; Sam Shapiro *et al.,* "Comparisons of Premature and Prenatal Mortality in a General Population and in a Population of a Prepaid Group Practice," *American Journal of Public Health* 48 (February 1958):170–87. A forerunner of these quality studies was the one sponsored by the Committee on the Costs of Medical Care, *An Outline of the Fundamentals of Good Medical Care and An Estimate of the Service Required To Supply the Medical Needs of the United States* (Chicago: University of Chicago Press, 1933).

57. Among those were Marie Jahoda, *Current Concepts of Positive Mental Health* (New York: Basic Books, 1958); George W. Albee, *Mental Health Manpower Trends* (New York: Basic Books, 1959); Gerald Gurin, Joseph Veroff, and Sheila Field, *Americans View Their Mental Health* (New York: Basic Books, 1960).

21

Incursions into Perceptions, Attitudes, and Decision Making

The influence of the public's perceptions and attitudes on their use of services was first studied by Earl L. Koos in the fifties in Rochester, New York.[1] He found that education and income were associated with perceptions of need and use: the lower a person's education and income, the lower the perception of symptoms and the lower the use of services. (This study was done before there was much voluntary health insurance.) Later research by sociologists would build on Koos' work.

Over the years, the American public has had a remarkably consistent and favorable attitude towards persons in the health services establishment. Despite horror stories from individual patients and critics in the mass media, there is a high degree of good will towards the enterprise, around 90 percent of adults reporting they are well- or reasonably well-satisfied regarding the treatment they receive and the quality of services.[2] Understandably, these attitudes vary considerably by income group, race, and residence. The lower the income, for example, the less favorable the attitude, although the majority attitude is still favorable. Thus managers and professional health personnel are serving a population that is well-disposed toward the health services, a fact that may result in their resting on their laurels. The relatively recent and rapid increase in malpractice suits by patients against physicians—particularly surgeons, orthopedists, and obstetricians and gynecologists—reveals some deep dissatisfaction on the part of an aggressive and aggrieved minority, which may be symptomatic of more pervasive problems such as lack of a personal physician and certainty of care.

Between 65 and 75 percent of adults feel there is a crisis in the health services. Probing reveals that the crisis consists mainly of high out-of-pocket costs and the difficulty of finding a physician during nights and weekends except in hospital emergency services; close to 40 percent of adults perceived these unfavorable aspects.[3] Objective data also reveal episodes of high costs paid directly by the patient and difficulty of access to physicians' care at certain times of the day and week, as well as long waits in physicians' offices. These data are very important to managers in that, given the reservoir of good will present, it behooves them to improve access and reduce high out-of-pocket costs. These goals seem to be fairly feasible: standby physician services could be arranged in private practice and hospitals, and health insurance benefits could be improved, thereby reducing or eliminating high-cost episodes.

People appear to insist on having insurance pay for all types of medical care episodes, whether small or large. This was cogently expressed at a Congressional hearing by a representative of labor who, on being asked, replied that he wanted coverage of both small and large costs. Insurance premiums would be cheaper if only relatively expensive episodes were paid in full, leaving intermittent and low-cost episodes to be paid for out-of-pocket.[4]

There are contrary opinions about the extent to which the public can be relied on to recognize and judge the severity of symptoms. An extreme view would be that an individual should see a physician at the slightest signs of swelling, headache, and tiredness, not to mention gashes, blood in the stool, sudden loss of weight, and pains in the chest. Approximately 20 symptoms have been delineated by physicians as signs that something is happening to the body. Over the years, several nationwide household surveys[5] have been conducted to investigate adults' perceptions of symptoms. In the late fifties, a nationwide study was conducted to test adults' knowledge of danger signals of cancer and heart disease. In the main, the public was well aware of the danger signals, revealing that dissemination of knowledge was having an effect. The usual differences among educational levels and income groups were noted, particularly education.

In subsequent studies,[6] up until the early 1970s, adults were queried as to (1) their recognition of around 20 symptoms, (2) the extent to which different symptoms would motivate them to see a physician, (3) whether they had experienced any such symptoms during the past year, and (4) if they had, had they seen a physician. A panel of physicians was asked to estimate the severity of each symptom and the urgency of seeing a physician if an individual had such a symptom. Researchers found reasonably close agreement between the physicians and the public. On some symptoms, such as sudden pain in the chest or a sore that would not heal, there was very close agreement—seek immediate attention. On other symptoms, such as a runny nose or a cough for a few days, there was also agreement—delay for a while. However, there was a decided discrepancy between recognition of the severity of a symptom and actually seeing a physician, whether because of time, cost or convenience. The more acute the symptom, such as shortness of breath, the more likely it was that the individual had actually seen a physician. There were differences in the expected directions among income groups and educational levels in perceptions of severity and urgency in seeing a physician.[7] My cautious conclusion is that the public is quite sophisticated in recognizing symptoms and knowing whether or not such symptoms warrant seeing a physician. The great increase in the proportion of the population seeing a physician since the 1930s seems to support this view.

The rising expenditures entailed by this increased demand were not regarded as a problem, and the increased use was welcomed as a sign of improved health. Recently, however, this increased use is being questioned as a sign of self-indulgence or dependency and a waste of resources. For example, Leon Kass, a physician, writes: "All kinds of problems now roll to the doctor's door, from sagging anatomies to suicides, from unwanted childlessness to unwanted pregnancy, from marital difficulties to learning difficulties, from genetic counseling to drug addiction, from laziness to crime."[8] At the same time, there is a great deal of criticism of physicians' wasteful use of tests and their use of technology at the margin of efficacy.[9] In any case, the managers of the health services enterprise are expected to assure adequate services equitably distributed. Measurements are so crude, however, that managers cannot possibly determine need and demand for or volume of services necessary as accurately as, say, an automobile manufacturer can calibrate the demand for automobiles. Confounding the problem for managers is the recognition that there is still an appreciable amount of unmet need in urban ghettos and rural areas, given current standards of desirable access; thus, if resources are not to be expanded, there must be increased use among some segments of the population and decreased use among others.

If planners and managers are to become interested in the nature of need and demand (or, in business parlance, "the market") beyond crude utilization data like hospital admissions and length of stay, they should realize that the American public has high demands and that these demands are based on reasonable perceptions, given the prevailing standard of living. The challenge then becomes one of filling unmet need and possibly even of trying to educate the public about which symptoms do not require a physician's care. If there were some way of separating necessary and unnecessary services, the necessary services could be publicly or privately financed through health insurance, and unnecessary services could be financed through a rider or special contract. This concept does not seem feasible, given current knowledge and the desire for comprehensiveness in health insurance benefits. Necessary services could be a public good, and unnecessary services could be a private good. This split is recognized in room differentiations in both public and private programs (ward, semiprivate, private). The split is also recognized in differentiating between elective surgery and urgent surgery.

Researchers continue to develop increasingly sophisticated measures of need, demand, and use, with the expectation that they will lead to greater predictability in managing the health services enterprise. Factoring out the various elements that should result in seeking services of a physician would seem important to public policy formulation and health services administration. So far, the most sophisticated model of need and demand is the one formulated by Ronald Andersen at the University of Chicago in the latter sixties and since refined by him and his staff. Other researchers have adopted this model, attesting to its general acceptance. Andersen classified the source of demand for health services into predisposing, enabling, and need. Since it is known that illnesses vary by age and sex, they are basic in predicting need and demand, the predisposing factor. The enabling factor involves the presence of the necessary services and the means to pay for them. The perception of need in the model is the element that triggers an individual to seek services. It is possible with this model to relate predisposing factors and perceptions of need to enabling factors in a variety of circumstances and delivery models.[10]

Since the formulation of this model, Andersen and Aday and their staff have been devising indicators of access to services by applying criteria of the severity of symptoms on a mass social survey basis. It is reasonable to assume that the severity of symptoms should be related to the time it takes to gain access and the type of personnel at the entry point.[11]

An important aspect of the closeness of fit between need and demand and the physician's services and decisions is the degree to which the patient follows the physician's directions. Assuming that the physician's diagnosis and recommended therapy are valid, the quality of service is determined by the understanding and compliance of the patient. I have mentioned that the public is generally sophisticated in recognizing symptoms and acting upon them; thus it seems reasonable to assume that the degree of compliance is a measure of how efficacious the therapy is—low compliance would indicate low efficacy. It seems, however, that the public's degree of compliance with physicians' orders is not as sophisticated as the public's knowledge about and action on symptoms. I make this observation cautiously because studies of compliance have been done on small and selected patient groups, not on national samples. Generally, a high proportion of patients do not follow the directions of physicians for taking medications.[12] An example is the tendency of persons with hypertension to slack off taking the indicated drugs as soon as they feel better. The reciprocal relationship between physician and patient is central to compliance, yet the relationship has rarely been explored with a view to improving the diagnostic and therapeutic process.

After almost 100 years of spontaneous expansion, there is a tremendous enterprise in place needing a means of management, control, and planning. Where are the control points and what means do we have of utilizing them? We know where the control points are, or, more specifically, the decision-making points, but we know little about how to manipulate them for intelligent management and control.

Let us start with the patient. In the old days, before insurance, the patient could not abuse the system, because the patient paid directly for the service. The accusation of abuse was heaped on the poor or near-poor, who received charity service. When voluntary insurance appeared in the thirties, the cost and use controls were the restrictions on the range and use of personal health services. For example, drugs outside the hospital were not a benefit, they were an unpredictable quantity. Physicians' office and house calls were normally not included because it was feared that they would be open-ended. The number of hospital days per person per year was limited in order to control the seemingly open-ended nature of hospital use. It was assumed that, if there were no charge for a bed, too many people would use the hospital as a hotel. Other controls on the patient were a waiting period after enrollment in the insurance plan before pregnancy or its exclusion altogether on the assumption that it was premeditated and not a risk like appendicitis! Certain conditions that a person might be suffering from at the time of enrollment, such as hernia or heart trouble, might be excluded altogether or subjected to a waiting period in order to control self-selection of enrollees. Extensive group enrollment eventually eliminated these restrictions, and maternity was normally included as a matter of policy. (The birthrate is quite easily predicted, given data on the number of women of childbearing age in an enrolled population.)

For all practical purposes there were no controls on the providers. Hospitals were paid costs or charges, whichever was lower; physicians were paid their usual and customary fees. The economy was expansive enough in the forties, at least for the burgeoning voluntary health insurance plans, that hard bargaining with providers was neither necessary nor practical. The funding sources went along. Although the health services enterprise has become a negotiated order between the parties at interest, there was nothing to negotiate or bargain about at that time. Rather, there was promotion and publicity and the problem of calculating risks (that is, use), but deficits could be made up. No Blue Cross or Blue Shield plans failed; although their management was generally not very good, it was apparently good enough for the purpose and time. Managers operated in an expansive environment.[13] Health insurance plans operated under state charters of incorporation, and their benefits, reserves, and premiums had to be approved by state commissioners. The major responsibility and legal concern of the insurance commissioners, however, was the solvency of the insurance agency: Could it deliver on the contract? The content of the contract was not really questioned.

This state of affairs lasted through the 1960s, after the passage of the Medicare and Medicaid acts. In the meantime, more controls were placed on the patient in the form of deductibles, for example paying part or all of the costs of the first day in the hospital or part of the fee for a visit to a physician's office. Another financial control was coinsurance, in which the patient paid a certain percentage of a hospital or medical bill. These types of controls on the patient were applied as a matter of faith. Research on their effectiveness has been inconclusive, to say the least. Very recently, however, the Rand Corporation has shown that use is reduced if deductibles are as high as $150.[14] There has been continuous and fruitless debate as to whether or not these financial controls on the patient inhibit "necessary" use rather than simply discouraging "unnecessary" use. There is some evidence that these controls reduce the use of services by low-income groups, which have relatively high need.[15] Interestingly, there was no evidence that immunizations for children were reduced by copayment requirements, although another study in the same state found that the use of preventive services was reduced.

The burden of controls was initially placed on the public not necessarily because of the self-serving intent of the providers, who were accorded by custom and law a virtual monopoly on personal health services delivery, but because of the intrinsic nature of a personal health service. The health services are a negotiated order largely because of lack of input and output measures. This is true regardless of ownership of the facilities, how personnel are paid, or where the money comes from. This characteristic is abundantly described in studies on the organization of the hospital and the structure and practices of the medical profession. An early study of the general hospital was given the earthy title of *The Give and Take in Hospitals* rather than the more pedantic "negotiated order."[16]

Later studies, such as one by Basil S. Georgopolous and Floyd C. Mann using sociometric and social psychological methods, concluded that the general hospital was the most complicated social institution in existence.[17] Sociologists were mystified that an institution with so few of the characteristics of a bureaucracy, as conceptualized by Max Weber, could actually function. They began to learn that informal structures are necessary to make seemingly formal structures work. Eliot Friedson explored the medical profession's need for discretionary authority and prerogatives, given the uncertainty inherent in their decision making. This need puts the profession outside the direct control of managers. What emerged in the hospital was a tripartite structure of board, administration, and medical staff, with the medical staff functioning collegially rather than hierarchically. Duncan Neuhauser concluded that this type of organization is appropriate for the hospital's tasks.[18]

There have also been many studies of the ambiguous role of the registered nurse, who must function in the crosscurrents of the administrator, the physician, and the patient. The nursing profession has been valiantly striving to establish its turf, but there is little evidence that its situation is changing appreciably.[19] Nurses seem to be incapable of combining the nurturing aspects of their profession with the high-status technical and esoteric knowledge characteristic of physicians. The difficult position of the nurse has been exacerbated by the gradual denigration of the service function in modern society. Service to the body, even though the body is a whole person, has low esteem, assuming that it ever enjoyed high esteem. Women have traditionally served as the major reservoir of unquestioned service, service as an end in itself. This reservoir is diminishing as women move into a wide range of jobs and at least commensurate pay.

It would be naive and patronizing to imply that managers were unaware of the organization of health services delivery before sociologists began studying it in the fifties. Sensitive managers responded more or less sensibly in adjusting to and coping with the many complex social situations involved. Successful hospital administrators, and there were many, would not have survived without being sensitive to what is necessary to operate an institution. They were not inclined, however, to generalize, at least in print, or to systematize their experiences and observations into training programs for would-be managers. Managerial lore was like the empirical medicine of the early days, when clinicians transmitted their experience by trying to add up their clinical impressions. Being able to tell patients that the hospital organization is a negotiated order and that a great deal of uncertainty is intrinsic to medical practice requires a certain managerial style, one suitable to the enterprise. Not long ago, it was commonly held that managers hated physicians because they were unmanageable and arrogant; physicians, in turn, hated managers because they were always trying to make the enterprise manageable in terms of budgets, patient flow, morale of patients, and a host of other matters. These notions persist in subtle forms.

Systematic studies of institutions should help in looking at management as a problem in understanding people without placing blame. What combination of circumstances is required to facilitate optimum performance on the part of a group of people trained as physicians? Similarly, what are the institutional requirements for nurturing people who are sick?

Freidson recognized that, to function adequately as professionals, physicians needed freedom.[20] Similarly, students of hospital organization recognized and appreciated that a hospital is not like a factory, which makes bricks of uniform sizes ready to be put into walls of predictable dimensions. The hospital manager needs to run the institution with a great deal of internal and external leeway. Until recently, the health services enterprise has been accorded this freedom de facto. Now that the costs of the enterprise are beginning to nudge other priorities, the extent of this freedom is being questioned. There is undoubtedly fat in the system, but nobody knows how much. Economists are certain there is a lot of fat because there are no incentives to relate demand to costs. Economic theory dictates that waste and inefficiency are inevitable in such a situation.[21] Physicians and sociologists might simply say that need is being met and the price system does not recognize need, only demand, which has to be calculated by the cost to the parties concerned.

In addition to controls on the patient through deductibles, coinsurance, and benefits, controls are now being exerted on the providers. Possibly physicians were the first to feel controls, however mild, through the clause in the Medicare Act mandating reviews of length of stay in hospitals. Hospitals would not be reimbursed by the federal government for Medicare and Medicaid patients unless they set up review committees. Although there was sparse evidence in subsequent years that utilization review committees did any good, the concept was expanded by Congress in 1972. The country was divided into 200 or so areas so that groups of hospitals could be reviewed regionally. These were called Professional Standards Review Organizations. The review committees were made up exclusively of physicians, as mandated by the law. The enforcement lever was reimbursement for Medicare and Medicaid patients, who were making up about 50 percent of all hospital income from patients.

Elaborate studies have been made of the impact of the PSRO mechanism on hospital use. Results have been mixed, calling into question whether or not the concept is worth the cost of application.[22] It is important to note, however, that even though evidence may show certain control mechanisms to be ineffective, their existence is regarded as a worthy end in itself; sociologists call this a latent function.

The attempt to move directly into the decision-making process and prerogatives of the physician was a radical one, both from the physician's standpoint and the manager's. The PSRO concept was a spillover from business management, which believes that procedures and outputs can be specified in any enterprise. Unlike Europeans, Americans have little faith in structuring health services so that the framework in which they are administered and financed is clearly delineated, with budget caps to show exactly how much money is available for the coming year. Whereas Europeans essentially leave it to the actors to reach some sort of equilibrium within the structure and the budget, Americans' dislike of structure drove them into the decision-making process of physicians. The hope was that, by making physician decision making more rational through peer review, the costs of health services could be more easily justified. Reasonable as this concept appears, there was (and is) no methodology for reviewing physician decision making, short of a few agreed-upon conditions that lend themselves to uniform and standard management.

Another control emerging on a voluntary basis among big buyers of services is the second opinion for surgery. Conventional wisdom has it that the rate of surgical operations in this country is excessive compared with that in other countries, particularly Great Britain. In fact, however, no one knows what constitutes a proper rate of surgery. For serious and costly operations, a second opinion would seem to be reasonable and presumably should result in fewer operations and more conservative decisions. The evidence collected so far, however, does not show conclusively that a second opinion results in fewer operations. We must rely on faith that a second opinion is a reasonable end in itself. The fact that there is peer review may reduce surgery (sentinel effect), but we do not know what this actually means for quality of care. Reduction of surgery is an end in itself.[23] Great Britain limits its supply of surgeons and puts them on a salary. We are less likely to do either, but we do encourage the patient to question the profession. We are more likely to manipulate the site of surgery, having as many as possible performed outside the hospital, congruent with safety and standards, thereby eliminating the costly per diem hospital charges.

A more recent control, devised by the Blue Cross and Blue Shield plans, was the elimination of payment for 20 or so medical procedures that have been declared obsolete by a committee of physicians. There is no evidence of how much this method is saving in costs, but it seems an eminently reasonable means of improving quality. In fact, it appears to be the simplest and least controversial means of monitoring quality.

The Hill-Burton Act had been so successful in increasing the supply of hospital beds, particularly in rural areas, that the United States began to have an excess supply. The annual occupancy rate fell below 80 percent, the generally accepted standard. A report issued by a National Institute of Medicine committee pondered the matter and concluded that the United States had an excess of 100,000 beds, close to 10 percent of all beds.[24] In the absence of scientifically derived standards, one must rely on the prestige of the source. The states were already beginning to pass legislation to control the supply of hospital beds through certificate-of-need laws, New York State as early as 1964. The intention was to limit demand by putting a brake on the supply. Roemer and Shain[25] pointed out that there was a positive relationship between the supply of hospital beds and use; this was hardly a startling finding, but it was picked up as the prime justification for limiting the supply. The question of what constitutes a proper supply remains, because the saturation point has not been tested: one is given to believe that if the supply of beds were unlimited, people would be in hospital beds rather than home or at work.

Certificate-of-need laws, whereby hospitals must justify the expansion, extensive renovation, or construction of a new hospital, are in effect in most states. Perversely, certificate-of-need laws seem to have had little effect on the number of hospital beds. Studies show mixed results at best. At worst, hospitals expand to include services not measured by beds.[26]

A method of regulating rates for hospital services naturally came to the fore (physicians' fees were regulated only during the short period of general price controls in the early seventies). The 20 percent of the medical dollar that went for physicians' services appeared small beside the 40 percent of the medical dollar attributed to hospitals. So regulators went after the obvious culprit, trying to control both supply of beds and price and, in effect, rationing demand for hospitals. In rather short order, state after state legislated review boards to approve or disapprove the rates desired by individual hospitals, usually on an annual basis. Rate setting is no simple affair, although it appears to be possible if certain arbitrary definitions of unit costs are adopted, such as depreciation, amortization, replacement value, and teaching costs; hospitals have no bottom line in a profit and loss sense and are supposed to serve all comers.[27]

Interest in methods of reimbursing hospitals, beyond the traditional and simplistic one of charges or costs, whichever was lower, grew up. Enter the federal government through Medicare and Medicaid, which are assumed to require greater accountability so that tax dollars are spent on what the law actually mandates. The basic method of reimbursement became what is called prospective reimbursement. Public hospitals had been operating with prospective reimbursement all along, only they called it annual budgeting. Various methods of reimbursement were tried under the aegis of the Bureau of Health Insurance of the Social Security Administration (now the Health Care Finance Administration). It is unclear which reimbursement methods worked or which ones were better than others.[28]

The regulation of hospital bed supply and rates and the inauguration of medical peer review surfaced at the same time as regulation of airline routes and rates, regulation of the trucking industry, and so on. All these enterprises have been under critical political scrutiny since the Nixon-Ford administrations. What is interesting is that the general disenchantment with regulation as a means of controlling rates somehow did not spill over to the health services enterprise. The health services have lagged behind other industries in the application of business trends to financial controls and accounting, personnel, management, unionization and supply and price regulation. Studies done by economists showing the ineffectiveness or, worse still, higher prices because of regulation were not taken seriously by persons who advocated regulating supply and price for the health services, specifically the hospitals.

Eventually, these various regulations and controls were combined into one stupendous national planning concept—the National Health Planning and Resources Development Act of 1975. Details of this act are presented in chapter 16. In addition to being de facto agents for the states and the federal government in advising on certificates of need, rate regulation, and peer review, local agencies were to encourage multiple hospital mergers, joint purchases of supplies, interhospital agreements on purchases of high-technology equipment, and group practice of physicians. These were regarded as cost-effective, but economists have a hard time determining economies of scale, cost effectiveness, and efficiency in the health field because of the paucity of input and output measures.[29]

The technology of planning itself is in its infancy. For that matter, planning may never mature beyond infancy because of the measurement problems relating need and demand to services.[30] The more candid personnel in planning agencies admit that health services planning is largely a political process of balancing need and demand, consumer and professional interest groups, and the generosity and relative power of the funding agencies. No country has really evolved a planning strategy beyond this level. Even if the technology were available and we could demonstrate systematically that a given input of resources would result in a given output at a given cost, the resolution of alternatives would remain a profoundly political problem.

Confounding further the possibility of managing and planning the health services is the confusion among economists as to whether physicians can create their own demand and, therefore, set target incomes.[31] A seeming paradox is that the greater the density of physicians, the higher their prices and incomes. Frank A. Sloan and Roger Feldman argue imaginatively that this is because a greater density of physicians is more likely to occur in areas that provide more amenities, more sophisticated technology, and generally greater specialization, all of which are associated with higher costs.[32]

Interest in the idea of competition rather than regulation, or a combination of the two, as a means of inducing efficiency and containing costs has grown considerably since the early seventies. The theory has it that there should be competition among groups of physicians rather than among insurance agencies and among individual physicians. The conceptual literature on this theory has approached a high level of sophistication.[33] The effects of competition, or, indeed, that competition in the laissez-faire economic sense is possible at all in the health services remains to be seen. Even worse, what also remains to be seen is the feasibility of evaluating competition itself.

A final and somewhat desperate attempt to reduce the overall cost of health services is to change life styles, which would lead to fewer heart attacks, cancer of the lungs, accidents, and other diseases associated with daily habits.[34] This suggestion goes all the way back to the Truman Commission report of 1952. Hedonistic habits are difficult to change, for many people believe they make life worthwhile. There certainly is evidence that life style is related to the above morbidities and that adopting a more healthful life style would result in an appreciable reduction in morbidity and deaths.[35] Only a minority—25 percent of the population would be an optimistic estimate—might embrace healthful living habits, and although there would be some impact on use (and lowered expenditures) it would not be enough to assuage the fundamental problem of rising costs. Perhaps the self-help movement would reduce the pressure on the health services by making people more conversant with what symptoms require physicians' services; a purported 80 percent of conditions cure themselves. This would still leave enough serious conditions, both acute and chronic, to require a large infrastructure of high-technology personal health services.

This brief, selective, global review of health services research has revealed that there is a great deal of information available on expenditure patterns and use of services and some insight into perceptions and attitudes. But can these help in the management and control of the health services enterprise? Yes, because increased knowledge of the "nature of the beast" contributes to a more rational appraisal of the possible and the impossible. So far, the proper relationship among need and demand, equity, and the health services infrastructure remains obscure. Proper information would promote more sophisticated decision making, particularly regarding the consequences of alternatives, but even if systematic indicators were formulated for the level of use and expenditures and the characteristics of the delivery system, decisions would still be political and market-driven, or, most likely, a combination of both.

NOTES

1. Earl L. Koos, *The Health of Regionville* (New York: Columbia University Press, 1964).
2. See, for example, Lu Ann Aday, Ronald Andersen, and Gretchen V. Fleming, *Health Care in the U.S., Equitable for Whom?* (Beverly Hills, Calif.: Sage Publications, 1980) pp. 141–84.
3. Ibid.
4. Odin W. Anderson and J. Joel May, *The Federal Employees' Health Benefits Program, 1961–1968: A Model for National Health Insurance?* Health Administration Perspectives No. A9 (Chicago: Center for Health Administration Studies, Graduate School of Business, University of Chicago, 1971), p.5.
5. See, for example, Jacob J. Feldman, *The Dissemination of Health Information: A Case Study of Adult Learning* (Chicago: Aldine, 1966).
6. Ronald Andersen, Joanna Lion, and Odin W. Anderson, *Two Decades of Health Services: Social Survey Trends in Use and Expenditure* (Cambridge, Mass.: Ballinger, 1976), pp. 10–12.
7. Lu Ann Aday and Ronald Andersen, *Development of Indices of Access to Medical Care* (Ann Arbor, Mich.: Health Administration Press, 1975), pp. 38–55.
8. Victor Fuchs, *Who Shall Live?* (New York: Basic Books, 1974); Leon R. Kass, "Regarding the End of Medicine and the Pursuit of Health," *The Public Interest*, no. 40 (Summer 1975):12.
9. Steven A. Schroeder, Alan Schiftman, and Thomas E. Piemme, "Variation Among Physicians in Use of Laboratory Tests: Relation to Quality of Care," *Medical Care* 12 (August 1974):709–13.
10. Ronald Andersen, *A Behavioral Model of Families' Use of Health Services*, Research Series No. 20 (Chicago: Center for Health Administration Studies, Graduate School of Business, University of Chicago, 1974) (reprint).
11. Aday, Andersen, and Fleming, *Health Care*, pp. 185–230.
12. For an excellent overview, see Bonnie L. Svarstad, "Physician-Patient Communication and Patient Conformity with Medical Advice," in *The Growth of Bureaucratic Medicine: An Inquiry into the Dynamics of Patient Behavior and the*

Organization of Medical Care, ed. David Mechanic (New York: Wiley, 1976), pp. 220–38.

13. See, for example, Odin W. Anderson, *Blue Cross Since 1929: Accountability and the Public Trust* (Cambridge, Mass.: Ballinger, 1975).

14. John Holahan, "Cost Sharing," in *Controlling Medicaid Utilization Patterns*, ed. John Holahan (Washington, D.C.: Urban Institute, 1977), pp. 1–27; Mark R. Chassin, "The Containment of Hospital Costs: A Strategy Assessment," *Medical Care* 16 Supp. (October 1978):1–55; Bruce Stewart and Ronald Stockton, "Control over the Utilization of Medical Services," *Health and Society* 51 (Summer 1973):341–94; L. Jay Helms, Joseph P. Newhouse, and Charles E. Phelps, *Copayments and Demand for Medical Care: The California Medical Experience*, Rand Corporation Publication No. R-2167–HEW (Santa Monica, Calif.: Rand Corporation, 1978); Emmett B. Keeler and John E. Rolph, *The Demand for Episodes of Medical Treatment: Interesting Results from the Health Insurance Experiment* (Santa Monica, Calif.: Rand Corporation, 1982).

15. Carl E. Hopkins et al., "Cost Sharing and Prior Authorization Effects on Medical Services in California: Part I, The Beneficiaries' Reactions," *Medical Care* 13 (July 1975):582–94; Earl W. Brian and Stephen F. Gibbens, "California's Medical Copayment Experiment," *Medical Care* 12 Suppl. (December 1974).

16. Temple Burling, Edith M. Lentz, and Robert N. Wilson, *The Give and Take in Hospitals: A Study of Human Organization in Hospitals* (New York: Putnam, 1956).

17. Basil S. Georgopoulos and Floyd C. Mann, *The Community General Hospital*. (New York: Macmillan, 1962).

18. Duncan Neuhauser, "The Hospital as a Matrix Organization," *Hospital Administration* 17 (Fall 1972):8–25.

19. This literature is very extensive, and it is difficult to select representative studies.

20. Eliot Friedson, *Professional Dominance: The Social Structure of Medical Care* (New York: Atherton, 1970).

21. Fuchs, *Who*; Mark V. Pauly, "Efficiency, Incentives, and Reimbursement for Health Care," *Inquiry* 7 (March 1970):114–31; Kong-Kyum Ro, "Anatomy of Hospital Cost Inflation," *Hospital and Health Services Administration* 22 (Summer 1977):75–88; Joseph P. Newhouse, "The Structure of Health Insurance and the Erosion of Competition in the Medical Marketplace," in *Competition in The Health Care Sector: Past, Present, and Future*, ed. Warren Greenberg, Proceedings of a Conference Sponsored by the Bureau of Economics, Federal Trade Commission, March 1978 (Germantown, Md: Aspen Systems Corporation, 1978) pp. 215–29;_____, "Toward a Theory of Nonprofit Institutions: An Economic Model of a Hospital," *American Economic Review* 60 (March 1970):64–74.

22. Overviews can be found in Odin W. Anderson and Mark C. Schields, "Quality Measure and Control in Physician Decision Making: State of the Art," *Health Services Research* 17 (Summer 1982):125–55; Michael J. Goran,

"The Evolution of the PSRO Hospital Review System," *Medical Care* 17 (Suppl.) (May 1979).

23. Paul M. Gertman et al., "Second Opinion for Elective Surgery: The Mandatory Medicaid Program in Mass.," *New England Journal of Medicine* 302 (1980):1169–74; Eugene G. McCarthy and Madelon Lubin Finkel, "Second Opinion Elective Surgery Programs: Outcome Status Over Time," *Medical Care* 16 (December 1978):874–994.

24. Institute of Medicine, Committee on Controlling the Supply of Short-Term General Hospitals, *General Hospitals in the United States: A Policy Statement,* Publication IOM: 76–03 (Washington, D.C.: National Academy of Sciences, 1976).

25. Milton I. Roemer and Max Shain, *Hospital Utilization Under Insurance,* Hospital Monograph Series, No. 6 (Chicago: American Hospital Association, 1959).

26. David S. Salkever and Thomas W. Bice, "The Impact of Certificate of Need Controls on Hospital Investment," *Health and Society* 54 (Spring 1976):185–214.

27. See, for example, David S. Abernethy and David A. Pearson, *Regulating Hospital Costs: The Development of Public Policy* (Ann Arbor, Mich.: AUPHA Press, 1979).

28. See pertinent chapters in Michael Zubkoff, Ira E. Raskin, and Ruth S. Hanft, eds., *Hospital Cost Containment: Selected Notes for Future Policy* (New York: Prodist, 1978), especially Harold A. Cohn, "Experience of a State Cost Control Commission," pp. 401–28.

29. Richard W. Foster, "Economic Models of Hospitals," *Hospital Administration* 19 (Fall 1974):87–93; Ralph E. Berry, Jr., "Cost and Efficiency in the Production of Hospital Services," *Health and Society* 52 (Summer 1974):291–313; and an early but still pertinent review article by Thomas R. Hefty, "Returns to Scale in Hospitals: A Critical Review of Recent Research," *Health Services Research* 4 (Winter 1969):267–80.

30. Robin E. Mac Stravic, *Determining Health Needs* (Ann Arbor, Mich.: Health Administration Press, 1980); Philip N. Reeves, David Bergwall, and Nina B. Woodside, *Introduction to Health Planning,* 2d. ed. (Washington, D.C.: Resources Press, 1979). For a very abstract point of view, see Henrik L. Blum, *Expanding Health Care Horizons: From a General Systems Concept to a National Health Policy* (Oakland, Calif.: Third Party Associates, 1976).

31. Uwe E. Reinhardt, *Physician Productivity and the Demand for Health Manpower* (Cambridge, Mass.: Ballinger, 1975), p. 107; Jack Hadley, John Holahan, and William Scanlon, "Can Fee-for-Service Reimbursement Coexist with Demand Creation?" *Inquiry* 16 (Fall 1979):247–58. Hadley et al. say: "While the potential for demand creation may be limited, the limits may occur at unacceptable levels of utilization. At this stage we simply do not know where the limits are," p. 257.

32. Frank A. Sloan and Roger Feldman, "Competition Among Physicians," in *Competition in the Health Care Sector: Past, Present, and Future,* ed. Warren

Greenberg, Proceedings of a Conference sponsored by the Bureau of Economics, Federal Trade Commission, March 1978 (Germantown, Md.: Aspen Systems Corporations, 1978), pp. 45–102.

33. See Alain C. Enthoven, *Health Plan: The Only Practical Solution to the Soaring Cost of Medical Care* (Reading, Mass.: Addison-Wesley, 1980) and Clark C. Havighurst, *Deregulating the Health Care Industry: Planning for Competition* (Cambridge, Mass.: Ballinger, 1982).

34. Institute of Medicine, Division of Health Promotion and Disease Prevention, *"Preventive Services for the Well Population,"* Summary of an April 13, 1978, meeting. This paper suggests standard preventive procedures by age groups. For estimated impact of selected diseases on mortality if preventive measures (that is, life styles) were carried out, see Gio B. Gori and Brian J. Richter, "Macroeconomics of Disease Prevention in the United States," *Science* 200 (1978):1124–30. Depending on the disease, the drop in mortality can be as high as 31 percent for cardiovascular-renal diseases.

35. Nedra B. Belloc and Lester Breslow, "Relationship of Physical Health Status and Health Practices," *Preventive Medicine* 1 (1972):409–21; Lester Breslow, "Risk Factor Intervention for Health Maintenance," *Science* 200 (1978):908–12.

22

The Escalation of Health Services Research

The previous two chapters on health services research reveal a rather steady and cumulative production of research in the broad spectrum of the development of the American health services, health insurance, financing, and public opinion and perceptions. These chapters brought health services research up to around 1980 and the beginning of the Reagan administration.

The escalation of research relevant to the policy issues and administrative problems of the health services during the 1980s is by all standards phenomenal. There is now an extraordinarily large infrastructure of qualified health services researchers based in universities, professional associations, the health insurance industry, and government. I will endeavor here to give some idea of the range of problems and issues being addressed, both profound policy issues such as equity, and technical administrative problems such as methods of cost containment and efficiency.

Duncan Neuhauser observed in a recent review article there have been three waves of studies.[1] One wave studied the application of the prospective payment concept not only to acute inpatient care but also to psychiatric, ambulatory, rehabilitative, and nursing home care. A second wave of studies was directed at severity-of-illness measures, trying to explain and control variance in costs and length of stay within DRGs in general hospitals. A third wave is documenting the effect of DRG payment on the delivery of hospital-based services.[2]

Robert L. Kane made a sweeping overview of health services research during the last 20 years.[3] He said that the priority of problems of concern for health services research was, until recently, access (i.e., equity) first, cost second, and quality third. Now the priorities have changed: cost is the first priority, quality is second, and access is third—equity now has a low priority.

Other areas that have become popular are long-term care of the elderly, medical-legal liability, medical ethics, the effects of competition, measurements of the quality and outcomes of care, and the extent of the uninsured segment of the population.

The research projects that appear to have aroused the most interest from policy makers and administrators are the Rand Corporation studies of the effect of deductibles and coinsurance on use of services and therefore as controls on volume and associated costs;[4] the Wennberg studies of the wide differences in surgical and hospital admission patterns among contiguous and small areas in New England;[5] and the studies by others of differences in costs and utilization between HMOs and the mainstream fee-for-service delivery system.

Estimates of the uninsured segment of the population have been made in one state after another. The conventional estimate now is that 37 million people in the United States lack any health insurance at all, and millions of others have inadequate insurance. The Robert Wood Johnson Foundation has sponsored surveys of the effect on the poor of recent fiscal reductions in Medicaid and other related programs.[6] The reduction in access to services for this population is real.

The effect of competition between HMOs and the mainstream fee-for-service insurance system, and among HMOs, continues to be elusive. As Victor Fuchs observed, policy makers in this country seem reluctant to try pure competition without a continuing reserve of regulatory threats.[7]

On the prevention side, the Prevention Research Center sponsored by *Prevention Magazine* has begun to publish an annual *Prevention Index: A Report Card on the Nation's Health,* for which Louis Harris and Associates interview a representative sample of adults. This interesting survey tries to measure the extent to which adults in this country are practicing 21 health-promoting behaviors, from not smoking in bed to maintaining the proper weight.[8]

The research style is toward micro studies by operations researchers and economists in physician decision making, hospital and HMO information systems, and fine-tuning interventions in administration and organization. Early in 1980 Paul Starr published his popular *Transformation of American Medicine* showing the shift in the practice of medicine from black-bag general practitioners to high-technology specialists, and the consequent restructuring of the profession into corporationlike arrangements.[9] Then in the middle of the decade, David Mechanic, another sociologist, took a macro look at the fundamental change in the

American health services delivery system resulting from the shift in the physician's role from that of patient advocate to that of allocator of resources.[10]

Shortly thereafter, the first edition of this book was published as *Health Services in the United States: A Growth Enterprise Since 1875*, a history of the transformation of the organization and financing of the health services delivery system.[11] About the same time there appeared by Anderson and associates a macro analysis of the health care delivery environment and the emergence of HMOs in two very different health services markets, the metropolitan areas of Minneapolis–St. Paul and Chicago.[12]

At the beginning of the eighties there appeared Avedis Donabedian's seminal work on the concept and measurement of quality of medical care.[13] It became the conceptual and theoretical framework for the development of quality measurement methodology.

The usual interest-group, liberal-democratic theory of the U.S. political process in the health field was goaded by a Marxist approach to the development of the health services delivery system both in this country and abroad by Vicente Navarro.[14] He appears to be the leading theorist for this school of thought, among a small, cohesive group of others.

It seems that at a certain stage in the development of an enterprise that is politically controversial and relatively expensive, in which attainment is difficult to measure, and in which trade-offs are agonizing for the public to make, books of an overview nature by sincere and sophisticated experts from a variety of disciplines and philosophies begin to appear. One such book on health care appeared in 1988, over two decades after the inception of Medicare, and deals with the problems and future of the Medicare program. In the foreword to this Harvard study, policy analysts Julius B. Richmond and David Blumenthal observe, "Compromises deemed necessary to secure passage of the legislation in 1965 have come back to haunt the program in the form of escalating costs and confounding regulations."[15] Indeed, while all legislation of a social service sort involves start-up compromises, the participants in this Harvard study feel that there is now such an obsession with cost constraints in the Medicare program that little consideration is paid to improvements that require little or no additional expenditure.

On the heels of the Harvard study, there appeared two books with capable and sophisticated contributors on the global problems of the cost of health services and equity issues. One of them, *The Medical Cost-Containment Crisis: Fears, Opinions, and Facts*, edited by Jack D. McCue, had as its starting point a symposium supported by the Kate

B. Reynolds Health Care Trust.[16] The other, *Care and Cost: Current Issues in Health Policy*, edited by Kenneth McLennan and Jack A. Meyer, was sponsored by the Committee for Economic Development with the assistance of the Robert Wood Johnson Foundation.[17]

Both of these overviews of the health services condition in the United States are wide-ranging and sophisticated. McCue's volume has an underlying liberal orientation; McLennan and Meyer's book has a rather explicit market orientation toward major solutions. The first is almost atheoretically pragmatic; the second draws on standard classical economic theory regarding such matters as financial incentives and competition. Both books are first-rate reviews, and both reveal frustrations as to how to deal with affordable care, equity of access, and other issues basic to health services delivery.

An earlier book, *Health Politics and Policy*, edited by Theodore J. Litman and Leonard S. Robins, comprises chapters by individual authors on health policy developments in the United States.[18]

Interest continues in this country in the experience of other developed countries—particularly the liberal democracies with some form of national health insurance—with the organization and financing of health services. In fact, interest has intensified of late, due to the continuing cost escalation in health care in the United States. Canada has become the subject of special scrutiny for a few years because it has stabilized its expenditures for health services relative to the GNP whereas other countries have not; at most, other countries have succeeded in slowing the escalation.

Cross-national comparisons of the organization and operation of health services delivery systems and their financing are complex endeavors, but three quite detailed studies appeared in the eighties: by Marshall W. Raffel,[19] Mark G. Field,[20] and Odin W. Anderson.[21] Generalizations from health care delivery systems in other countries are not easy to apply to the United States. Let it be said, however, that all countries—whatever their expenditures as a percentage of GNP—complain that they are spending too much money for health services in relation to other national priorities. Frustration with the cost of health care is a characteristic emotion everywhere.

A specific recent cross-national interest is that of how developed and developing countries are managing the health and social care of the elderly, a proportion of the population that is increasing everywhere. The first book to examine this question is a useful one, edited by Teresa Schwab and written by authors well acquainted with each country from China to Sweden.[22] The book describes the struggles of various countries to adapt acute-care-oriented health services delivery systems to long-term care problems. In all countries there is a gray area between the biomedical model of care and the psychosocial medical model; these two models have not been adequately bridged.

The standard measurement of the level of health of a country has been the mortality rate translated into the average length of life. Admittedly, this is a gross measure; it is difficult to attribute to specific causes the great decrease in general mortality rates which have resulted in a greater average length of life—up into the 70s. A generation ago the average life span was in the 60s or less. There is a persistent belief, lacking any other measure, that since the rate of increase in average longevity is slowing down, expenditures for personal health services are now receiving a very marginal return and hence money is being wasted.

This description, oversimplified for the sake of brevity, is probably enough to suggest another measure to justify expenditures for personal health services. Such a measure would show the contribution of personal health services to the quality of life. Methods and criteria could be devised to quantify the degree to which living is enhanced by such efforts as cataract operations, hip replacements, and other restorative surgery, not to mention the more subjective efforts toward mental health amelioration and pain relief. Odin Anderson and Ellen M. Morrison made a conceptual and empirical attempt to describe such a measure, hoping to stimulate thinking and research toward this objective far beyond their own.[23]

Finally, a policy blockbuster was published in the form of a book by ethicist Daniel Callahan. Callahan argues courageously that it is time to consider the possibility and the humanity of setting limits on the heroic attempts of medical high technology to prolong life in elderly patients who are clearly terminal and in a near-vegetative state or comatose.[24] The book dealt with many other issues of growing old, but the foregoing was central. Callahan raised a storm of controversy which is salutary to the consideration of life prolongation as an end in itself. This issue, of course, has a clear relationship to the concept of the quality of life.

To return to the health services research establishment—a notion which is now almost reality—there are now 1,200 members in the Association of Health Services Research (AHSR), which was organized only in 1981. The association meets annually, and there appears to be great esprit among the members, all of whom are professionals engaged in one line of health services research or other. The members represent a wide spectrum of disciplines: economists, sociologists, political scientists, epidemiologists, biostatisticians, public health experts, clinicians, statisticians, and operations researchers.

A pervasive concern in health care is the interface between health services researchers and those on the firing line—policy makers, administrators, planners, caregivers—whose desire for information and facts is keen. Researchers trained to place data in a framework or context are dismayed at this desire for simple facts: the number of persons who are uninsured, the number of unfilled nursing positions, the Medical Price Index last week. By the time a study relevant to policy is completed, its results are too late to be useful—policy makers have already had to make their decisions. Political reality is a variable researchers frequently overlook. Academics do not take kindly to "quick and dirty" research or even "quick and clean."

I wrote in 1966 and it continues to be true that health services research follows policy, has in general little influence on policy except after the fact.[25] Senator Daniel Moynihan, an avid user of research data, believed indeed that the reasonable and legitimate function of social research is to evaluate after the fact.[26] In my view a primary, legitimate, and practical function of research is to provide a context in which to think about and solve problems. This is called the enlightenment model and differs from the model according to which physical science and social engineering research is conducted—the type of research that got us to the moon. As Eric Severeid remarked, we got to the moon because there were no people in between.[27]

Of course, if policy makers, administrators, planners, and caregivers want simple facts, these can be provided; we have tremendous and efficient data machines that can grind out facts. Indeed, many establishments have their own data machines and personnel to gather internal intelligence. Sometimes, however, the people on the firing line want results bearing the imprimatur of a respected, university-based research center. The federal government itself, through its Agency for Health Care Policy and Research (formerly the National Center for Health Services Research and Development and Health Care Technology Assessment), sponsors a great deal of health services research, much of it evaluative. The Health Care Financing Administration sponsors additional research within, from the viewpoint of academicians, rather bounded protocols.[28]

What is a new and anomalous development from the standpoint of health services researchers and social researchers is the apparent expectation that health services researchers should lobby for federal research funds like any other self-seeking entrepreneurs. William L. Roper, formerly chief of HCFA and healtn care consultant to the President and now director of the Centers for Disease Control, recommended this course of action,[29] and the recommendation would seem to cast the researcher in the role of policy maker by virtue of advocating research directed along lines of policy pleasing to one or another politician.

AHSR is already engaging in lobbying activities, although it might be more accurate to describe the effort as informing the Congress. In this instance Uwe Reinhardt, then president-elect of AHSR, together with representatives of the American Medical Association and the American Medical Peer Review Association, testified before a congressional committee on the need for broad discretionary funds to support a variety of research on medical care outcomes. Reinhardt, an ideal person to offer testimony, also emphasized that "the development and implementation of a sustained, well-funded, multidisciplinary agenda is the only way to attract the best minds to this field and build a knowledge base over the next decades that will be useful for health professionals, consumers, payors, and policymakers."[30] He was careful not to promise any quick fixes, the usual hope and expectation of funding sources looking for some way to control costs.

Probably it is inevitable that academicians be drawn into the interest-group-lobbying style of politics in this country. The style is suitable and functional for many groups of people, but presumably neutral researchers should consider carefully before they wade into charged, politically controversial waters. This development should be watched carefully. A further caution is that researchers and their professional associations do not have the money needed for effective lobbying.

Finally, it is of interest to note the proliferation of scholarly journals relating exclusively to the health services establishment and its broad range of problems, from lifestyle change to "DRG creep." The market for these journals seems to be large and specialized. Not long ago there were only the venerable *American Journal of Public Health* and *Milbank Memorial Fund Quarterly*. The *Journal of the American Medical Association* and even the *New England Journal of Medicine* rarely published anything on health services economics except articles that were critical of contemporary developments in health insurance, group practice prepayment, and government intrusions.

Now *JAMA* and the *New England Journal of Medicine* publish scholarly articles on many problems relating to health care delivery, and the *Journal of Gerontology* has added sections on the psychological and social sciences. Furthermore, in the 1960s, five whole new journals appeared. In 1960 the American Sociological Association established what has become the *Journal of Health and Social Behavior*. In 1963 the Blue Cross Association (now the Blue Cross and Blue Shield Association) launched *Inquiry*, directed to practitioners and policy makers. The Hospital Research and Educational Trust started *Health Services Research* in 1966 (in the 1980s it became the official journal of the AHSR), and *Social Science & Medicine* and *Medical Care* first appeared in 1967.

The 1970s saw the advent of the *International Journal of Health Services* in 1970, the *Journal of Health Politics, Policy and Law* in 1971, and the Institute of Society, Ethics and the Life Sciences' indispensable *Hastings Center Report* also in 1971. In 1973 the Milbank Memorial Fund revised its quarterly and named it *Health and Society* (renaming it the *Milbank Quarterly* in 1983).

Seven journals made their debuts in the 1980s, starting in 1980 with the Group Health Association of America's *GHAA Journal*, directed to HMO developments nationally. The Project Hope Foundation followed in 1981 with the broad-ranging *Health Affairs*. Economists inaugurated the *Journal of Health Economics* in 1982, and the *International Journal of Technology Assessment in Health Care* appeared in 1985, to deal exclusively with health care technology. Another international journal began publication in 1985, the *International Journal of Health Planning and Management*. Covering current developments in the health services, *Healthweek* has appeared since 1986, joining the long-established *American Medical News* (formerly *AMA News*) of the American Medical Association and *AHA News* of the American Hospital Association. The latest entrant into the market for health care delivery journals is *Health Services Management Research*, which the Association of University Programs in Health Administration started in 1988. The 1990s may bring more journals still.

NOTES

1. Duncan Neuhauser, "The Future of Health Care Research in Cost Containment," in Jack D. McCue, *The Medical Cost-Containment Crisis: Fears, Opinions, and Facts* (Ann Arbor, Mich.: Health Administration Press, 1989), pp. 285–93.
2. Viola B. Latta and Charles Helbing, "Medicare Short-Stay Hospital Services, by Leading Diagnostic Related Groups, 1983 and 1985," *Health Care Financing Review* 10 (Winter 1988):79–107.
3. Robert L. Kane, "The Link between Cost and Effectiveness in Patient Care and Program Management," paper delivered at the Eighth Annual Symposium on Geriatrics and Gerontology, St. Louis, Mo., September 14, 1989.
4. Emmett B. Keeler, Joan L. Buchanan, John E. Rolf, Janet M. Hanby, and David M. Reboussin, *The Demand for Episodes of Medical Treatment in the Health Insurance Experiment* (Santa Monica, Calif.: Rand Corporation, 1988).
5. John E. Wennberg, "Dealing with Medical Practice Variations: A Proposal for Action," *Health Affairs* 3 (Summer 1984):6–32.
6. Robert Wood Johnson Foundation, *Access to Health Care in the United States: Results of a 1986 Survey*, Special Report No. 2 (Princeton, N.J.: The Foundation, 1987). The survey was conducted by the Survey Research Laboratory,

University of Illinois, and Wisconsin Survey Research Laboratory, University of Wisconsin–Madison. The 1986 survey is the seventh in a series of national household surveys of access to health care. The first five were conducted by the Center for Health Administration Studies of the University of Chicago. The sixth was conducted by Louis Harris and Associates, Inc., with secondary analyses carried out by the Center for Health Administration Studies. See also Lu Ann Aday, Gretchen V. Fleming, and Ronald Anderson, *Access to Medical Care in the U.S.: Who Has It, Who Doesn't?* University of Chicago Center for Health Administration Studies, Research Series 35 (Chicago: Pluribus Press, 1984).

7. Victor Fuchs, "The 'Competition Revolution' in Health Care," *Health Affairs* 7 (Summer 1988):5–24.

8. Prevention Magazine, *The Prevention Index: A Report Card on the Nation's Health, 1988* (Emmaus, Pa.: Rodale Press, 1988), p. 3.

9. Paul Starr, *The Social Transformation of American Medicine* (New York: Basic Books, 1982).

10. David Mechanic, *From Advocacy to Allocation: The Evolving American Health Care System* (New York: Free Press, 1986).

11. Odin W. Anderson, *Health Services in the United States: A Growth Enterprise Since 1875* (Ann Arbor, Mich.: Health Administration Press, 1985).

12. Odin W. Anderson, Terry E. Herold, Bruce W. Butler, Claire H. Kohrman, and Ellen M. Morrison, *HMO Development: Patterns and Prospects,* University of Chicago Center for Health Administration Studies, Research Series 33 (Chicago: Pluribus Press, 1985).

13. Avedis Donabedian, *The Definition of Quality and Approaches to Its Assessment. Explorations in Quality Assessment and Monitoring,* Vol. I (Ann Arbor, Mich.: Health Administration Press, 1980).

14. Vicente Navarro, *Health and Medical Care in the United States: A Critical Analysis* (Farmingdale, N.Y.: Baywood Publications, 1977).

15. David Blumenthal, Mark Schlesinger, and Pamela Brown Drumheller, eds., *Renewing the Promise: Medicare and Its Reform* (New York: Oxford University Press, 1988).

16. Jack D. McCue, *The Medical Cost-Containment Crises: Fears, Opinions, and Facts* (Ann Arbor, Mich.: Health Administration Press, 1989).

17. Kenneth McLennan and Jack A. Meyer, eds., *Care and Cost: Current Issues in Health Policy* (Boulder, Colo.: Westview Press, 1989).

18. Theodore J. Litman and Leonard S. Robins, *Health Politics and Policy* (New York: Wiley, 1984).

19. Marshall W. Raffel, *Comparative Health Systems: A Descriptive Analysis of Fourteen National Health Systems* (University Park, Pa.: Pennsylvania State University Press, 1984).

20. Mark G. Field, ed., *Success and Crisis in National Health Systems: A Comparative Approach* (New York: Routledge, 1989).

21. Odin W. Anderson, *The Health Services Continuum in Democratic States: An Inquiry into Solvable Problems* (Ann Arbor, Mich.: Health Administration Press, 1989).

22. Teresa Schwab, ed., *Caring for an Aging World: International Models for Long-Term Care, Financing, and Delivery* (New York: McGraw-Hill, 1989).
23. Odin W. Anderson and Ellen M. Morrison, "The World of Medical Care: A Critique," *Medical Care Review* 46 (Summer 1989):121–56.
24. Daniel Callahan, *Setting Limits: Medical Goals in an Aging Society* (New York: Simon & Schuster, 1987).
25. Odin W. Anderson, "Influence of Social and Economic Research on Public Policy in the Health Field: A Review," *Milbank Memorial Fund Quarterly* 44 (July 1966, Part 2): 11–51.
26. Daniel P. Moynihan, *Maximum Feasible Misunderstanding: Community Action in the War on Poverty* (New York: Free Press, 1969), p. 193.
27. Eric Severeid made this observation during a television broadcast shortly after Americans reached the moon.
28. In fact there is a great deal of evaluation research going on. See, for example, Lu Ann Aday, M. J. Aiken, and Donna Hope Wegener, *Pediatric Home Care: Results of a National Evaluation of Programs for Ventilator-Assisted Children,* University of Chicago Center for Health Administration Studies, Research Series 36 (Chicago, Pluribus Press, 1988).
29. William L. Roper, in his remarks upon receipt of the President's Award, at the Sixth Annual Meeting of the Association for Health Services Research, Chicago, June 19, 1989.
30. Association for Health Services Research, *HSR Reports.* (June 1989):1.

PART VI
Epilogue

23

Epilogue

In the health care field pluralistic, interest-group, American-style democracy—or what an English observer once called "riotous pluralism"
rather than the more structured pluralism of other liberal democracies—
appears to be stalemated less on goals than on how to achieve them.
The goals are cost containment, which can result in "affordable" costs
(that much repeated and meaningless concept); adequate quality; and
the coverage of the uninsured in some form or other without dipping
into general revenue. These goals are incompatible without an overall
national health policy to synthesize them. Central to that policy should
be universal coverage and facing up to the need for tapping more general revenue, politically infeasible as it seems to be now.

In this connection I agree fully with Don Herzog's observation:

> I have been endorsing ambiguity and conflict, and skeptically assaulting
> drives to enshrine shining principles for what should happen, or simple
> theories of what does. Some may indignantly respond that this is a ratio-
> nale for leaving ourselves hopelessly muddled, and surely the point of
> theory is to illuminate the world. My response, predictably, would run
> this way: There are muddles and muddles, some inarticulate and con-
> fused, some nuanced and precise. If anything is to be made of policy as
> the science of muddling through, we need to replace our baffled and
> inarticulate muddles—and our neatly precise but false accounts—with
> more precise and accurate ones. If we want "to strive for imperfection,"
> we need to confront moral conflicts and to correct our images of how the
> world works. Finding a reasonable health policy, if there is one, will
> depend on getting our "values" and "facts" straighter than they are now.[1]

This is, of course, asking for some interest-group convergence on a
national health policy and its implementation. The goal of cost containment is apparently embodied in competition as previously described.

Nevertheless, the costs are still rising rapidly. Perhaps they would have risen more rapidly without the competition, such as it is.

Serious challenges to the viability of competition are now being raised. Economist Victor R. Fuchs wrote a cogent article in *Health Affairs* that questioned whether competition is working and showed appropriate data. He questioned whether Americans really want to try competition, because HMOs, Medicare, and Medicaid continue to be hemmed in by regulations and seemingly arbitrary reimbursement levels to hospitals via DRGs and freezing physicians' fees for Medicare. There is fear of letting competition run wild, as it has, say, in the airline industry. Health care does not lend itself to competition; it is not a commodity.[2]

On the other hand, sociologist Jeff C. Goldsmith has faith in competitive bidding. He writes, "Though critics who wish to see competition fail have been quick to herald a return to the failed strategies and tired rhetoric of the past, competitive forces in the American health system continue to offer the most promising avenue of health system reform." He expects another "violent tremor" by the end of the Nineties.[3]

A most thoughtful examination of the concept of competition, by political scientist Lawrence D. Brown, appeared in 1988 in an issue of the *Journal of Health Politics, Policy and Law* that reviewed a number of articles on the growth of competition in the health services with retrospective and prospective views on it. Brown was the editor of the issue, and excellent as the papers in it were, he reflected in his "Afterword" that "In some respects, however, the meanings, workings, and consequences of competition remain mysterious."[4] He observed that, ten years after the publication of the Federal Trade Commission study and fifteen years after the Nixon administration's initial enthusiasm for a competitive approach (Chapter 16), there seems to be little agreement on what is meant by "competition" or a "market approach" to containing health costs.

Brown delineated three different meanings of competition. The first, he said, emphasizes individual cost sharing; the prerequisites of competition are present and the erosion of the market is arrested or reversed to the degree that *individual* consumers must make choices as to their own willingness to pay before seeking services. A second meaning of competition is that *organizations* offer consumers different product mixes, that is, HMOs, PPOs, and traditional insurers that compete by marketing different mixtures of quality, access, and cost. A third meaning is that organizations vie for subscribers within *detailed rules of the game*, rules that may (or should) constrain such matters as benefit ranges and levels, premiums, and enrollment practices.

To quote Brown,

Two reasons why it has been difficult to sell policymakers on a broad, procompetition approach are the clear presence of these diverging denotations [of the word competition] and uncertainty as to whether and how they can be made consistent. . . . Is there a central core of meaning—much less a unified theory—of competition in health services? If so, what is it? If not, what do these variations and somewhat inconsistent meanings imply for competitive policy strategies and the political prospects of achieving them?

The *workings* of competition, as Brown put it, remain an institutional black box: "In the real world of complex formal organizations with traditions, ideologies, structures, constituencies, and environmental constraints as well as competitors—what does competitive behavior mean concretely and what practical meanings would it have to assume if competition were to work?"

To my mind, Brown moved into the crux of the problem with this at-least-suggested conclusion: "Perhaps the real issue is not competition after all, but rather the fragmentation of financing. Perhaps the real solution is not enlarged competition (which aggravates that fragmentation) but rather firm, comprehensive budgetary controls, for which one looks not to the market but to government." It is apparent, for example, that business coalitions have so far been unable to coalesce for unified budget controls. The government is, of course, trying for budget controls for Medicare. All foreign health services systems have eventually adopted politically determined budget caps through the negotiating and bargaining process.

Another attempt to control physicians' costs by regulation is the official endorsement by the Physician Payment Review Commission (PPRC) for Medicare, Part B, which is to establish expenditure targets (ETs), another addition to the numerous acronyms in health care. ETs are regarded as a rational way to apportion limited funds for physician services as well as hospital care. PPRC anticipates that a national ET will eventually be applied to multiple targets. This method sounds like the budget cap methods that have been used in Canada, Great Britain, and other countries for years.

Philip Lee, chairman of the PPRC, quite rightly asserts that Congress should not enact a fee schedule without some mechanism to limit volume. Lee also testified before the House Ways and Means Health Committee that there is so much "fat" in the health care system that ETs would not deny beneficiaries access to necessary and appropriate care. He asserted, as have others, that some 20 to 30 percent of all medical procedures are not necessary or have marginal benefit, and "if we first reduce some of those, we would save all the money we needed."

This is quite an assertion given the current lack of systematic professional criteria of "unnecessary procedures."[5] It would seem the politicians should be informed more candidly of the state of the art of professional judgment and standards. On the other hand, there are important efforts underway to establish protocols for diagnosing and treating diseases and to assess the efficacy of various technologies. The Joint Commission on Accreditation of Healthcare Organizations, for example, has established Clinical Indicators task forces to study and publish approved protocols, and the American College of Physicians has just published its second edition of a volume called *Common Diagnostic Tests: Use and Interpretation.*[6] One element in the state of the art is the public's own perceptions of need and demand given the current emphasis on consumer sovereignty.

Summarizing a number of observations from health experts and policy makers in a 1989 issue of *Health Management Quarterly,* Eli Ginzberg presented eight challenges to the current, felt muddle in health care to make the system more effective and efficient. I paraphrase:

1. The uninsured—the ranks of the uninsured will increase given the demise of community rating and given that large- and medium-sized employers are opting for self-insurance. What is becoming clear, according to Ginzberg (and alluded to earlier), is that the fracturing of the insurance pool through self-insurance is eroding the prospects of providing coverage at an acceptable cost for two segments of the population, the high-risk and employees in small firms.

2. Cost containment—premium rates are still going up.

3. Medicare reimbursement—although many hospitals had a "bonanza" during the early period of DRGs, during the last few years Medicare reimbursements have failed to cover costs. If this continues, hospital care will deteriorate.

4. Surplus beds—there are not authoritative figures for the number of excess beds, partly because of the lack of criteria. The fall in occupancy, however, is beyond dispute.

5. Physician surplus—people want more physicians, and Congress will likely control physician fees.

6. Medicaid shortfalls—one-half of the "poor" are not covered.

7. Administrative costs—they are too high, pushing 20 percent.

8. Conflicting expectations—public opinion surveys show that Americans want more and better health care. There is no sup-

port for rationing. Organ transplants should be available as needed. The big buyers of services, government and employers, may now be reaching a point of no return; that is, the "deep pocket" is no longer deep.[7]

With the above as a backdrop, Richard Reece, a physician who left his practice and turned writer and spokesperson for the medical profession, described in 1989 the turmoil that has emerged in health care delivery in the Twin Cities of Minneapolis–St. Paul. In the last 15 years there, the provision of health services has been transformed from mainline fee-for-service and insurance to managed care.

He asked, "What kind of system has emerged in a largely middle class, relatively affluent, mostly white and well-educated metropolitan area [of 2 million people and with over 50 percent HMO penetration] where major industries have backed managed care as the 'rational solution'"? His conclusions are that among the "principal players"—patients, physicians, hospitals, payers—there are no clear winners. Costs have not gone down; quality is about the same; demand for services remains high, and physicians are unhappy. As a matter of fact physicians for three of the four major HMOs have been in court or are arbitrating with HMO management. Further, "corporate lawyers" in Reece's words, "are quietly dismantling [the HMO concept] by shifting to self-funding and by transferring risks to patients."[8] What has happened is a compromise or stand-off between fee-for-service and managed care. The people want, in effect, everything: the best that both HMO and fee-for-service have to offer. Most physicians want to remain in fee-for-service practice but realize that they have to accept HMO patients. Employers want to satisfy their employees yet control their costs.

What has happened is that the Twin Cities market has shifted from fee-for-service to HMOs, and then from HMOs to managed care systems in which HMOs offer fee-for-service or PPO options. Reece concluded, reasonably, that in the end people want choice—choice of physicians, choice of hospitals, and choice of best care. He believes that many people are willing to pay for that choice as an 80/20 option (80 percent of the cost covered, 20 percent paid out-of-pocket) or even as a 70/30 option or a 60/40 option.

Reece reported also the unhappiness of physicians across the country who are going through what can be called a transition period:

> In the last six weeks (early 1989) I have visited with physicians in Kansas City, Long Island [New York], New Orleans, Chicago, San Diego and in small towns and medium-sized cities. Everywhere I hear uneasiness about the directions medicine is headed—the discounting of fees, demands for

accountability, the disappearance of practitioners in organizations, the intrusion of managed care, the explosion of utilization review, the erosion of traditional values, physician-bashing by politicians and a decline in patient loyalty.

And in addition, "the patients and payers [are] in confusion as they try to sort out the confusing alternatives."[9]

With eloquence and bitterness, Reece went on to say that the biggest discontinuity of all for physicians has been the transformation from "organized medicine"—a loose agglomeration of independent physicians in solo practice or small groups—to "organizational medicine" in which physicians are integrated in a variety of ways into large organizations. In the Twin Cities the 6,000 or so physicians work either as employees of or as contractors for four HMOs, three PPOs, four hospital systems, one large remaining independent hospital, academic centers, or organized medical groups. Reece predicted that physicians will regroup and stabilize and regain power. "In the future, physicians will be part of management teams of medium to large organizations. If we play our cards right, I believe we will be leaders of those teams."[10]

Hospital administrators also have their spokespersons and feel themselves to be under siege. The late David M. Kinzer, formerly chief executive officer of two hospital associations and later associated with the faculties of Harvard, Duke, and Arizona State universities, kept in touch with many hospital CEOs and described how their positions changed from the precompetition days. In 1989 he wrote,

> Factionalism has divided membership constituencies, both nationally and locally. There is big trouble here, and you get chapter and verse on this in private conversation with any [hospital] association executive. It was an emerging problem when I left my job in 1985, but now it is a lot worse.
>
> Everyone I speak to seems pretty clear on why this is happening. At the root of it is the widespread acceptance, within the health provider sector, of the competitive strategy for controlling health care costs. With the blessings of Ronald Reagan, we bought into this as a field and, until further notice, it seems like we will have to live with it.[11]
>
> So our health care managers are going through very hard times. They have terrible jobs. In some of the circles where I now move, there is a declining respect for such jobs and the people holding them. They are being criticized for being "too business-like" with all the negativism that the word implies. This is happening not long after everyone was saying that CEOs were not "business-like enough."[12]

Kinzer went on to observe that as long as we are not sure whether health care should be a business or service, we can expect more of the same. A lot of political decision makers are convinced that all hospitals care about is money, which was not so true before.

Robert M. Cunningham, Jr. added another woeful view in 1989. Cunningham, a long-term editor and publisher of hospital journals and an editorial consultant to the Blue Cross and Blue Shield Association and contributing editor to *Hospitals*, has written:

> The emotional tone of the entire hospital environment is notably different from what it used to be. Charity, generosity, and love have lost ground to efficiency, systematization, and speed. . . . This isn't a business like any other business, and we'll keep on losing as long as we keep on pretending we're something we're not. Calling ourselves CEOs instead of hospital administrators comforted us and made us feel like business bigshots.[13]

Finally, from the hospital standpoint it is pertinent to cite Edward J. Connors in a speech he delivered as he was installed as the chairman of the board of trustees of the American Hospital Association in January 1989:

> Our current system is characterized—accurately—by diffuse and competing interests with strongly held philosophical views that are not always compatible with one another.
>
> The changes required are likely to be *systemic* [Connors's emphasis] in nature, considered to be radical by some, and will not be responsive if they merely tinker at the edges of our current system of care.

He continued,

> The principles of pluralism and freedom of choice should be strengthened and preserved *insofar as practical* [my emphasis]—freedom for the patients to choose sources of care; freedom for practitioners to choose the type of location and practice; and pluralism in funding sources and institutional ownership in order to promote creative responses and to avoid monolithic mediocrity.[14]

Apparently what Connors is hoping for is a more structured pluralism, with freedom of choice "insofar as practical" as the constant goal rather than the "riotous pluralism" through which the American health services are now passing.

I close under the broad mantle of Daniel Callahan, a philosopher in bioethics and director of the Hastings Center. Callahan is reported as saying that the crisis in the health field is philosophical, that of setting limits. The public is demanding and expecting too much; the physicians are going to medical technological extremes: "What does not work can be—even if painfully—eliminated. Now we are going to be forced to eliminate or scale down that which works. We can only do that by changing some of our most cherished hopes and values. This is the task to which we need to turn."[15] Insofar as I can infer from Callahan's writing, he means we must start with reducing heroic and expensive use of medical high technology for bizarre life prolongation.[16]

WHAT OF THE FUTURE?

Futurology is popular in this country. In 1987 the American College of Healthcare Executives collaborated with Arthur Andersen and Company to conduct a Delphic forecasting process in which panels of experts considered issues and made predictions regarding particular problems. In this study the problem was the future of health care up to 1995.[17] Five panels were made up from 1,600 "national health care leaders and astute observers." The panels were: (1) health care executives; (2) hospital trustees; (3) physicians and nurses; (4) payers and government, including insurance companies, legislators, and regulators; and (5) consumer advisory groups.

The predictions, as reported in the study, do not seem to be particularly startling:

1. Quality will be even better by 1995, but not everyone will see this improvement firsthand because of fiscal restrictions.

2. Health care's share of the GNP will increase to over 12 percent, but access will not improve for everyone.

3. Marketplace incentives, rather than a comprehensive national health insurance plan, will guide the system, and approximately 700 hospitals will close by 1995.

4. The private sector—physicians, hospital executives, and the Joint Commission on Accreditation of Healthcare Organizations—will define the quality of care, but the "highest" quality of care will be replaced in the public agenda by a goal of "adequate" quality.

5. The responsibility to fund care for the medically indigent will fall to government, but indigent care costs to hospitals will increase 80 percent.[18]

Perhaps the notable perceptions are that health care's share of the GNP will continue to increase, and that there will be no comprehensive national health insurance plan. Equity of access for the uninsured will have to be met in other ways.

All panelists ranked the top five national health care issues in 1995 as follows:

1. The growth in the elderly population in proportion to the younger population
2. Government payment decisions
3. The cost of providing care to the medically indigent
4. The AIDS epidemic and other catastrophic diseases
5. The size of the federal deficit[19]

Curiously, the top five issues did not include differences in access based on ability to pay and increased demand for long-term care, although these issues were listed.

My own predictions follow, with a three-year advantage over the Andersen-College survey. The pace of change is so swift that even a three-year advantage may be helpful. I will, however, extend my predictions to the year 2000.

1. In general, public demand for access to services, particularly the high-technology variety, will continue. This demand may well necessitate rationing for such procedures as renal dialysis, vital organ transplants, and heroic measures for life prolongation. It is likely that rationing will apply to the "frail" elderly, but given current trends (e.g., Oregon), rationing may also apply to Medicaid patients. Allocation decisions will vary between public and private sources of funding. Medicare patients will also experience some rationing, or certainly more conservative treatments.

2. Some of the seeming hardheartedness of rationing will be mitigated by the general public's gradually increasing acceptance of "appropriate" dying and the finite span of a human life.

3. The mix of services between inpatient care and ambulatory care in outpatient departments, physicians' offices, surgicenters, nursing homes, and hospices, not to mention other settings, will be changing, as is already apparent. The general hospital will be for very sick people. Still, while the volume of acute hospital care will be reduced as to number of days, there will be no significant reduction in laboratory services, which are perversely costly relative to the other components of health care. Reductions in hospital use are already leading to significant expansions in outpatient services—the so-called pressed-balloon effect. The entire health care system will expand and cost more; I will hazard an estimate of 15 percent of the GNP by 1995 and 20 percent by 2000.

4. The health care delivery system will continue to take on more corporate characteristics. Horizontal and vertical organizations will manage and deliver most health services. These large centers are already becoming the basic health services planning entities. Overall so-

cial planning for the health field died in 1983 when the Reagan administration ceased appropriating funds for the Health Resources and Planning Act of 1974.

5. Competition will be intensifying between the fewer and fewer HMOs and the variants of managed systems. The market will be increasingly fragmented, particularly with the continuing growth of employer self-insured plans. This trend will relegate a larger and larger segment of the population to underinsurance (contraction of range of benefits) or no coverage at all. The apparent solution now is mandating employers to cover the uninsured or underinsured employed. Where the benefits for alcoholism, chemical dependency, and psychiatric services have been cut back or even eliminated, they will be thrown on the government.

6. Managed care of one kind or another will be the predominant method of insuring and delivering services. It is no longer feasible financially to foster an open-ended service as before the 1970s, except for the very rich. However, managed care will likely emerge in three levels of convenience in terms of access to primary, elective, and acute or emergency care in hospitals and choice of physicians, both generalists and specialists. The American health services market is fantastically large and diverse, like nowhere else in the world. The degree of affluence of the majority of the population may give rise to three levels of managed care. The first (and lowest) level of managed care will include relatively quick access to primary care, quick access to acute and emergency services in hospitals, and waiting lists for whatever may be regarded as elective surgery. Entry to the system, even for primary care, will be monitored by nurses or other professionals, and there will be no choice of specialist outside the system except in extreme cases. The second level of managed care—the broad middle class level—will feature quick access to primary care, no waiting lists to speak of for elective surgery, and quick access to acute and emergency care in hospitals. Access to specialists outside the system will be more flexible. The third level will offer luxury, in terms of choice of physician, convenience, and amenities. Each of the three levels of care will have a premium price commensurate with its features. These levels are emerging in Europe and Scandinavia and on the Continent—in incipient form, but emerging. The much-talked-about concept of basic care may be taking form, a level of care above which people will pay extra.

7. Differences in premiums for more or less the same services among managed care plans will narrow and possibly even disappear, correcting for such variables as deductibles and coinsurance. Overall costs from all sources will flatten out as the health care system is squeezed financially more and more; the limits will soon be reached as

the country learns what the rock-bottom cost of adequate health care is. The cost differential among delivery options will not be great enough to include shifts among employees for that reason alone.

8. Expenditures for health services will continue to increase from all sources because of sustained demand, new and horrendously expensive technology, the aging of the population, the low pain-and-anxiety threshold, and the general unwillingness to die. As I predicted above, the percentage of GNP devoted to health services will have to go up as far as 15 percent and even more.

9. There will never be universal compulsory health insurance in the United States on the pattern of European countries and Canada. Never, however, is a long time. It will likely take a generation or so to cover the various segments of the uninsured by the usual salami-slicing technique of tackling one segment at a time (e.g., the employed uninsured) with one source of funding or another, the usual source being the "deep pocket" of employers. After a generation or so, as we look at this "riotous pluralism" of population segments and sources of funding, we may think it reasonable and more efficient to consolidate these segments and their funding. Other liberal-democratic countries have followed this course as they eventually evolved national insurance systems combining general revenue, employers, and direct pay from the public.[20]

10. Apropos of the above, it is likely that employers will become restive enough to lobby Congress to have general revenue share some of the burden of the cost of employee health insurance. Industrial firms face differential profit margins in large part because of the contributions they make to employee health insurance as a result of collective bargaining. Employers are also facing competition from firms abroad, where the cost of health insurance is borne largely by the general revenue tax structures, thus relieving foreign firms of much of the health insurance burden.

11. The so-called physician surplus will vanish as more and more physicians are capitated and salaried and fees are regulated. The great increase in the numbers of women physicians will underscore this trend. Both sexes are and will be working shorter hours. As for nurses and related care personnel, there will probably even be enough given the dynamics of aging, long-term care, home care, and hospices. Their relationship to the informal support network is still not fully understood. Undoubtedly, if the informal support network were to disappear, the formal health services infrastructure would collapse.

12. The last prediction is that in time the medical profession now being fragmented into competing entities will regroup across entities as professional labor unions, to bargain as a collegial professional asso-

ciation. The issues will be freedom to diagnose and treat according to adequate (and high) standards of care—in other words, professional working conditions—plus the bread-and-butter issue of what is perceived in all walks of life as adequate pay. In this connection, the Minnesota Medical Association has requested the state legislature of Minnesota to enact legislation for the profession to engage in collective bargaining. Physicians in countries with government health insurance are organized nationally (in Canada, by provinces) to bargain with the sources of funding.

NOTES

1. Don Herzog, "How to Argue about Health Care," *Medical Care Review* 44 (Spring 1987):11–36. The phrase "to strive for imperfection" is a quote from Amy Gutmann, "For and Against Equal Access to Health Care," in Ronald Bayer, Arthur L. Caplan, and Norman Daniels, eds., *In Search of Equity: Health Needs and the Health Care System* (New York: Plenum Press, 1983), p. 66.
2. Victor R. Fuchs, "The 'Competition Revolution' in Health Care," *Health Affairs* 7 (Summer 1988):5–24.
3. Jeff C. Goldsmith, "Competition's Impact: A Report from the Front," *Health Affairs* 7 (Summer 1988):173, 163.
4. Lawrence D. Brown, "Afterword," *Journal of Health Politics, Policy and Law* 13 (Summer 1988):361–63. All subsequent quotations are from these three pages.
5. Michele L. Robinson, "PPRC Endorses ETs to Reform Part B," *Hospitals* 63 (May 20, 1989):20.
6. Harold C. Sox., Jr., ed., *Common Diagnostic Tests: Use and Interpretation*, 2d ed. (Philadelphia: American College of Physicians, 1990).
7. Eli Ginzberg, "Harder Than It Looks," *Health Management Quarterly* 11 (Second Quarter 1989):19–21.
8. Richard Reece, "Publisher's Note: Physicians and Business, Part Two. From Schizophrenia to Discontinuities in Medical Care: The Minnesota Experience," *Reece Report* 4 (April 1989):1–3. See also Odin W. Anderson, Terry E. Harold, Bruce W. Butler, Claire H. Kohrman, and Ellen M. Morrison, *HMO Development: Patterns and Prospects* (Chicago: Pluribus Press, 1985).
9. *Reece Report*, ibid., p. 3.
10. Ibid.
11. David M. Kinzer, "The Future of the Hospital Association Mission," *Hospitals* 63 (May 20, 1989):26.
12. Ibid., p. 27.
13. Robert M. Cunningham, Jr., "The Last Word: A Reason for Living in the Past: A Better Time," *Hospitals* 63 (June 5, 1989):72.
14. "Changes in Health Care to be Slow but Profound," *AHA News* 25 (February 6, 1989):8, adapted from speech by Edward J. Connors.

15. Daniel Callahan, "Solving the Crisis in Health Care Requires Changing Philosophy," *Healthweek* 2 (December 27, 1988):18.
16. See his controversial but necessary problem-posing work: Daniel Callahan, *Setting Limits: Medical Goals in an Aging Society* (New York: Simon & Schuster, 1987), especially the section "Can There Be A 'Natural Life Span,' and a 'Tolerable Death'?" pp. 65–76.
17. Arthur Andersen and Company and the American College of Healthcare Executives, *The Future of Health Care: Changes and Choices* (Chicago: Arthur Andersen and the American College of Healthcare Executives, 1987).
18. Ibid., p. 1.
19. Ibid., p. 3.
20. Odin W. Anderson, *The Health Services Continuum in Democratic States: An Inquiry into Solvable Problems* (Ann Arbor, Mich.: Health Administration Press, 1989).

Index

Abrams, Morris B., 249
Aged, health care of, 19–20, 161–80,
253, 320, 339; Catastrophic Coverage Act, 255–56; Eldercare (AMA),
175–78: National Committee on
Health Care for the Aged, 173–74;
old age assistance, study of, 296;
Old Age, Survivors, and Disability
Insurance (OASDI), 120, 142, 153,
161, 162, 165, 166, 169–78, 297; private sector activity, 166–68; studies
of other countries, 322–23; White
House Conference on Aging, 168,
170, 297
Aged, health care of: federal legisla-
tion (1952–1960), 161–68; (1960–
1965), 168–80
Agricultural Extension Service, 288
AIDS (acquired immuno-deficiency
syndrome), 263, 339
Aid to Families with Dependent Chil-
dren (AFDC), 179–80, 247
Agency for Health Care Policy and Re-
search, 324
Allen, John J. (R-Cal.), 163
Allied health personnel, shortage of,
262
Allman, David B., 149
Altman, Stuart, 214
American Academy of Pediatrics, 240

American Association of Foundations
for Medical Care, 221
American Association for Labor Legislation (AALL): admininistrative
council, members of, 68n; /AMA activities, 72, 75–77, 92; background,
67–73, 91–93; CCMC reports and,
103; Committee on Social Insurance, 69, 70, 71–72, 76–77, 82, 97,
89; studies, 96
American Catholic Hospital Association, 231
American College of Healthcare Executives, 338–39
American College of Obstetrics and
Gynecology, 240
American College of Physicians, 334
American College of Radiology, 240
American Dental Association, 97, 167
American Drug Manufacturers' Association, 88
American Economics Association, 67,
72
American Federation of Labor (AFL):
compulsory health insurance and,
74, 80, 85–86, 167; reinsurance,
149–50
American Hospital Association
(AHA), 54, 85, 88–90, 128, 135n1,
189, 212–13, 273, 326; and the aged,

About the Author

ODIN W. ANDERSON is Professor of Sociology on the faculty of the University of Wisconsin, Department of Sociology and the Program in Health Services Administration. He was on the faculty of the University of Chicago, Graduate Program in Health Administration, Graduate School of Business, where he was Director of both the program and The Center for Health Administration Studies. Earlier in his career he taught at the University of Western Ontario, New York University, and Columbia University. Dr. Anderson earned his Ph.D. at the University of Michigan in Sociology. He is a Fellow of the American Sociological Association, the American Public Health Association, the American Association for the Advancement of Science, and the Institute of Medicine, and an Honorary Fellow of the American College of Healthcare Executives. He has an Honorary Doctorate (Faculty of Medicine) from Uppsala University, Uppsala, Sweden. Dr. Anderson has published many books and journal articles.